W9-AWU-276

CONTENTS

Contents

9 • INFECTIOUS DISEASE

10 • KIDNEY, BLADDER, AND LIVER HEALTH

Contents

PREFACE

We are proud to bring to you *The Ultimate Women's Guide to Beating Disease and Living a Happy, Active Life 2023*. This essential volume features trustworthy and actionable life-saving information from the best health experts in the world—information that will help women beat the most deadly conditions.* In the following chapters, you'll find the latest discoveries, best treatments and scientifically proven remedies to keep you living a long, happy and active life.

Whether it's heart care, the latest on breast cancer prevention and treatment, breakthrough treatments for hot flashes or cutting-edge nutritional advice, the editors at Bottom Line Books talk to the experts—from top women's health doctors to research scientists to leading alternative care practitioners—who are creating the true innovations in health care.

Over the past four decades, we have built a network of literally thousands of leading physicians in both alternative and conventional medicine. They are affiliated with the premier medical and research institutions throughout the world. We read the important medical journals and follow the latest research that is reported at medical conferences. And we regularly talk to our advisors in major teaching hospitals, private practices and government health agencies for their insider perspective.

In this 2023 edition, we've gone beyond diseases and have included several chapters of life-enhancing health information on pregnancy, depression, fitness, nutrition, quality medical care, pain relief and aging...all of which are essential to living a happy, active life. And it's all backed by breaking studies and top health experts.

The Ultimate Women's Guide to Beating Disease and Living a Happy, Active Life 2023 is a result of our ongoing research and connection with these experts, and is a distillation of their latest findings and advice. We trust that you will glean new, helpful and affordable information about the health topics that concern you most...and find vital topics of interest to family and friends as well.

As a reader of a Bottom Line book, be assured that you are receiving well-researched information from a trusted source. But please use prudence in health matters. Always speak to your physician before taking vitamins, supplements or over-the-counter medication...stopping a medication...changing your diet...or beginning an exercise program. If you experience side effects from any regimen, contact your doctor immediately.

Be well,
The Editors, Bottom Line Books
Norwalk, Connecticut

---

*"Leading Causes of Death in Females," Centers for Disease Control and Prevention (*http://www.cdc.gov/women/lcod/2017/index.html*).

Chapter 1

AGE WELL: STAYING YOUNGER LONGER

Tired? Forgetful? Rising Cholesterol? Think Thyroid

Low inside the front of your neck lies a gland that produces hormones to help regulate the energy use and cell function in every system and tissue of your body. When that gland underperforms, the effects can be widespread. But while the condition, called hypothyroidism, is easy to treat, it's not always easy to diagnose.

Numerous studies suggest that up to 14 percent of older people have undiagnosed hypothyroidism, likely because people tend to display fewer symptoms after age 60—often just one. If cognitive dysfunction is the only symptom, for example, few physicians will think to test the thyroid. The condition is more common in women than in men.

A Host of Symptoms

Further complicating diagnosis, many of the possible signs of hypothyroidism can be easily attributed to other causes. *If you're experiencing one or more of the following symptoms, talk to your doctor about having your thyroid tested...*

•**Fatigue.** People with an underactive thyroid may feel tired, listless, and lacking in energy to perform daily tasks.

•**Weight gain.** A sudden unexplained weight gain is a good reason to check in with your doctor.

•**Constipation.** As digestive processes slow, you may notice more gut discomfort and difficulty with bowel movements.

•**Dry skin.** You may also have more brittle hair and nails.

•**Cold intolerance.** People with a slowed metabolism may feel chilly all the time and find it difficult to get warm in cold conditions.

•**Mental fogginess.** Some people with underactive thyroid feel more forgetful or have trouble concentrating.

•**Hair loss.** Disruptions in thyroid hormones can affect hair follicles, leading to gradual or sudden hair loss.

•**Eyebrow thinning.** A distinctive loss of hair on the outer third of your eyebrows can be a sign of an underactive thyroid.

Victor Bernet, MD, chair of the division of endocrinology at Mayo Clinic in Jacksonville, Florida, and past president of the American Thyroid Association.

• **An enlarged thyroid gland.** Both under-active and overactive thyroids can enlarge, creating a visible lump on the neck called a goiter.

• **Rising cholesterol levels.** Thyroid hormones help to clear low-density lipoprotein (LDL) cholesterol particles from your bloodstream. When too little is cleared, that so-called "bad cholesterol" rises, along with overall cholesterol levels, leaving you more vulnerable to a buildup of plaque in your arteries.

• **Elevated diastolic blood pressure.** The lower number in a blood pressure measurement may rise in people with hypothyroidism.

Getting a Diagnosis

If you suspect that your thyroid may be underperforming, make an appointment with your physician for a workup. He or she will assess your symptoms, ask about your personal and family history, and run some blood tests. Those tests usually include one for thyroid-stimulating hormone (TSH) and one for a hormone called thyroxine (T4). TSH is a hormone produced by the pituitary gland that stimulates the thyroid to make T4 and, in lesser amounts, another hormone called triiodothyronine (T3).

An elevated TSH level is the clearest sign of an underactive thyroid: It suggests that your brain is detecting low thyroid hormone levels, so TSH is rising to correct the imbalance. When you have a clearly elevated TSH level combined with a clearly reduced level of T4, you meet the criteria to be diagnosed with hypothyroidism.

However, results aren't always that clear. If your hormone levels are just slightly abnormal, your doctor might want to rerun the lab work because levels can shift, and you don't want to treat a problem you don't have.

In other cases, TSH levels are clearly elevated but T4 levels appear normal. In that case, your doctor may diagnose you with subclinical hypothyroidism, or a mildly underactive thyroid.

Treatment

If you have a clear case of hypothyroidism, your doctor will usually prescribe synthetic T4. If you are diagnosed with subclinical hypothyroidism, many doctors take a more individualized approach, considering the severity of your symptoms, your family history, and other factors to decide whether you are likely to benefit from treatment.

Older patients may need to start with a lower dose of medication and slowly work up to the full dose to avoid putting too much stress on the heart and central nervous system. If, after starting on the medication, you notice an increase in angina, shortness of breath, or confusion, or have a change in sleep habits, let your doctor know right away.

Your symptoms may not disappear overnight, but they typically improve gradually over several weeks to months. Your dose may need to be adjusted a few times to achieve target TSH and free T4 levels as well as improvement in symptoms.

One caveat: Because the symptoms associated with an underactive thyroid can have multiple alternate causes, you may find that some symptoms don't disappear because they're being caused by another underlying issue.

Dietary Support

In addition to medication, you can support your thyroid by eating a healthy, well-balanced diet with a few tweaks. Several foods and medicines interfere with thyroid medication absorption, so take your medication with water only. Wait at least 30 to 60 minutes before drinking coffee, tea, or milk. Wait at least four hours to eat soy-containing foods (tofu, soy sauce, soy milk). If you have an iodine deficiency, limit your intake of Brussels sprouts, kale, cabbage, cauliflower, turnips, and bok choy to no more than 5 ounces per day. These cruciferous vegetables may block the thyroid's ability to use iodine.

Dance After Menopause for Better Health

Study titled "Dance Practice Modifies Functional Fitness, Lipid Profile, and Self-Image in Postmenopausal Women," by researchers at São Paulo State University, Brazil, published in *Menopause*.

Warning: Menopause can be hazardous to your health. The drop in estrogen that occurs during and after increases a woman's risk for weight gain, LDL ("bad") cholesterol, and heart disease. Menopause also increases the risk of osteoporosis, falls, and fractures. Menopause happens to most women around the age of 51. The years during and after menopause can be a difficult ride, both physically and emotionally.

Dance Practice: A Fun Exercise

A new study published in the North American Menopause Society journal *Menopause* has found a safe, inexpensive, and effective remedy for improving health after menopause. It's called dance practice. And it's as enjoyable as it sounds.

Study details: A team of researchers from several university physiotherapy programs enrolled 36 postmenopausal women in dance classes. Their average age was 57. Before dance classes began, the researchers recorded the women's body composition (body fat and lean mass), cholesterol, triglycerides, coordination, agility, aerobic fitness, and self-esteem levels. They measured overall fitness using a test called the general functional fitness index (GFFI).

The women took three 90-minute dance classes each week for 16 weeks. They learned and practiced Samba, Funk, Zumba, and a few other Latin dances. All the dances required a certain amount of balance and agility. The dances were also active enough to be considered aerobic exercise, which is exercise that moves the arms, body, and legs enough to increase oxygen and blood supply to the heart and muscles. *At the end of the 16 weeks, this is what the research team found...*

- **Triglycerides went down by 25 points.**
- **Good cholesterol went up by 4.5 points.**
- **Coordination, agility, aerobic capacity and GFFI scores all improved.**

As an added bonus, mental health also improved. The women reported higher levels of self-image and self-esteem.

Exercise Curbs the Hazards of Menopause

Women who do not get enough exercise or are not physically active after menopause may also be at higher risk for high blood pressure and type 2 diabetes. They are more likely to suffer from back pain, poor sleep, poor circulation, and depression. Aerobic exercise helps improve mood and mental health by releasing those "feel good" hormones *endorphins*. Endorphins can improve a person's mood for several hours after exercise. Other good aerobic exercise choices for women include walking, jogging, swimming, and biking.

Takeaway: Other studies have called out the benefits of exercise after menopause. This study confirms many of those benefits. But regular exercise can seem like another bit of drudgery for some women. Dancing offers an enjoyable, safe, inexpensive, and effective option for aerobic exercise that also improves coordination and balance. It also provides a social element missing from many forms of exercise. The improved health and shared experience of dance can boost both body...and mind.

Sample routine: For an online dance-fitness class that samples several beginner dance moves, go to Youtube.com and search 20 Minute Dance Workout for Seniors or 20 Minute Beginner Dance Workout 375 Dance Studio.

Longevity Science: Old-School Hacks That Work

Seema Bonney, MD, founder and medical director of the Anti-Aging and Longevity Center of Philadelphia. Dr. Bonney is board-certified in emergency medicine and anti-aging and regenerative medicine.

You may already know some of the tweaks in daily habits and lifestyle choices that scientists tout to reduce inflammation and thwart the effects of aging. Along with certain types of preemptive testing and other vigilance, some biohacks may seem like a decidedly old-school approach. But if we've learned anything during the recent pandemic, it's that keeping our bodies strong can help guard against unwanted outcomes.

Remember the adage that living longer is a marathon and not a sprint. It's a long game that challenges us to make small, regular changes that can add up to longevity and vitality. *Here's a menu of evidence-backed options...*

• **Health and history audit.** Take a thorough look at medical conditions you've had and any new symptoms you're experiencing now. Review these with your primary care doctor to make sure you're doing all you can to manage any existing health concerns.

• **Genetic tests.** Using your health history, genetic testing might determine if certain genes or enzymes further predispose you to serious diseases. A genetic specialist could tease out, for example, if certain cancers or Alzheimer's disease are likelier for you and point the way toward more aggressive preventive measures that you can take now.

• **Blood tests.** Simpler than genetic tests, blood panels can detect key imbalances in nutrients, hormones, or inflammatory markers such as C-reactive protein or homocysteine that can indicate simmering problems in your cardiovascular or central nervous systems, among others.

• **Intermittent (or longer) fasting.** Consuming all your daily calories within a six- or eight-hour window each day may be challenging at first, but this current weight-loss fad does more than help shed unwanted pounds: Long hours without processing glucose act as an anti-inflammatory clean-out, ridding the body of damaged cells and proteins. Fasting for even longer periods, such as having only clear liquids for 48 hours once a month or eating 75 percent fewer calories two days a week, expands these evidence-backed anti-aging benefits even more.

• **Less red meat.** Even small amounts of red meat can have a negative effect on longevity. Eating more than 18 ounces of beef, pork, or lamb each week significantly increases colorectal cancer risk, and cutting consumption dramatically reduces all types of inflammation.

• **More beans.** Sweeping research conducted by the World Health Organization called consumption of beans and other legumes the most important dietary predictor of longevity. Every 20-gram daily increase (less than an ounce) in legume consumption was linked to an 8 percent reduction in death risk. Soy, tofu, miso, red beans, peas, lentils, chickpeas, and white beans all provide powerful health benefits across global cultures.

• **More movement.** This is also no big revelation, but the importance of exercise on longevity cannot be overemphasized. It's not just any exercise: Vigorous movement confers the most life-extending benefits. It reduces the risks of heart disease, diabetes, and other health conditions, and it wards off obesity. Aerobic activity should be supplemented with one key anti-aging exercise: squats. Research shows definitively that older adults who can rise from sitting without support are less likely to die in the short term than those who can't. Strength training (weightlifting or resistance training) is also highly correlated to longer life because stronger muscles help protect age-vulnerable bones and joints.

• **Out and about.** Among other lessons from the pandemic is just how important in-person connections are to our mental health.

Social engagement is also integral to longevity: Research shows that survival rates are highest among seniors who leave their homes daily for any reason, and lowest among those holed up and cut off from others. Bonus points if you mix the social and physical realms by playing sports like tennis or pickleball.

• **Deep breathing.** Take three minutes each day to lower your cortisol, a pro-inflammatory stress hormone, by practicing 4-7-8 breathing. Breath through your nose to a count of four, hold your breath to a count of seven, and exhale to a count of eight. Ideally, repeat twice a day for four breath cycles.

Reduce the Toxins That Cause Premature Aging

Ann Louise Gittleman, PhD, CNS, a holistic nutritionist based in Post Falls, Idaho, and *The New York Times* best-selling author who has written more than 35 books, including *Radical Longevity: The Powerful Plan to Sharpen Your Brain, Strengthen Your Body, and Reverse the Symptoms of Aging.* AnnLouise.com

---

Wouldn't it be nice if those headlines about living vibrantly to age 100 were true? And, even better, if it didn't require voodoo or new-age machinery to do it? Well, it is…and it doesn't. You just need to understand the root causes of deterioration as we age, most of which are because the body accumulates pro-aging toxins faster than it can eliminate them.

A Primer on Premature Aging

At the cellular level, aging is caused by free radicals, unstable molecules that break down our bodies' cells and damage DNA. By doing this, they create a sort of cellular chaos—called oxidative stress—that can hasten aging and fuel the development of disease.

Most approaches to fighting oxidative stress involve antioxidants—restorative vitamins and minerals in food and supplements—to counter the effects of free radicals.

But all the kale in the world won't help you keep pace with the alarming rate with which free radicals infiltrate the body.

Best defense: Integrate smart, science-backed strategies into your daily life to reduce the amount of pro-aging toxins that enter your body and eliminate the ones that do get in.

STRATEGY #1: **Reduce consumption of advanced glycation end products (AGEs).** AGEs are inflammatory compounds formed when high-heat cooking methods (grilling, broiling, browning, roasting, frying) alter the fat and proteins in food. AGEs also are created when proteins and fats in certain foods—particularly animal-based fats (butter, meat, cheese) and processed foods—mix with fructose and glucose in the bloodstream. The resulting "sticky" molecules promote oxidative stress and signs of aging in the body, from the skin (that sagging skin on your upper arm) to the heart (arteries stiffened by AGEs can nearly double the chance of dying from heart disease). *Self-defense…*

• **Choose the right fats**—olive oil and avocados…and avoid the wrong ones—bacon and fried foods. You can eat nuts and seeds raw or lightly toasted—roasting can double their AGE content.

• **Eat plant-based foods.** Fruits and veggies are low in AGEs and rich in detoxifying enzymes, fiber, antioxidant vitamins and minerals. Avoid high-fat animal products such as bacon and cheese.

• **Limit "high and dry" cooking methods,** such as grilling and roasting. Go for low-heat, wet cooking methods including simmering, braising, steaming, poaching, and slow-cooking to maximize nutrients while limiting AGEs. If you grill, first marinate the fish or meat in an acidic medium such as citrus juice, organic grass-fed broth, apple cider vinegar—even olive oil will work. Per pound of meat or fish, use four to six tablespoons of liquid (plus enough water or other ingredients to cover the food), and add herbs and spices for flavor. This can slash AGE formation in half.

***STRATEGY #2:* Minimize heavy metals and misbehaving minerals.** Metals and minerals such as aluminum, mercury and copper suppress the immune system, speeding aging and development of degenerative diseases.

•**Aluminum** increases osteoporosis risk and is linked to neurodegenerative diseases, such as Parkinson's and Alzheimer's. It enters the body in aluminum-containing medicines and foods cooked using aluminum products. *Self-defense…*

•Minimize use of aluminum-containing medications and products. Many antacids, antidiarrheals, OTC painkillers and deodorants contain aluminum.

•Use parchment paper instead of aluminum foil when cooking.

•Replace aluminum pots, pans and cookie sheets with stainless steel, glass, Pyrex, and ceramic nonstick cookware.

•**Mercury** exposure occurs through consumption of certain fish and seafood…medications and personal-care products…and dental amalgams (mercury fillings). Mercury damages nerves' protective covering, which impacts cognitive function and may lead to Alzheimer's. It also can cause tinnitus (ringing in the ears) and hearing loss. *Self-defense…*

•Avoid eating large fish (swordfish, ahi tuna, orange roughy, king mackerel and shark).

•Skip mercury-containing self-care products, including Preparation H and some contact lens solutions.

•Consider having mercury fillings removed. Mercury vapors may be released from fillings. Visit the website of the International Academy of Biological Dentistry and Medicine (IABDM.org/location) to find a dentist trained in mercury filling–removal protocols.

•**Copper** comes in two forms—*monovalent*, or food-based (found in avocado, asparagus, mushrooms, nuts, liver and chocolate)…and *divalent*, or synthetic (mostly in environmental sources such as drinking water from copper pipes, multivitamin/mineral supplements, copper-lined cookware and copper IUDs). Monovalent copper is essential for healthy bones, connective tissue, red blood cells and the immune system. But divalent copper accumulates over the years and is highly inflammatory, paving the way toward the destruction of brain cells and possibly leading to Alzheimer's disease. *Self-defense…*

•Test levels of copper in your drinking water. It should be a conservative 0.01 ppm (0.01 mg/L) or less. Home-testing kits are available at WaterCheck.com. If the copper level is over 0.01 ppm, install a copper filter (such as a reverse osmosis filter) on the tap used for drinking and cooking water.

•Avoid copper-containing supplements. Multivitamin/mineral supplements often are enriched with copper.

•Supplement with resveratrol, a plant compound that binds and removes copper. I like the Longevinex brand (one to two capsules per day).

***STRATEGY #3:* Reduce exposure to "smart" radiation.** Cell phones, smart devices (including smart thermostats and doorbells), Wi-Fi and cordless phones emit electromagnetic fields (EMFs), a form of radiation linked to fatigue, migraines, back pain, cognitive issues, problems with the heart, digestive system and sleep, cataracts—even brain tumors and cancer. They also raise levels of the stress hormone *cortisol*, which can accelerate aging, disrupt sleep, and increase risk for cardiovascular disease. *Self-defense…*

•Hard wire your home using Ethernet cables instead of Wi-Fi. If you have Wi-Fi, turn it off at night to slash exposure while you are sleeping. Keep cell phones away from your head—instead use a speaker phone or an air-tube headset, rather than wireless ear buds. Keep your phone off or on airplane mode when not in use, and never leave it next to your bed when you're sleeping. If you need an alarm clock, get a battery- or electricity-powered one. Try to limit cell-phone or smart-device use to areas that have excellent reception—these devices use more power (and emit more radiation) in areas with poor reception. Avoid 5G-enabled devices. Until now, the wavelengths of all generations of wireless telecommunications technology, including 4G, have traveled along the surface of the skin, but 5G wavelengths are absorbed by the skin.

•Eat hemp seeds, rosemary, and miso soup, all of which absorb radiation and mitigate its effects in the body.

•Supplement with magnesium, which helps offset the effects of EMFs. Take 5 mg of magnesium per pound of body weight per day.

•Decorate with plants that absorb electromagnetic radiation—snake plants, aloe vera, rubber plants and cacti.

Gardening May Lead to Longer Life

Roundup of studies by environmental and health researchers in the UK, the US and the Netherlands, reported at CNBC.com.

In communities worldwide where many people are age 100 or older, residents have been consistently found to do gardening well into old age. Gardening may increase well-being and longevity by keeping people connected with sunlight, fresh air, and plant life…providing an ongoing form of physical activity…giving people who grow fruits and vegetables a source of super-fresh, high-nutrition plant foods…keeping the mind sharp by requiring planning and problem-solving…and establishing a form of meditative mindfulness by keeping gardeners centered in the moment.

Older Adults Are Mentally Sharpest and Less Distracted in the Morning

Researchers are not sure why this is so but believe it may have to do with circadian rhythms. If you need to do a cognitively challenging activity, tackle it first thing in the morning, when you're at your best.

Mind, Mood & Memory, reported in Harvard Heart Letter.

Keep Your Driving Skills Sharp as You Age

William Van Tassel, PhD, manager of driver-training programs at the national office of the American Automobile Association (AAA) in Heathrow, Florida, where he is also three-time chair of The Association of National Stakeholders in Traffic Safety Education, funded by the National Highway Traffic Safety Administration (NHTSA). He has published peer-reviewed articles in various journals relating to public health and safety. AAA.com

Americans are living longer these days, and we want to maintain our independence and mobility for as long as possible. By staying current with new car technology, keeping driving skills up to date and caring for our bodies and minds, we don't have to lose that independence.

Driving expert William Van Tassel's tips to extend our safe-driving years…

The Elements of Driving

Driving consists of three components—perception, decision, and action. You perceive a car braking ahead of you…you decide to decelerate…and you act by tapping your brakes. *To maintain your skills in each of these three areas…*

•**Perception.** Our eyesight begins to diminish as early as our 40s. We start losing some of our peripheral vision…our ability to see well in low light declines…and cataracts, macular degeneration and other conditions can make things even worse. *Steps to keep your perception sharp…*

•Get screened. Every senior driver should have his/her vision tested at least once a year and, of course, stay on top of eyewear prescriptions and any new vision problems.

•Drive only when visibility is good. Many seniors are retired and therefore have flexible schedules. Take advantage of that by being selective about when you drive to avoid crowded roadways and poor weather conditions.

• Brighten your headlights. You might be surprised at the improved visibility after simply changing to a new set of factory bulbs. Xenon or high-intensity discharge (HID) bulbs are especially good for seniors because they can improve visibility at night.

Also: Be sure to clean your headlights regularly.

• Modify your rig. If your peripheral vision has diminished, you can install special mirrors that help you see better out to the sides. If your neck hurts when you turn around to back up, have a rear-view camera installed.

Caution: These cameras can take some getting used to—be sure to practice in a safe, off-street location before using a camera for actual backing-up and parking maneuvers.

Important: These cameras are no substitute for looking directly at the area into which you are backing.

• Use a spotter. Many older drivers wisely venture out only with a passenger to act as a second set of eyes.

• **Decision.** Thanks to the wisdom that comes with years of driving, seniors actually have a leg up on younger drivers when it comes to decision-making. They recognize threats, anticipate the moves of other motorists, and know how to react effectively. *Still, those skills can be maintained throughout your life…*

• Stay up to date. All drivers—not just seniors—should consider taking a classroom-based refresher course every few years. These are available from AAA, AARP, National Safety Council and driving schools around the country, with courses typically taking six-to-eight hours total. Traffic laws, vehicle technology, signage, roadway design and driving techniques continue to evolve.

Examples: Roundabouts used to be rare in the US but now are springing up in many areas. While they're much safer than traditional intersections—because all drivers are moving in the same direction, and no drivers are turning left in front of others— many drivers panic the first few times they encounter them. Even basics such as how to hold the steering wheel have changed—driving instructors used to train people to grasp the wheel at the 2:00 and 10:00 positions, but now the safest grip is considered to be the 9:00 and 3:00 positions.

There are refresher courses specifically for seniors that focus on maneuvers that have proven statistically problematic for older drivers, including left turns, merges, right turns from a dedicated lane and lane changes.

• **Action.** It's no secret that our reflexes get slower with time, and a loss of flexibility and mobility make it more difficult to maneuver a vehicle. *Steps to keep your mobility in top shape…*

• Modify. Make your vehicle as comfortable as possible so that you will feel confident when driving. Adjust the height of your seat and steering wheel and also your seatbelt. Add a seat cushion that allows you to easily swivel your legs when you need to look over your shoulder. Wrap an ergonomic grip around the steering wheel.

• Maintain. Keep your car in top running order. Spongy brakes, bald tires and poor acceleration are just a few of the maintenance issues that can severely disrupt your ability to drive safely. If your budget allows, consider buying or leasing a latest-model vehicle that will provide you with the newest safety features.

• Practice. If you do get a new vehicle with unfamiliar safety technologies, spend time with the salesperson becoming familiar with the features. Then take the car to an empty parking lot and drive around to get used to the new bells and whistles.

Caution: Don't become overly reliant on safety tech—it could make you less vigilant over time. Instead, continue to drive as if the vehicle did not have these new technologies—and use them to back you up if needed.

More Ways to Stay Safe

• **Exercise your body and your brain.** A fit person is a fit driver. Whether it's pickleball, Ping-Pong or yoga, any activity that helps you maintain balance, strength and flexibility also will help you behind the wheel.

Also: Computer games can keep your mind sharp and help your hand-eye coordination.

• **Watch your meds.** Senior drivers are less likely to fall asleep behind the wheel than younger drivers. But many older drivers take prescription drugs, some of which can cause drowsiness or brain fog. Ask your doctors which of your medications have such side effects and arrange your schedule so you do not need to drive after taking them.

Face Change Head On

Older drivers don't deserve their reputation for being dangerous. Statistically speaking, per mile driven, teens are more likely to be involved in a crash than older drivers. But around age 75, crash rates involving seniors start to rise.

Instead of waiting for loved ones to intervene or until you have an accident, monitor your own driving habits. Have you noticed other drivers honking at you a lot lately? Have you gotten a ticket for driving too slowly? Have you had some near misses? If so, that doesn't necessarily mean you need to hang up your keys, but it does mean that you should take an honest look at your situation.

Start with a professional in-car assessment of your driving skills. Your local driving school or AAA should be able to help you find one. Someone will ride with you for about 45 minutes, noting any deficits, and then will make recommendations that might include taking a class, in-car training or, if your situation warrants it, a clinical evaluation by a physician.

If you feel like your driving career is nearing its end, start planning now for how you'll get around.

How to Deal with Age-Related Night-Vision Problems

Harvard Health Letter. Health.Harvard.edu

Get regular eye exams to keep prescriptions current and identify any diseases. *Get treatment for other vision issues,* such as dry eyes and cataracts. *Use a flashlight or flashlight app* on a smartphone when out walking in dark areas. *Turn on more lights indoors,* and consider installing night-lights throughout your house. *Keep eyeglass lenses clear*—wash the lenses regularly, and have an optician buff out any small scratches. *Keep your car's windshield and headlights clean*—that will help with driving at night and when the sun hits your windshield during the day. Keep windshield-washer levels topped up. *Adapt to night driving by dimming dashboard lights* and using the night setting on your rearview mirror.

New and Improved Cataract Care

Ravi Goel, MD, a comprehensive ophthalmologist, cataract, and refractive surgeon at Regional Eye Associates in Cherry Hill, New Jersey, an instructor at Wills Eye Hospital, Philadelphia, and a spokesperson for the American Academy of Ophthalmology.

For hundreds of years, cataract removal surgery was only that—removal of the clouded lens that impaired vision. In 1949, Sir Harold Ridley invented the first artificial lens to replace the one that was removed in surgery, but it wasn't a widely accepted practice for decades.

Now, not only are lenses replaced, but patients aren't limited to a basic, one-size-fits-all approach: Several lens choices offer the opportunity to improve vision. (You might even be able to ditch those reading glasses you've needed for years.)

Early Cataracts

About half of all people will develop cataracts by age 80, but the process starts sooner than you think. Proteins can begin to build up on the lens in your 40s, though they likely won't cause any noticeable effects until your 60s or later. If you notice that colors seem faded, lights look too bright or have haloes, or your night vision is declining, make an appointment with an ophthalmologist. A comprehensive eye exam can identify cataracts as well as other dangerous eye conditions that become more common with age.

When It's Time for Surgery

In the early stages of cataracts, you can try a variety of stopgap measures to improve your vision (see sidebar). When those measures are no longer sufficient, it's time to have your cloudy lenses replaced with clear ones.

Cataract surgery is an outpatient procedure. Your eye will be numbed, so you won't feel any discomfort, and you may also be given medication to help you relax. In the most common procedure, the surgeon will make a tiny incision and use ultrasound waves to break the cataract apart, remove it, and then replace it with an intraocular lens (IOL). *There are several options…*

• **Fixed-focus monofocal IOLs.** These lenses will give you clear vision at a distance, but you'll still need reading glasses to see up close. If you have cataract surgery in both eyes, you might choose a lens that provides near vision in one eye and a lens that pro-

vides far vision in the other, a combination called monovision.

• **Accommodating monofocal IOLs.** Using the natural musculature around the eye, you can shift these lenses from near to far vision. Distance and middle-distance vision are typically excellent with this newer choice, but close-up vision may not improve.

• **Toric IOLs.** These lenses are used for people with astigmatism, a flaw in the eye's curvature that causes blurred distance and near vision. By bending light more efficiently, toric lenses provide focused vision at a single distance, correcting astigmatism so distance glasses are no longer needed.

• **Multifocal IOLs.** These lenses work like progressive or bifocal glasses, with different sections geared for distance, middle, and near vision. Your brain and eyes work together to decide which part of the lens you need at any given time. Multifocal lenses are the most versatile.

What to Expect

If you have cataracts in both eyes, expect to have two separate surgeries. Two procedures separated by mere weeks may seem inconvenient and even wasteful, but there are distinct advantages to this approach. By staging your second surgery once the first eye has healed and vision is stable, you can determine how the new lens behaves. If tweaking seems appropriate, the power of the second lens can then be fine-tuned. Most health insurers cover cataract surgery, though your out-of-pocket costs will vary.

Want to ensure you're among the nine in 10 people for whom cataract surgery spells success? While the odds of complications

---

Boost Your Vision

If your eye doctor diagnoses cataracts, it doesn't mean you need surgery right away. You may be able to use these stopgap measures to significantly boost vision:

• **Use brighter lights or a magnifying glass** to read, knit, or do other detailed tasks.

• **Wear anti-glare sunglasses.** Protecting your eyes from sunlight can also slow cataract progression.

• **Ask your doctor if dry eye might be aggravating your symptoms.** With 70 percent of the power to bring an image into focus relying on healthy tear film in your eyes, dry eye can significantly cut vision clarity. Over-the-counter or prescription tear replacement drops might help.

—Dr. Ravi Goel

---

such as infection, pain, or vision loss are low, your actions in the days and weeks after the procedure influence the outcome. The main goal is preventing infection. You'll need to use antibiotic eye drops several times a day and keep water out of your eyes. You may also need to wear a bandage or shield to stop yourself from rubbing and keep specks of dust or debris from getting in your eye.

Light daily activities are fine as your eyes heal, but avoid bending over, jogging, or lifting heavy objects. You'll schedule follow-up visits with your eye surgeon for the day after the procedure, as well as a week or two later and a month after that.

Cataract Surgery Lowers Risk for Dementia

Cecilia S. Lee, MD, Klorfine family associate professor of ophthalmology at University of Washington, Seattle, and lead researcher for a study of 3,000 people with cataracts published in JAMA Internal Medicine.

Study participants who had their cataracts removed were nearly 30 percent less likely to develop dementia compared with participants with cataracts who did not have the surgery. The restored vision improves stimuli to the brain by allowing higher-quality sensory input and light to reach the retina. Better engagement with the world also might be brain protective.

Sight Stealer: Ocular Hypertension

Michael A. Kass, MD, Bernard Becker Professor of Ophthalmology and Visual Sciences at Washington University School of Medicine in St. Louis, Missouri.

Glaucoma is called the silent thief of sight. Open-angle glaucoma, the most common type, doesn't have symptoms until late in its course. The key risk factor for glaucoma is ocular hypertension, or elevated eye pressure.

At the start of a study, 46 percent of participants had evidence of glaucoma in one or both eyes, but only 25 percent had vision loss when examined 20 years after the study's launch. So not everyone needs preventive treatment—monitoring may be enough.

A prediction model that takes a set of variables into account can help determine if your risk is low, medium or high. The variables are age…level of intraocular pressure…thickness of the cornea…thickness of the rim of the optic nerve (glaucoma causes changes in the rim)…and the results of standard eye exam tests. If needed, an imaging test called *optical coherence tomography* (OCT) can provide information or a baseline from which to look for changes in the future.

Using this approach allows the eye doctor to outline a patient's potential risk for glaucoma and make an informed decision about whether or not to begin treatment to lower eye pressure.

If you choose to monitor ocular hypertension at first, eye-exam frequency will depend on your risk—for low risk, you might see the doctor yearly…for high risk, two or three times a year. Other factors that make more frequent exams necessary are having diabetes, having cataracts at a younger-than-usual age and your age—eye diseases, in general, are more common in people after age 60.

Connection between glaucoma and sleep: A separate study presented at the 2021 Annual Meeting of The Association for Research in Vision and Ophthalmology highlighted the high prevalence of sleep disorders among people with glaucoma. The exact connection between the two conditions isn't fully understood, but one theory is that glaucoma can impair certain cells involved in the body's sleep-regulating system, throwing off circadian rhythms. If you suspect that you have a sleep disorder, talk to your doctor about doing a sleep study to find out if a CPAP machine or cognitive behavioral therapy would help.

The Leading Cause of Vision Loss

Chris Iliades, MD, retired ear, nose, throat, head, and neck surgeon who now dedicates his time to patient education through medical writing.

Age-related macular degeneration (AMD) is more common than glaucoma and cataracts put together, and it's the leading cause of vision loss in people over age 50. Once you have it, there is no cure, but you can take steps now to reduce your risk.

The macula is the central part of the retina at the back of the eye. Light-sensitive cells in your macula are responsible for central vision, what you see in front of your face. When your macula starts to degenerate, you begin to lose your central vision: what you need to drive, read, see faces, and work with your hands. AMD does not affect your peripheral vision, so you will not be completely blind, but loss of central vision is a handicap.

Controllable Risk Factors

The biggest risk factor for AMD, as you might expect from the name, is age. AMD starts to occur after age 50. After age 75, about one-third of people will have some amount of AMD.

Genes appear to play a role, too. Researchers estimate that 75 percent of people carry the genes for AMD, which can be passed down through families. But many people never get AMD, so we know that there are clearly other contributing factors. *Controlling these is the key to reducing your chances of developing AMD…*

• **Quit smoking.** If you smoke, you are up to five times more likely to get AMD.

• **Exercise and maintain a healthy weight.** Being obese doubles your risk of AMD.

• **Get high blood sugar, high blood pressure, or high cholesterol under control.**

• **Wear sunglasses.** There is some evidence that ultraviolet rays from the sun can cause AMD, especially if you have blue eyes. Sunglasses also reduce your risk of cataracts.

• **Eat a healthy diet rich in antioxidants,** such as leafy green vegetables and other colorful vegetables and fruits. Oxidative stress, which occurs when unstable molecules called free radicals damage cells, may play a role in causing AMD. Antioxidants capture these free radicals and prevent cell damage.

The Role of Supplements

Two National Eye Institute studies, called the Age-Related Eye Disease Studies (AREDS and AREDS2), found that high doses of antioxidant supplements could delay and possibly prevent the progression of AMD. The recommended supplements are vitamins C and E, the minerals zinc and copper, and the antioxidants lutein and zeaxanthin. These

The Stages of AMD

AMD has three stages…

• **Early stage.** Your vision is still normal, but an eye specialist can look into your eye with a special lens and see early changes of AMD.

• **Intermediate stage.** You start to have symptoms, such as blurred vision, blank or dark spots in your central vision, or seeing straight lines as wavy or curvy. One way to test for early symptoms of AMD is with a visual test called the Amsler Grid, which you can find on the American Macular Degeneration Foundation website at Macular.org/amsler-chart. If you see any dark, blank, blurry, or wavy areas on the grid, let your doctor know.

• **Late stage.** You have complete loss of central vision. AMD does not affect your peripheral vision.

—Dr. Chris Iliades

supplements are combined into a product called AREDS2 that you can get at drug or health food stores. The National Eye Institute recommends taking AREDS2 if you have intermediate AMD in one or both eyes to help slow down the vision loss.

Types of AMD

There are two types of AMD, and the cause and treatment for each type is different...

• **Dry AMD is the most common type.** It happens when a type of protein builds up beneath the macula, causing the macula to become thin and dry. Symptoms of central vision loss are gradual, and complete loss of central vision rarely occurs. The only treatment for dry AMD is AREDS2. Treatment may slow down dry AMD, but it does not cure it.

• **Wet AMD is less common.** In this type, abnormal blood vessels grow under the macula and leak, causing rapid degeneration of the macula and a rapid loss of vision. The main treatment for wet AMD is an injection of a substance called anti-vascular endothelial growth factor directly into the macula. This treatment may reduce the growth of the abnormal blood vessels or even stop the growth for a while, but the injections need to be repeated. Like dry AMD, wet AMD cannot be cured.

Regular Checks Lower Risk

You can reduce your risk of AMD, but you can't completely prevent it. That's why the most important step is to get regular eye exams. The American Academy of Ophthalmology recommends a complete eye exam that includes looking at your retina and macula for everyone at age 40. If you are over age 65, you should get the exam every one or two years. An eye doctor can diagnose AMD before you have symptoms.

Diabetes Drug May Protect Against Glaucoma

Qi N. Cui, MD, PhD, assistant professor of ophthalmology, University of Pennsylvania, Philadelphia, Pennsylvania.

Researchers looked at retrospective data on more than 6,000 patients with diabetes. While 1.3 percent of people in a nonmedicated control group developed glaucoma, just 0.5 percent of those taking a glucagon-like peptide-1 receptor agonist, such as *dulaglutide* (Trulicity) or *semaglutide* (Rybelsus), did.

Caffeine Can Increase Glaucoma Risk

Louis Pasquale, MD, professor of ophthalmology at Icahn School of Medicine at Mount Sinai, New York City, and leader of a study of more than 120,000 adults, published in *Ophthalmology*.

According to a recent study, compared with people who had low genetic propensity for high intraocular pressure (IOP) and who consumed little caffeine, those who had the highest genetic tendency for high IOP and consumed more than 320 mg of caffeine daily (about three cups of coffee) had a 3.9-fold increased risk for glaucoma. If glaucoma runs in your family, limit coffee to two cups a day.

Eyedrops Could Replace Your Reading Glasses

Eric Donnenfeld, MD, ophthalmologist and eye surgeon, Ophthalmic Consultants of Long Island, Garden City, New York, commenting on studies of 750 participants presented to the American Academy of Ophthalmology.

Pilocarpine HCL ophthalmic solution (Vuity), a prescription eyedrop medication recently approved by the FDA for people whose near vision has become blurry with age (presbyopia), helped 35 percent of participants read three additional lines on a vision chart. Vuity works by constricting pupil size, increasing depth of focus without disrupting distance focus.

Cost: About $100 for a month's supply. Check with your eye doctor whether Vuity is appropriate for you.

Red Light Therapy Can Improve Eyesight

University College London

Three minutes of morning exposure to deep red light can improve color vision by 12 to 17 percent, a new study shows. As cells in the back of the eye age, they produce less of an energy molecule called adenosine triphosphate (ATP). Red light appears to boost ATP production, improving vision for up to a week.

Don't Ignore Your Hearing Loss

Carrie Ali, editor, *Bottom Line Health*. BottomLine Inc.com

If you've noticed that your hearing isn't as sharp as it used to be, you're not alone. About 2 percent of people begin to have hearing loss by age 55. By age 70, half of the population is affected. By age 80, it rises to 80 percent.

Hearing loss is more than an inconvenience: Research shows that it can lead to social isolation and is associated with cognitive impairment, dementia, a greater risk of hospitalization, and reduced independence.

There's a seemingly simple solution that 86 percent of hearing-impaired Americans go without—hearing aids. Part of the problem is

Look Out for These Signs of Hearing Loss

Buzzing or ringing that comes and goes—this can indicate nerve damage, often caused by using headphones at too-high volumes. *Balance problems*—the inner ear sends signals to the brain to help the body balance, so stumbling more often could indicate ear damage. *Forgetfulness*—difficulty hearing makes remembering harder. The brain uses more energy to process sound and devotes less to thinking and memory. *Pain from loud noises*—some irritation caused by sirens, car horns and similar loud sounds is normal, but actual pain may indicate hearing loss. *Trouble hearing in places with background noise*—this could be caused by poor acoustics or by the ear's decreased ability to differentiate among sounds. If you have any of these worrisome symptoms, talk to your doctor.

Roundup of otolaryngologists reported on The Healthy.com.

stigma, or the belief that hearing loss is untreatable, but for many people, it simply boils down to price. Hearing aids cost from $1,000 to $4,000 per ear, and they last for only four to six years. Insurance coverage is spotty at best.

But relief is on the horizon: In 2022, the FDA published new regulations that allow over-the-counter hearing aids to come to market. The National Academies of Sciences, Engineering, and Medicine, an organization that has been pushing for access to OTC devices for several years, expects those devices to be much more affordable and accessible.

That doesn't mean you have to wait until next year to get help with your hearing. *Here are some strategies you can implement right now…*

• **Talk to a hearing health professional** who may be able to help you find discounts that you didn't know existed.

• **Bargain.** A *Consumer Reports* survey found that 40 percent of people were able to bargain for a better price on their hearing aids.

● **Check your insurance.** Coverage is constantly changing.

● **Consider hearing assistive technologies** that help with talking on the phone, watching television, or participating in one-on-one or small-group conversations. Personal sound amplification products may provide some of the technological features that hearing aids have even though they are not FDA-approved to be marketed as such.

What Is a Cochlear Implant?

Virginia Ramachandran, AuD, PhD, adjunct assistant professor of communication sciences and disorders, Wayne State University, Detroit, Michigan.

A cochlear implant is surgically inserted into the inner ear and receives signals from a speech processor that is typically worn on the ear, much like a hearing aid. Electrical impulses generated by the implant directly stimulate the auditory nerve, which sends signals that the brain recognizes as sound. The implant bypasses the damaged inner ear, so many people experience better hearing with an implant than with hearing aids. With a cochlear implant, the brain must learn to use the signals that are received. A speech-language pathologist can help you learn to interpret these sounds.

Not Enough Americans Are Getting Their Hearing Checked

Michael McKee, MD, associate professor, department of family medicine at University of Michigan, Ann Arbor, and leader of research published as part of the National Poll on Healthy Aging.

A mong Americans over age 50, 80 percent have not been asked about their hearing by their primary doctors within the past two years, and 77 percent have not been checked by a hearing specialist.

But: Research shows that around half of older adults have some degree of hearing loss, which has physical and mental health repercussions, including higher rates of depression, falls and cognitive decline.

This Device Can Reduce Ringing in the Ears

Science Translational Medicine

In a clinical trial, 326 people with tinnitus tried the Lenire (Neuromod) device, which plays sequences of audio tones layered with wideband noise through headphones while also sending electrical stimulation pulses to the tip of the tongue. After 12 weeks, 86 percent of the participants who used the device for at least one hour each day reported an improvement in their tinnitus symptoms.

High Blood Pressure? Intensive Treatment Could Save Your Life

Study titled "Trial of Intensive Blood-Pressure Control in Older Patients with Hypertension," by researchers at the Chinese Academy of Medical Sciences, et al., published in *The New England Journal of Medicine*.

If you have high blood pressure, lowering it is one of the most important things you can do to reduce your risk of cardiovascular disease (CVD). This is especially important for the elderly, since 70 percent of people ages 65 and older have hypertension, according to the American College of Cardiology. That number is expected to rise as the population ages.

How Low Do You Go?

Experts all agree that treating hypertension in seniors reduces the risk of death from CVD—the big question is, how low do you go? The most important number for lowering blood pressure is the higher systolic number. This is the pressure inside arteries when your heart beats. It is measured in millimeters of mercury (mmHg). *These are the current hypertension treatment guidelines for the systolic number...*

- **130 mmHg or less** (American Heart Association and American College of Cardiology)

- **140 mmHg or less** (The European Society of Cardiology and European Society of Hypertension)

- **150 mmHg or less** (American College of Physicians and American Academy of Family Physicians)

A 2015 study, called the Systolic Blood Pressure Intervention Trial (SPRINT), found intensive treatment to get the systolic blood pressure under 130 mmHg in hypertensive patients at or over age 65 improved risk for CVD. Now, researchers from China support the SPRINT study, confirming lower is better.

The aim of the study was to find the appropriate target for systolic blood pressure to reduce CVD risk in older patients with hypertension, a number that has remained unclear. The study was published in *The New England Journal of Medicine* and was also presented at the 2021 meeting of the European Society of Cardiology.

This was a large trial conducted at many treatment centers in which patients were randomly selected to receive standard or intensive blood pressure treatment. There were about 8,500 patients in the trial, and they were about equally divided into the two treatment groups. The age of the patients ranged from 60 to 80.

Lower Systolic Numbers Mean Fewer Heart Attacks

The primary goal of the study was to see which treatment group had fewer CVD events. CVD events included stroke, heart attack, hospital admission for angina, heart failure, a procedure to open a heart artery (coronary revascularization), atrial fibrillation or death from any CVD cause.

In the intensive treatment group, the goal was a systolic blood pressure from 110 to under 130 mmHg. In the standard treatment group, the goal was a systolic blood pressure from 130 to under 150 mmHg. The key finding was that the risk of a CVD event was about 25 percent lower in the intensive-treatment group compared to the standard-treatment group.

The corresponding author of the Chinese study says that these findings and the SPRINT study could unite the guidelines to recommend a lower target for systolic blood pressure in elderly people with hypertension.

For ways to reduce high blood pressure: Visit the American Heart Association website at Heart.org/en/health-topics/high-blood-pressure/commit-to-a-plan-to-lower-your-blood-pressure/lower-numbers-start-here.

Stay Active as You Age

University of California, San Francisco

When elderly people stay active, their brains have more proteins that enhance the connections between neurons to maintain healthy cognition. The protective effect is found even in people whose brains have toxic proteins associated with Alzheimer's and other neurodegenerative diseases.

Just 10 Minutes of Exercise Helps You Live Longer

Study of nearly 5,000 adults by researchers at National Cancer Institute, Rockville, Maryland, published in *JAMA Internal Medicine*.

Recent finding: More than 110,000 lives could be saved by adults over age 40 if they added just 10 minutes of moderate-to-vigorous activity to their daily routines. Even more lives would be saved if they increased that activity by 20 or 30 minutes daily. Research shows that even a very small amount of moderate-to-vigorous exercise can have a big impact on health.

The Longevity Vitamin

Traci Mitchell, MA, MS, a health and nutrition consultant based in Chicago, Illinois, and author of the book *The Belly Burn Plan*.

Would you like to lower your odds of dying by about 20 percent? Then get plenty of vitamin K. That's the recent and remarkable finding from a team of scientists at the Jean Mayer USDA Human Nutrition Research Center on Aging at Tufts University. In their analysis of health data from more than 4,000 Americans ages 54 to 76, they found that those with the lowest level of vitamin K were 19 percent more likely to die during the 13 years of the study.

Vitamin K was discovered in 1929 by European scientists who realized it played a crucial role in blood clotting or coagulation—*koagulation* in German, hence "vitamin K." Since then, researchers have discovered a growing number of ways that vitamin K can protect you against the chronic diseases of aging, and against dying from them. *Here's what the latest science shows…*

• **Chronic inflammation.** Vitamin K blocks the production of inflammatory components in the immune system called cytokines. In a paper published in *Current Nutrition Reports*, researchers cite several studies that link higher dietary intake of vitamin K to lower levels of several inflammatory biomarkers.

• **Osteoporosis.** Vitamin K is essential for your body to form *osteocalcin*, a protein that binds calcium to bone, increasing bone mineral content and ensuring bone strength. In a review published in the journal *Medicine*, scientists analyzed five studies (involving more than 80,000 people) on vitamin K and fractures. They found that those with the highest intake of the vitamin were 24 percent less likely to break a bone.

Fractures can be deadly in seniors: A hip fracture doubles the risk of dying in older women and triples it in older men. Even minor fractures, like breaking a wrist, are linked to a higher risk of dying within five years.

• **Atherosclerosis.** Vitamin K activates *matrix Gla*, a protein that keeps calcium away from your arteries—helping prevent atherosclerosis, the buildup of calcified plaques that can block an artery and trigger a heart attack or stroke.

• **Cardiovascular disease (heart attack and stroke).** Menopausal women who took 180 mcg of vitamin K2 for three years had a decrease in arterial stiffness, a cause of high blood pressure and a risk factor for heart attack and stroke. In a 10-year study published in *BMJ Open* in 2020, Norwegian scientists

Poor Mobility and Disability

Getting enough vitamin K can even help you maintain mobility and independence in old age, according to a study published in *The Journal of Gerontology: Medical Sciences*. Researchers looked at more than 1,300 adults ages 70 to 79 and found that those with low levels of the vitamin were 1.5 times more likely to develop mobility limitation (difficulty walking a quarter of a mile or climbing 10 steps without resting), and twice as likely to develop mobility disability (a lot of difficulty or inability to walk or climb stairs).

—Traci Mitchell

analyzed data from nearly 3,000 people and found that those with the highest dietary intake of vitamin K2 were 48 percent less likely to develop heart disease.

• **Osteoarthritis.** Studies show that people with low blood levels of vitamin K are 1.5 to 2.6 times more likely to develop osteoarthritis, a disease that causes pain, stiffness, and decreased range of motion. It is the most common cause of disability in the United States.

• **Chronic kidney disease (CKD).** Approximately 37 million Americans have chronic kidney disease, which causes high blood pressure, and most of them develop fatal heart disease. Research shows that CKD patients have very high rates of vitamin K deficiency.

• **Cognitive decline.** Vitamin K also appears to help keep brain cells alive as we age. A study published in the *Frontiers in Neurology* shows that in people ages 65 and older, low dietary intake of vitamin K is linked to poor cognitive performance. Another study, published in the *Journal of the American Dietetic Association*, shows that early-stage Alzheimer's patients consume less vitamin K than "cognitively intact" older adults.

• **Emphysema.** A study published in *Frontiers in Nutrition* in 2020 shows that people who consume adequate vitamin K have a 39 percent lower risk of emphysema, a progressive disease that causes shortness of breath, persistent cough, and fatigue.

Boost Your Vitamin K

Vitamin K is a family of compounds that includes *phylloquinone* (vitamin K1) and *menaquinone* (vitamin K2). Vitamin K2 comprises 10 subtypes, the most biologically active of which is menaquinone-7 (MK7).

Vitamin K1 is mainly found in green vegetables, such as kale, spinach, Brussels sprouts, broccoli, green beans, and green peas. It's also found in vegetable oils, soybean oil, and olive oil. Vitamin K2 is found in fermented foods such as yogurt, hard cheeses, sauerkraut, and kimchi. (The best source is natto, or fermented soybeans.) It's also generally found in full-fat dairy products. Try to get a

daily serving of food from each group. You can also supplement your diet with 90 to 120 micrograms (mcg) of MK7.

Benefits of Not Wearing Makeup

Less acne—makeup sits on top of skin, creating a barrier that can increase oil production, leading to clogged pores and pimples. **Fewer fine lines**—powder makeup rests in wrinkles and fine facial lines and makes them more prominent, especially around the eyes. **Fuller eyelashes**—mascara can cause lashes to break and fall out, so eliminating it can allow lash density to increase, making lashes look fuller after about a month.

Roundup of dermatologists reported on Womens HealthMag.com.

Anti-Aging Skin Care— Hope or Hype?

Jessica Weiser, MD, a board-certified dermatologist in New York City and assistant clinical professor of dermatology at Columbia University.

When it comes to skin care, fantastic promises are everywhere. Creams that range from $10 to several hundred dollars promise sunny, youthful faces, while procedures that can cost thousands offer relief from fine lines, wrinkles, and scars.

The vast array of products and procedures can leave you with more questions than answers. *Here's a quick guide to what you can realistically expect in the world of anti-aging skin care…*

Over-the-Counter Products

Products that you buy at the drugstore or beauty counter may soften fine lines, reduce pore size, and lessen crepe-like texture to the skin, but they won't do anything for deep lines and folds. *Here are the ingredients you're likely to see…*

• **Antioxidants.** Just as a diet filled with antioxidant-rich fruits and vegetables is good for overall health, antioxidants applied to the skin can help reduce signs of aging caused by unstable molecules (free radicals) that damage collagen, the protein that keeps skin plump. This process is called oxidative stress. Antioxidants stabilize free radicals by giving them an extra electron. Some of the antioxidants that you'll see in skin-care products include vitamin C, green tea extracts, polyphenols, niacinamide, and coenzyme Q10.

• **Alpha hydroxy and other acids.** In non-prescription strengths, these acids, which also include lactic, glycolic, and salicylic acids, are mild exfoliating chemicals. They're designed to create some skin-cell turnover, so you'll see some improvement in skin quality over a period of months when used twice a week. But because you're not abrading a layer of skin, you're not getting a true peel with these products. The strength required to abrade skin would be dangerous to use at home and is only available professionally.

• **Peptides.** When formulated as small molecules, these proteins can penetrate skin and stimulate cell turnover, often with less irritation than retinols.

• **Retinols.** These vitamin A derivatives, when found in OTC products, are milder than the prescription tretinoin, which means they provide both milder improvement and milder side effects. Keep in mind that there are different types of retinol and it's hard to tell what you're getting in typical products.

The products you choose and when you use them depends on what you're trying to accomplish.

If you want to combat wrinkling, use an antioxidant product in the morning to shield skin and a retinol-based one at night for skin renewal. (Retinol makes skin vulnerable to the sun, so you don't want to use it during the day.) If you want to soothe dry and sensitive skin, use a product with glycerin or hyaluronic acid to help skin retain moisture.

More expensive does not guarantee more effective when it comes to skin-care products. The key is finding the active ingredients that create the best results on your skin type, which will vary significantly from person to person. Oily skin will be more tolerant of retinol and acid treatments, while dry, sensitive skin will respond better to humectants and heavier emollients to help restore the skin barrier.

Light Therapy

Another way to get some mild skin firming and cell turnover is to try LED therapy. This treatment uses different wavelengths of light to reduce inflammation, heal wounds, and promote anti-aging effects. The strongest devices are limited to dermatologists' offices, but the U.S. Food and Drug Administration has approved several LED light devices for home use. The verdict is still out on their effectiveness, but the American Academy of Dermatology considers the therapy to be safe as long as you are not on any medication that makes you sensitive to sunlight.

Professional-Grade Results

To get more noticeable results, you'll need to visit a dermatologist who can determine your skin type and its needs, listen to what bothers you most about your appearance, and know what products and procedures will be most effective. You might be surprised by all the possible treatments that exist.

Not only can you get stronger light therapy, but you'll also unlock access to creams like *tretinoin* (Retin-A), a form of vitamin A that can boost collagen production when applied at least two times per week, leading to smoother, younger-looking skin. Tretinoin can cause redness and flaking as it starts to work and is not a replacement for all other skin products.

For both daily care and rejuvenation, there are now many specialty skin-care formulas that have gone through rigorous clinical testing. They're made with slightly different active ingredients and often more effective

Healthful Skin Habits

Lifestyle habits can have a big impact on skin quality. Think of these steps as part of your anti-aging skincare.

● **Use sunscreen daily.** The ideal product is a true sunscreen, rather than a tinted moisturizer or foundation with SPF. To get the full SPF protection from makeup, you'd need to apply an amount equal to a nickel, and that's more than most people are willing to put on their face. Choose a physical barrier sunscreen with at least 10 percent zinc oxide and/or titanium dioxide. There are many health reasons to avoid chemical-based sunscreens, including that they can increase the risk for oxidative skin damage.

● **Do not sunbathe.** The less sun you get, the longer your skin will stay youthful. There's still no such thing as a healthy tan.

● **Don't smoke.** The smoke itself triggers the destruction of collagen and, on a surface level, the repeated squinting reaction creates or deepens lines around eyes and lips.

● **Avoid home peel kits that include microneedling rollers.** Designed to help active ingredients in products get deeper into the skin, professional-quality devices can be effective in the hands of a dermatologist. However, the needles in home products are not long enough to achieve that goal yet are long enough to break the skin and cause infection and scarring. Never use anything that breaks the surface of your skin.

—Dr. Jessica Weiser

combinations than what you'll find in drug- or beauty-store brands, so some of them can travel down pores and help activate stem cells to get robust skin turnover. While these medical-grade brands are not prescription items, you can buy them only from a dermatologist.

Fillers and Procedures

Among the most visible and immediate skin-rejuvenating treatments are injectable dermal fillers that build volume where tissue has been lost, such as in deep creases or hollow cheeks. They can soften folds, enhance the jawline, and bring back body to the lips. Fillers are usually injected in the doctor's office and don't require surgery or downtime. *They can be made of a variety of substances…*

● **Those made from hyaluronic acid** last for six to 12 months before the body dissolves the molecules.

● **Fillers made of calcium hydroxylapatite** are calcium-based molecules that may last for about 12 months for most patients. Poly-L-lactic acid has been used for many years in medical devices, such as dissolvable stitches. It is a small particle suspended in sterile water that stimulates the production of collagen to smooth fine lines. The water is resorbed a few days after treatment, leaving a matrix of particles to stimulate collagen production over a period of many weeks.

Your dermatologist may suggest a range of other nonsurgical options as well…

● **Chemical peels.** In this procedure, the doctor will apply a solution to your skin to remove the top layers. Peels may be used to treat wrinkles, discolored skin, and scars.

● **Radiofrequency microneedling.** These devices use insulated needles that deliver high-intensity radiofrequency energy into the skin to stimulate new collagen growth and re-texture all skin types safely.

● **Laser therapy.** In this therapy, the doctor will apply a low-level laser to the skin. Many types of lasers can be used to address fine lines and wrinkles, uneven pigmentation such as age spots or rosacea, acne scars, and skin tightening.

Results May Vary

Word of mouth is a great way to find a dermatologist, but keep in mind that a specific procedure that worked for a friend or colleague might not be the right one for you. Research the doctor's credentials—he or she should be board certified in dermatology—

and investigate what's offered at a practice. Generally, more options are better. Having just one type of laser, for instance, often indicates that the doctor isn't as tech-savvy as he or she could be.

You want to establish a rapport with someone you can trust and who will educate you about choices rather than just tossing names of procedures at you. Also, looking at a dermatologist's personal aesthetic may help you decide who you feel comfortable with. According to research published in the *Journal of Cosmetic Dermatology*, a dermatologist's appearance, which can be very natural or very dramatic, often reflects their approach to rejuvenation.

To Reduce Under-Eye Bags and Other Facial Swelling

Real Simple

Freeze your daily facial toner into cubes, then rub a cube on your face after cleansing—start at your forehead and work down. The cold will help reduce swelling, including bags under eyes. You also can chill face masks—in the refrigerator, not the freezer—for a similar effect.

Caution: Freezing may reduce the potency of toners that contain retinol, vitamin C, salicylic acid, and glycolic acid.

Ageism: A Threat to Your Health

Charles B. Inlander, consumer advocate and health-care consultant. He is author or coauthor of more than 20 consumer-health books.

There is an old joke in the medical world: An elderly woman goes to the doctor with pain in her left knee. The doctor examines the knee and says, "What do you expect? Your knee is 90 years old." The patient looks him in the eye and says, "But so is my right knee, and it doesn't hurt a bit."

One of the most overlooked threats to our health is a medical bias against elderly patients. This bias, known as ageism, can be found in a variety of situations. For example, most clinical trials of new drugs or treatments include few, if any, patients over 60. In the doctor's office or hospital, many health-care providers speak louder, more slowly, or with a condescending tone to older patients. Ageism was also obvious in how health authorities set up the distribution of the COVID-19 vaccine. While people over 65 were placed in high-priority groups, little thought was given to their ability, or lack thereof, to access and use computers to set up appointments.

Fight Back

Just because you are older, it doesn't mean you are less likely to benefit from a medical procedure or should be treated like a child. *Here are some tips to help you avoid and even fight back against health-care ageism…*

Talk It Out

If you feel that you are being ignored or spoken down to, stop the session and tell the health-care professional how you feel. Don't hold back in expressing yourself. Quite often, he or she may not even realize it's happening. If your doctor sloughs off your feelings or gets irritated by your complaint, it may be time to find a new practitioner.

Take Someone with You

I have long recommended that you have a family member or friend with you in a medical examination room. For older patients, this is vitally important. When you are in pain or not feeling well, it can help to have another person to help ask questions or seek clarification about a diagnosis or treatment options. Your companion can also note if you're being treated in a condescending way and quickly intervene.

More from Charles B. Inlander...

Screening Tests and Age: Should You Get a Mammogram in Your 80s?

Here is how to make sure you are not just a statistic when it comes to decisions about medical testing or treatment...

●**Understand what's happening.** For the past 30 years, there has been widespread debate on when women should start getting mammograms (between 40 and 50 years of age), and the same thing about at what age a woman might stop routine testing. The guidelines now recommend stopping at age 75 if a woman is of average risk or has a life expectancy of 10 years or less. But as a healthy woman, you could live another 30 years!

●**Talk with your doctor.** It's important that you and your doctor(s) are on the same page when it comes to testing or treatment. The two of you need to frankly assess your current health status and your health history. Does breast cancer run in your family? Would you live longer or feel better if treated for a major condition?

The two of you should review the guidelines on a specific test, but the ultimate decision should be yours. Studies show that treatment of serious conditions such as breast cancer in otherwise healthy women who are in their 80s or 90s is often extremely effective and beneficial.

Consider a Geriatrician

If you are older than 65, consider using a geriatrician as your primary care provider. Geriatricians are physicians who are trained to diagnose and treat issues that affect older adults. As our population ages, more geriatricians are coming into practice. One way to find a geriatrician is to call hospitals that service your area and ask for affiliated geriatric professionals. You can also do a computer search for geriatric physicians in your area.

LVADs Are OK for People Over Age 70

Joanna Chikwe, MD, founding chair of the department of cardiac surgery in the Smidt Heart Institute at Cedars-Sinai, Los Angeles.

Many cardiologists shy away from using left ventricular assist devices (LVADs) in heart-failure patients in their 70s and beyond because of the fear of complications. Now, a new study shows that newer LVAD devices lead to fewer device failures, less blood clotting, and lower rates of infection and stroke than previous devices. Patients older than 75 experienced even fewer LVAD-related complications than their younger counterparts.

Older Adults Who Have Gained a Little Weight Live Longest

Study of more than 8,000 adults ages 31 to 80 by researchers at The Ohio State University, Columbus, published in *Annals of Epidemiology*.

People who live longest enter their 50s with a normal body-mass index (BMI, 18.5 to 24.9) but then take on an overweight but not obese BMI (25.0 to 29.9) over the next few decades. Next longest lived are those who stay at a normal BMI throughout their lives...followed by those who are overweight throughout their lives. Not surprisingly, the least long-lived are those who started out obese (BMI of 30.0 and above) and gained more weight through the years.

Improve Your Functional Fitness

Karl Knopf, EdD, retired director of adaptive fitness at Foothill College in Los Altos Hills, California. He is author of more than 17 books on functional fitness including *Resistance Band Workbook* and *Injury Rehab with Resistance Bands*.

Have you stopped riding a bike, bowling, or playing golf or tennis because these activities are too hard to perform? Do your muscles sometimes struggle when you're going up the stairs? Or raising yourself up from a low chair, the toilet, or the car? Do you find yourself losing your balance more often than you used to? These all are telltale signs that you need to improve your functional fitness—the ability to perform everyday tasks that use multiple muscle groups and require balance, strength, and dexterity.

Although our physical capabilities naturally decline with age, our increasingly sedentary lifestyle also significantly impacts our strength and flexibility. If you have trouble carrying groceries into your home or feel winded after a short brisk walk, this decline in physical function can mean the loss of the ability to live independently as you age.

But it doesn't have to be this way. *Starting a functional fitness program can improve your ability to live a full life...**

Creating Your Routine

To design your routine, start by assessing which activities you do regularly that you find challenging. Then choose from the exercises described on these pages. Start with two or three repetitions of each exercise, rest and then repeat several times, eventually working up to two to three sets of 10 or 15 repetitions.

Important: Maintaining proper form and posture through each exercise is critical to its effectiveness.

*Note: Get clearance from a doctor before starting any exercise program to determine if you have an underlying dysfunction that is contributing to your limitations.

These exercises require only exercise bands (buy at least two—one that is open and one that is a closed loop) and dumbbells (start with one- to three-pound weights depending on your current strength). Resistance bands normally come in sets of low-, medium- and high-resistance. Experiment to see what's right for you. When you get comfortable, challenge yourself with more resistance, more weight and/or more repetitions.

If you have trouble going up stairs or getting up from a chair or if your legs are weak, you need to strengthen the leg and core muscles. *Doing so can help to reduce the load on your knees and possibly reduce knee pain...*

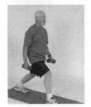

Lunges

1. Stand up tall on a nonslip surface holding a dumbbell in each hand at your sides or while wearing a weighted vest. Inhale.

2. As you exhale, lunge forward with your right leg while keeping your left leg stationary. Only lunge forward as far as comfortable and be sure to keep your front knee aligned with your ankle.

3. Inhale and step back to your starting position. Repeat. Then switch sides. Be sure to maintain erect posture as you do each repetition.

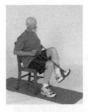

Leg Presses

1. Sit in a chair, and wrap an exercise band around your left foot. Hold on to both ends of the band with your elbows bent and shoulders relaxed.

2. Exhale and slowly extend the left leg forward. Do not lock your knee.

3. Inhale and return your leg to the starting position. Repeat, and then switch sides.

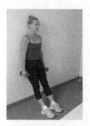

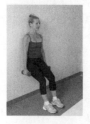

Wall Squats/Slides

1. Lean your back against a wall with your feet about 12 to 18 inches away from the wall. Hold a dumbbell in each hand with your arms at your sides. Inhale.

2. Exhale as you slide yourself down along the wall, going no farther than feels comfortable or until your thighs are parallel with the floor. Do not let your knees extend beyond your toes.

3. Inhale and return to the upright position...or for greater challenge, hold for a count of five before inhaling and returning to the starting position. Keep your head straight and eyes looking forward.

Note: Skip this exercise if you have heart or blood pressure issues. Instead, try a Mini Chair Squat. Just stand in front of a chair or tall stool to hold onto for balance and only lower yourself slightly, rather than doing a full squat.

If you have trouble opening heavy doors or carrying groceries, you need to strengthen your arms and shoulders...

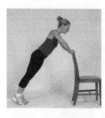

Chair Push-Ups

1. Stand behind a sturdy chair or countertop. Lean forward, and place your hands on the chair back/countertop shoulder-width apart. Extend your arms fully, without locking your elbows, as you walk your legs back until your body is at a 45-degree angle to the floor. Your heels will be raised slightly. Keep your legs straight but not locked. Inhale.

2. Exhale and slowly lower your chest to the chair. Keep your elbows close to your body and your torso in a straight line with your legs.

3. Inhale and press your body away from the chair, fully extending your arms without locking them, returning to the starting position.

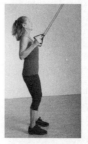

Pull-Downs

1. Tie a knot in the middle of an open exercise band, and anchor it at the top of a closed door, leaving both ends hanging down. Sit in a chair or stand and reach overhead, arms straight, to grasp each end of the band at a point that will provide resistance when stretched. Inhale.

2. Exhale as you pull your elbows back, bringing your hands to shoulder level. Be careful not to arch your back and to keep your shoulders down.

3. Inhale. Return to starting position.

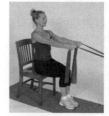

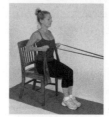

Shoulder Retractions

1. Position a chair near a closed door. Tie the middle of an open exercise band around the doorknob leaving two long ends. Grasp an end in each hand about halfway up so you feel a comfortable level of resistance. Inhale and suck in your stomach to stabilize your back.

2. Exhale and slowly pull your elbows back toward your sides. Keep your shoulder blades together throughout.

3. Inhale and return to the starting position.

Bow and Arrow

1. Stand with your feet about hip-width apart. With your left hand, grab one side of a closed-loop exercise band and extend that arm out to your side at shoulder height. Now grab the opposite side of the band with your

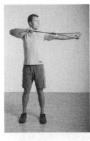

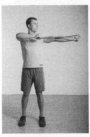

right hand, keeping your right hand near your left shoulder and your right elbow at shoulder height. You should be positioned as though holding an archery bow.

2. Inhale and stretch the band back across your chest with your right hand as if you were pulling a bow. Your right elbow will be bent, left arm extended. Keep shoulders relaxed/down.

3. Exhale. Return to the starting position. Repeat and switch to the other side.

If you have trouble reaching things on high shelves, you need to stretch and strengthen the arms and shoulders…

Walking Fingertips

1. Stand sideways to a wall about an arm's distance away…or stand facing it.

2. Reach out to the wall. Slowly walk your fingertips up the wall as high as you can.

3. Crawl your fingers down to the starting position, repeat and switch sides.

Wall Circles

1. Stand facing a wall with one arm extended touching it at shoulder level.

2. Draw small circles clockwise, increasing to larger circles as feels comfortable. Repeat, and switch sides.

Apple Picker

1. Stand tall with your hands on your shoulders.

2. Reach your right hand up to the ceiling, stretching as high as is comfortable.

3. Return your right hand to your shoulder, and reach up with your left hand.

Exercise photos courtesy of Karl Knopf.

What to Do with Ugly Nails

Jonathan D. Rose, DPM, a podiatrist in private practice in Baltimore.

Thickened, yellowed nails happen often with age. One of the most common causes is a fungal infection called onychomycosis, which strikes about 50 percent of people over age 70.

Small cracks in the nail or the skin around it allow the fungus to enter the nail, and closed-toe shoes then provide a warm, moist environment for the fungus to thrive.

Treat the Infection

You can try treating the infection with over-the-counter antifungal nail creams and ointments, but if you have a persistent infection or have diabetes, immune system disorders, or poor circulation, it's important to see your primary care doctor, dermatologist, or podiatrist.

Prescription treatments may include oral antifungal drugs such as *terbinafine* (Lamisil) and *itraconazole* (Sporanox), antifungal nail polish or creams, and/or removal of the damaged part of the nail in a process called debridement.

Prevent Infection

Use these steps to minimize the risk for fungal infections…

- **Dry between your toes after a shower.**
- **Wear flip-flops in public showers.**
- **Use an antifungal powder.**
- **Allow your shoes to dry after wearing them.**
- **Clean inside shoes with vinegar and water or spray with a disinfectant.**
- **Wear socks that wick away moisture,** such as those made from acrylic, wool, nylon, or polypropylene.

• **Keep your nails trimmed to help prevent nail trauma,** which makes it easier for fungus to get under the nail and flourish.

Varicose Veins Can Be Repaired Instead of Removed

Dominic Mühlberger, MD, attending physician, vascular surgery department, St. Josef Hospital, Ruhr-Universität, Bochum, Germany.

In severe varicose vein disease, damaged veins are usually removed or destroyed, but that means that those large blood vessels can no longer be used if patients later need coronary artery bypass surgery.

Recent alternative: A thin sheath placed around a defective vein can alleviate symptoms and save the vein in 95 percent of cases.

Seniors Are Susceptible to Hypothermia— Even Indoors

Luke K. Hermann, MD, associate professor of emergency medicine, Icahn School of Medicine at Mount Sinai, New York City, reporting in *Focus on Healthy Aging.*

The body's natural temperature-regulation system becomes less effective after about age 65, so it becomes harder to maintain normal body temperature as temps drop outside.

One-Stop Shop for Age-at-Home Products

Home-improvement chain Lowe's partnered with AARP to launch Livable Home in 2022—a program that offers products, services, and DIY expertise to help seniors stay in their own homes instead of moving to assisted-care facilities. The program includes specially trained Lowe's employees wearing AARP-branded badges available to help customers with products and information for installing shower grab bars, nonslip floors, wheelchair ramps, and walk-in bathtubs. The program is in 500 stores in 50 metro areas.

Information: Lowes.com (search "liveable home").

CNBC.com

Other factors also make seniors more vulnerable to hypothermia (internal body temperature below 95°F): Reduced mobility can keep seniors from moving around enough to generate body heat. And certain medications and medical conditions compromise the ability to generate body heat—and the ability to recognize temperature changes. There is even risk indoors—temperatures at 60°F to 70°F can be dangerously low for at-risk seniors. Hypothermia symptoms to watch for include shivering, confusion, slurred speech and being drowsy and/or unsteady. These symptoms can creep up gradually.

Self-defense: Wear several light layers when it's cold out, even if it's just chilly, including a hat and gloves.

Also keep in mind: Body temperature drops quickly if clothing is wet, especially in windy conditions.

Chapter 2

BRAIN HEALTH AND STROKE ALERTS

Eat for Your Brain

What we eat affects our weight, our energy levels, our susceptibility to diseases and, we now know, our cognition, too.

But while a poor diet can set off a chain reaction that leads to memory loss, all evidence suggests that we may be able to improve and protect cognition by swapping foods that compromise our gut bacteria—which directly affects the neurochemicals involved in memory—with foods that enhance it. Diet may even prevent or slow down cognitive decline and conditions like Alzheimer's disease (AD).

First, Do No Harm

Both high-fat and high-glycemic-index foods (those that cause a rapid rise in blood glucose) can alter brain pathways that are necessary for learning and memory. Neurons in the hippocampus—the part of the brain most involved in remembering things such as a new acquaintance's name or facts about the world—are particularly sensitive to diet. High-fat and high-sugar consumption can hamper the expression of critical growth factors and other hormones that promote healthy function in the hippocampus and can affect insulin signaling and insulin sensitivity in the body's tissues. The traditional fatty, sugary, and processed Western diet can even cause the hippocampus to shrink.

Research is showing that neuro (brain) inflammation has been linked to both age-related cognitive decline and the risk of developing AD.

The MIND Diet

Thankfully, it appears that dietary changes can halt these processes and even reverse them, protecting against cognitive decline. For five years, a team of researchers from Rush University Medical Center and the Harvard School of Public Health studied the link between diet and cognition. They concluded that a combination of two established dietary plans, the Mediterranean diet and the Dietary Approaches to Stop Hypertension (DASH), provided clear and significant cognitive benefits. They named the combination of the two the MIND diet (short for the Med-

Uma Naidoo, MD, instructor in psychiatry at Harvard Medical School, director of nutritional and lifestyle psychiatry at Massachusetts General Hospital, and author of *This Is Your Brain on Food: An Indispensable Guide to the Surprising Foods That Fight Depression, Anxiety, PTSD, OCD, ADHD, and More.*

iterranean-DASH Intervention for Neurode-generative Delay).

The investigators discovered that people who followed the MIND diet the most closely were 7.5 cognitive years younger than those who followed more of a standard American diet. They showed better episodic memory (long-term recall of personal facts), working memory (short-term recall of information that is still being acted upon), semantic memory (memory of facts and knowledge about the world), visuospatial ability (the ability to see and understand the size and space of their surroundings), and perceptual speed (how quickly things are seen). The effects were most pronounced with episodic memory, semantic memory, and perceptual speed.

The MIND diet was also associated with a reduced incidence of AD. The higher the adherence to the MIND diet, the slower the rate of cognitive decline. In 2019, another research team reported that the diet was also associated with a reduced incidence and delayed progression of Parkinson's disease.

Brain-Boosting Foods

The basic tenets of the diet are simple. *Strive to base your diet on 11 foundational foods...*

1. Green leafy vegetables (kale, collards, greens, spinach, lettuce, tossed salad, microgreens): six or more servings per week

2. Other vegetables (peppers, squash, carrots, broccoli, celery, potatoes, tomatoes, tomato sauce, string beans, beets, corn, zucchini, summer squash, eggplant): one or more servings per day

3. Berries (strawberries, blueberries, raspberries, blackberries): two or more servings per week

4. Nuts: five or more servings per week

5. Whole grains: three or more servings per day

6. Fish (not fried, particularly high-omega-3 fish such as salmon): one or more meals per week

7. Beans, lentils, soybeans: more than three meals per week

8. Poultry: two or more meals per week

9. Wine: one glass per day

10. Fruit: at least one or two servings per day

11. Use olive oil as your primary oil

At the same time, there are some foods you should limit or eliminate...

• **Margarine or butter-like spreads:** less than 1 tablespoon per day

• **Cheese:** less than once per week

• **Fried food:** less than once per week

• **Red meat and pork:** a few times per week

• **Limit sweets** such as ice cream, cookies, brownies, snack cakes, donuts, and candy.

Additional Food Research

Outside of the MIND diet, researchers have identified some specific foods that may add even more protective benefits...

• **Coffee.** Caffeine, which increases the neurotransmitters serotonin and acetylcholine, may stimulate the brain and help stabilize the blood-brain barrier. The polyphenols in coffee may prevent tissue damage by free radicals. Trigonelline, a substance found in high concentration in coffee beans, may activate antioxidants that protect blood vessels in the brain.

Research suggests that three cups of coffee per day may lower the risk of cognitive decline, dementia, and AD. Keep your overall caffeine consumption (which includes chocolate, cola, tea, and guarana) under 400 milligrams per day.

• **Turmeric.** The active ingredient of this spice is curcumin, which has antioxidant, anti-inflammatory, and neuron growth-promoting properties. A 2019 review of curcumin studies showed that consumption of curcumin improved attention, learning, overall cognition, and memory. It improves cognitive

Beat Brain Fog

Brain fog occurs when you struggle to concentrate, think clearly, or multitask. It can also affect both short- and long-term memory. Experts believe it comes from excessive brain inflammation and suggest that it can be alleviated by following a whole-foods diet, such as the MIND diet, and avoiding processed, fatty, and sugary foods. *Some additional nutrients may help too...*

- **Luteolin** is an antioxidant and anti-inflammatory agent that prevents toxic destruction of nerve cells in the brain. You can find it in Mexican oregano, juniper berries, fresh peppermint, sage, thyme, hot and sweet peppers, radicchio, celery seeds, parsley, and artichokes.

- **Citicoline.** If your brain fog is due to acetylcholine and dopamine depletion, foods such as beef liver and egg yolks may help.

- **Phosphatidylserine** is required for healthy nerve cell membranes and coverings, and its protective effects can prevent brain fog. You can find it in soybeans or supplements.

- **Probiotics** are often beneficial, but sometimes they can cause slower digestion that leads to brain fog. If you're taking a probiotic and finding your thoughts sluggish, consider switching supplements. Better yet, get your probiotics from dietary sources like plain yogurt with active cultures.

- **Gluten.** After consuming gluten, some people find themselves thinking less clearly and wanting to sleep all day. If you are suffering from brain fog, cut out gluten to see if you improve. It may turn out that you have celiac disease or non-celiac gluten sensitivity.

function in people with AD and may help prevent it.

When you consume plain turmeric or curcumin, however, very little of it is absorbed into the blood. Boost absorption by combining it with black pepper or a fat such as olive oil. Cooking with it also makes it easier for your body to use.

- **Black pepper and cinnamon.** Black pepper and cinnamon suppress inflammatory pathways and may act as antioxidants. They increase the availability of acetylcholine, which improves memory, and help clear amyloid deposits. (A build-up of these deposits is a hallmark of AD.)

- **Saffron.** Several studies suggest that saffron has cognitive benefits, from enhancing memory to increasing cognition in people with AD. It has antioxidant and anti-inflammatory properties. Saffron can be used in cooking or taken as a supplement.

- **Ginger.** Ginger has been shown to enhance working memory in middle-aged healthy women. In animals, it has increased the levels of adrenaline, noradrenaline, dopamine, and serotonin contents in the cerebral cortex and hippocampus, so it may work through these brain chemicals to enhance memory.

These first four spices work well together in a variety of savory dishes, including Indian curries. (This stew-like dish with meat or vegetables in a spiced gravy is not the same thing as the spice called curry.) That may be part of the reason why the incidence of AD for people ages 70 to 79 is four times lower in India than in the United States.

- **Rosemary.** One study found that the aroma of rosemary changes brain waves so that people become less anxious, more alert, and better able to compute math problems. Rosemary can also boost acetylcholine, which is instrumental in memory. You can use it in cooking (try it on roasted potatoes or chicken) or aromatherapy.

- **Sage** decreases inflammation in the brain, reduces amyloid deposits, decreases oxidative cell damage, increases acetylcholine, and helps neuronal growth. It can enhance memory, attention, word recall, and speed of memory in healthy adults. It can make people feel more alert, content, and calm. You can use it in cooking or aromatherapy.

Don't Let These Treatable Conditions Rob You of Your Cognition and Memory

Marc E. Agronin, MD, an adult and geriatric psychiatrist and affiliate associate professor of psychiatry and neurology at the University of Miami Miller School of Medicine and author of *How We Age*.

Alzheimer's disease (AD) and dementia stand out as the most feared health conditions that can strike as we age. But if you notice that your memory or cognition isn't what it used to be, put the brakes on that panic: Memory loss and cognitive challenges can come from a host of other disorders, the majority of which are treatable. Because the myth that memory loss is a normal part of aging persists, even among some health-care professionals, you may need to advocate for yourself or your loved ones to rule out the following common causes of reversible cognitive impairment.

Adult ADD or ADHD

People associate attention-deficit disorder (ADD) and attention-deficit hyperactivity disorder (ADHD) with children, but these conditions also affect 2 to 4 percent of adults—and most are never diagnosed. This neurobiological disease makes it difficult to focus or pay attention and, as a result, difficult to learn and remember new information. People with ADD are easily distracted, may have a history of work problems, and often don't follow through on tasks at home. (*Editor's note*: See page 117 for a detailed look at adult ADD/ADHD.)

Memory fix: These symptoms are reversible with stimulant medications such as *methylphenidate* (Ritalin) and *amphetamine-dextroamphetamine* (Adderall).

Who to see: Some primary care doctors will screen and treat patients for ADD/ADHD, but you may want to see a neurologist for a more thorough examination and treatment.

Obstructive Sleep Apnea

In this common sleep disorder, the muscles in the back of the throat relax too much and block the airway. When oxygen levels drop, the sleeper wakes up just enough to move and take a breath. These episodes can occur hundreds of times per night, but most sufferers don't know they're happening. Diminished nighttime oxygen and excessive daytime sleepiness can impair memory and concentration. Patients with sleep apnea also have a higher risk for stroke and heart disease.

Warning signs include gasping, snorting, or loud snoring during sleep, a dry mouth in the morning, morning headaches, and/or difficulty staying alert during the day. People who are overweight or who have thick necks have an elevated risk, but sleep apnea can strike anyone.

Memory fix: Obstructive sleep apnea can be treated with a small bedside device called a continuous positive airway pressure machine that delivers mild air pressure through a hose to help keep the airways open.

Who to see: Your primary care doctor can refer you to a sleep specialist to arrange for testing and treatment.

Medication

If you're taking codeine or another opioid medication for pain, you expect to be a little groggy, but some of the drugs that affect memory aren't the ones that most people are aware of or think to discuss with their doctors. These include statins to lower cholesterol, benzodiazepines to treat anxiety, antiseizure drugs, antidepressants, and dopamine agonists for Parkinson's disease (see table on next page). Over-the-counter decongestants and antihistamines, recreational drugs, and alcohol can cause cognitive problems, too.

Memory fix: Tell your doctor if your cognitive symptoms seem to get worse after

Drugs With Cognitive Side Effects

DRUG CLASS	USE	EXAMPLES
Benzodiazepines	anxiety disorders, agitation, delirium, muscle spasms, seizures, insomnia	*alprazolam* (Xanax), *chlordiazepoxide* (Librium), *clonazepam* (Klonopin), *diazepam* (Valium), *flurazepam* (Dalmane), *lorazepam* (Ativan), *midazolam* (Versed), *quazepam* (Doral), *temazepam* (Restoril) and *triazolam* (Halcion)
Statins	high cholesterol	*atorvastatin* (Lipitor), *fluvastatin* (Lescol), *lovastatin* (Mevacor), *pravastatin* (Pravachol), *rosuvastatin* (Crestor) and *simvastatin* (Zocor)
Antiseizure drugs	seizures, nerve pain, bipolar disorder, mood disorder, mania, migraine	*acetazolamide* (Diamox), *carbamazepine* (Tegretol), *ezogabine* (Potiga), *gabapentin* (Neurontin), *lamotrigine* (Lamictal), *levetiracetam* (Keppra), *oxcarbazepine* (Trileptal), *pregabalin* (Lyrica), *rufinamide* (Banzel), *topiramate* (Topamax), *valproic acid* (Depakote) and *zonisamide* (Zonegran)
Tricyclic antidepressants	depression, anxiety disorders, eating disorders, obsessive-compulsive disorder, chronic pain, smoking cessation, hormone-mediated disorders	*amitriptyline* (Elavil), *clomipramine* (Anafranil), *desipramine* (Norpramin), *doxepin* (Sinequan), *imipramine* (Tofranil), *nortriptyline* (Pamelor), *protriptyline* (Vivactil) and *trimipramine* (Surmontil)
Narcotic painkillers	pain	*fentanyl* (Duragesic), *hydrocodone* (Norco, Vicodin), *hydromorphone* (Dilaudid, Exalgo), *morphine* (Astramorph, Avinza) and *oxycodone* (OxyContin, Percocet). These drugs come in many different forms, including tablets, solutions for injection, transdermal patches and suppositories.
Dopamine agonists	Parkinson's disease, pituitary tumors, restless legs syndrome	*apomorphine* (Apokyn), *pramipexole* (Mirapex), and *ropinirole* (Requip)
Beta-blockers	high blood pressure, congestive heart failure, abnormal heart rhythms, chest pain (angina), migraines, tremors, glaucoma	*atenolol* (Tenormin), *carvedilol* (Coreg), *metoprolol* (Lopressor, Toprol), *propranolol* (Inderal), *sotalol* (Betapace), *timolol* (Timoptic) and some other drugs whose chemical names end with "-olol"
Nonbenzodiazepine sedative-hypnotics	insomnia, sleep problems, mild anxiety	*eszopiclone* (Lunesta), *zaleplon* (Sonata) and *zolpidem* (Ambien)
Anticholinergics	overactive bladder, urge incontinence	*darifenacin* (Enablex), *oxybutynin* (Ditropan XL, Gelnique, Oxytrol), *solifenacin* (Vesicare), *tolterodine* (Detrol) and *trospium* (Sanctura). Another oxybutynin product, Oxytrol for Women, is sold over the counter.
Antihistamines (first-generation)	allergy symptoms, motion sickness, nausea, vomiting and dizziness, and anxiety or insomnia	*brompheniramine* (Dimetane), *carbinoxamine* (Clistin), *chlorpheniramine* (Chlor-Trimeton), *clemastine* (Tavist), *diphenhydramine* (Benadryl) and *hydroxyzine* (Vistaril)

starting a new medication. You might need to change drugs or take a lower dose. The cognitive effects can be amplified when you take multiple drugs, so make sure all of your physicians have a complete list of the drugs you take.

Who to see: Talk to any physician who prescribes medication for you. Your pharmacist can also tell you if any of the medications you are taking, or have been prescribed, has cognitive side effects.

Mental Health

When you meet people at a party, do you remember their names? Or are you so nervous that their names don't register? Anxiety and stress cause distraction, and it's difficult to form memories when you're not paying attention. Some people become so worried about memory problems that every slip causes them to freeze and stop paying attention to what's happening around them.

Depression is also linked to cognitive lapses, especially since it interferes with concentration, interest in activities, and sleep, all essential factors for good memory.

Memory fix: These conditions can be treated with medication, therapy, and lifestyle changes, such as getting more exercise and practicing relaxation techniques.

Who to see: If you notice a problem with stress, anxiety, or depression, talk to your primary care doctor or a mental health provider for a thorough evaluation to assess your mood, thinking, and behavior.

Thyroid Disease

Cognitive dysfunction is a little-known effect of thyroid disease and one that can easily be missed, especially since people over age 60 may have no other symptoms of thyroid disease.

Memory fix: Medication can restore proper thyroid levels and cognitive performance.

Who to see: Your primary care doctor can use a simple blood test to look at how your thyroid is functioning.

Vitamin B12 Deficiency

People who don't eat animal foods and those who take medications called proton-pump inhibitors for acid reflux have a higher risk of developing a vitamin B12 deficiency, which can cause confusion and memory loss.

Memory fix: The cognitive effects of a B12 deficiency are reversible by restoring your levels of the vitamin.

Who to see: Your primary care doctor can check your B12 levels with a blood test and recommend supplementation.

A Good Listener Can Boost Your Brain Health

Study titled "Association of social support with brain volume and cognition," published in *JAMA Network Open*.

Researchers at NYU Langone have discovered that people who can count on someone to listen when they need to talk have greater cognitive resilience, a measure of the brain's ability to function better than would be expected at a set age or disease state.

In the study, researchers used MRI scans to measure participants' brain volume and neuropsychological assessments to measure cognition. A cognitive resilience score was assigned based on the relative effect of brain volume on cognition. Lower brain volume is generally associated with lower cognitive function.

But among the more than 2,000 study participants, people who reported having strong social supports, specifically the availability of a friend or loved one they could count on to listen, had better cognition than would be expected from their brain volume alone.

These findings could have important implications for people ages 65 and older who have or who are at risk for developing Alzheimer's disease, notes lead researcher Joel Salinas, MD, assistant professor of neurology at NYU Grossman School of Medicine.

But younger people should pay attention to their social support systems, too. The study showed that people in their 40s and 50s who did not have a supportive listener had a cognitive age that was four years older than those who did.

Concerned About Alzheimer's? Meditation May Beat Medication

Dharma Singh Khalsa, MD, president and medical director of the Alzheimer's Research and Prevention Foundation in Tucson, Arizona, and prevention editor of *Journal of Alzheimer's Disease*.

Just as physical fitness is recognized for its ability to protect brain health, an active spiritual or religious life is known to reduce rates of mild cognitive impairment (MCI) and Alzheimer's disease (AD).

These days, spirituality and religion are separate concepts. The word "spirituality" increasingly is used to represent a person's search for a higher power or something sacred or divine within themselves. In recent years, many Americans have begun viewing themselves as spiritual but not necessarily religious.

Regardless of your views, engaging in some form of meditative thought—prayer, meditation, deep breathing, or guided imagery—reduces activity in areas of the brain associated with stress while simultaneously enhancing cognition and focus. Stress is a risk factor for AD. The more stress you have, the more *cortisol* (a stress hormone) your body produces. Chronically elevated cortisol levels may promote brain shrinkage, inflammation, and cognitive decline.

Spiritual fitness meditations, which involve focusing attention on a specific mantra, phrase, song, or object, do more than reduce cortisol levels. They also lower heart rate and blood pressure, and enhance immune function by reducing stress, which is immunosuppressive. All of these have brain-protective effects—they reduce risk for heart disease, cancer, and other chronic diseases, too.

Spirituality and religion also help people cultivate a sense of meaning or purpose in life, which, research suggests, independently helps slow AD.

Fascinating: In a study conducted by Rush University researchers, individuals who scored high on a "purpose in life" (PIL) assessment were 2.4 times more likely to remain free of AD than individuals with low PIL.

Spiritual fitness also may reduce depressive symptoms and engender positive emotions. And people who practice religion or spirituality are less likely to engage in unhealthy practices.

A 2019 study by Korean researchers published in *American Journal of Alzheimer's Disease & Other Dementias* found that religious practice positively affects cognitive functioning. And when European researchers analyzed 51 studies exploring a link between religious practice, spirituality and AD, 50 of them yielded positive correlations. Many involved the benefits of spirituality on caretakers of those with AD or on helping patients with AD find meaning in their diagnosis. There's even a research field called *neurotheology* that examines how various meditative practices affect the brain.

Meditation May Be the Key

One type of meditation—Kirtan Kriya—shows promise in terms of counteracting the effects of stress on our brain. Practiced for thousands of years as part of the Kundalini yoga tradition, Kirtan Kriya involves singing a mantra of four sounds—*Saaa, Taaa, Naaa, Maaa*—while performing repetitive finger poses, or mudras. Traditionally practiced for 12 minutes a day, Kirtan Kriya has been shown to reverse memory loss, and neurological studies reveal it increases blood flow to, and activation of, anatomical areas important for memory function and emotional regulation. Research on Kirtan Kriya also suggests benefits related to anxiety, depression, sleep and mood.

How to do it: Sit up straight in a chair or on the floor. For two minutes, sing out loud *Saaa, Taaa, Naaa, Maaa*, which means "my truest self" in Sanskrit. As you sing, touch your thumb to each fingertip—*Saaa* (index to thumb), *Taaa* (middle finger to thumb), *Naaa* (ring finger to thumb), *Maaa* (pinky finger to thumb). Repeat the practice for two minutes while whispering instead of singing. Next, spend four minutes repeating the mantra silently, followed by two minutes of whispering and two final minutes of singing. The fingertip mudras are performed the entire time. As you sing, try to imagine the sound flowing in through the tip of your head, sweeping through your brain and exiting through the forehead. End the practice with a deep, centering breath.

Recent finding: A new review published in *Journal of Alzheimer's Disease* shows that Kirtan Kriya increases blood flow to key brain areas after a single session, with improvements building after eight weeks of daily practice.

Any type of meditative thought has the potential for stress reduction and improved brain function. But unlike, say, Transcendental Meditation, in which you silently focus on a mantra, Kirtan Kriya integrates singing and finger poses. It reduces cortisol levels and triggers the release of endorphins, which relieve stress, regulate mood and improve immune function…and, when the tongue touches the roof of the mouth while singing, it triggers the hypothalamus, key to maintaining hormone/chemical balance. The fingertip poses stimulate blood flow to the brain.

Recent study: My research team assigned 161 women, most of whom had reported cognitive decline or mild cognitive impairment (MCI), to one of two groups. One group performed Kirtan Kriya for 12 minutes a day for eight to 12 weeks. The other listened to music or underwent a memory-training program.

Result: Those in the Kirtan Kriya group showed larger improvements in blood flow to the brain, cognitive functioning, and markers of brain health. They also showed a greater increase in the length of *telomeres* —the caps at the end of chromosomes that prevent DNA from deteriorating. Shorter telomeres are associated with poor immune function, inflammation, accelerated aging and AD,

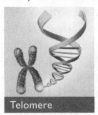

Telomere

while longer telomeres usually correspond to a longer life with a clearer mind. Women who began the study with the worst cognition experienced the most improvement in telomere length.

A Brain-Healthy Lifestyle

Spiritual fitness is just one spoke on the wheel of cognitive health. In 2014, the Finnish Intervention Study to Prevent Cognitive Impairment and Disability showed that a brain-healthy lifestyle with specific dietary guidelines (heavy on produce, fish and whole grains)…physical activity (aerobic, strength and balance)…cognitive stimulation…social activity…and managing heart health—can slow cognitive decline.

What About the New AD Drug?

At first blush, the FDA's recent approval of the first treatment for early-stage Alzheimer's disease (AD) since 2003 offers a glimmer of hope for the six million Americans with AD. Marketed under the name Aduhelm, *aducanumab* removes amyloid, a sticky compound often found in the brains of people with AD. Amyloid can clump and form plaques that disrupt cell-to-cell communication.

Theory: By removing amyloid, you may be able to slow or reduce cognitive decline. Aducanumab is not a cure, and it cannot bring back lost cognitive function. One year of aducanumab, given intravenously every four weeks for 45 to 60 minutes at a time, costs $28,000.

Concerns: The new drug was approved via an accelerated approval pathway, meaning that despite uncertainty about its efficacy, the FDA wanted to provide access to a treatment that it believes is "reasonably likely" to help. This approval came after trials of the drug were initially halted because it seemed aducanumab wasn't working as well as hoped. Subsequent reanalysis of the data suggested some potential, and, despite the FDA's own advisory committee being against it, the accelerated approval happened.

Aducanumab has some side effects, including headaches, brain swelling and increased risk of falling.

Note: The Cleveland Clinic and the Mount Sinai Health System do not plan to carry aducanumab due to safety and efficacy concerns.

Perhaps even more important is that more and more high-level AD researchers now suggest that amyloid deposits may not be the only cause of AD. Many patients live long, cognitively healthy lives despite having those plaques. Amyloid may be a marker of aging, but many holistic- and integrative-minded brain experts believe that AD results from lifestyle factors, including stress, poor diet, lack of exercise, lack of mental stimulation, lack of meditation and more.

Is Your Forgetfulness Normal?

NeuroscienceNews.com

The Self-Administered Gerocognitive (SAGE) test gives doctors a baseline of a patient's cognitive function. Taking the test again later allows changes to be evaluated for possible signs of problems. The test was developed at Ohio State University's Wexner Medical Center, College of Medicine and College of Public Health, and has been shown effective in identifying when mild cognitive impairment is likely to progress to dementia. The test is free and easy to take on your own. You can bring the results to your doctor, who can keep it as part of your medical record.

Download the SAGE test: WexnerMedical. osu.edu/SAGE.

Loss of Pleasure Signals Early-Onset Dementia

Study titled "Uncovering the Prevalence and Neural Substrates of Anhedonia in Frontotemporal Dementia," by researchers at the University of Sydney, Australia, published in *Brain*.

Imagine if you lost the ability to enjoy simple life pleasures, such as watching a sunset or eating a fine meal. It's possibly the most tragic symptom of dementia, known as *anhedonia*. Unfortunately, loss of interest in pleasurable activities is common among individuals with depression and Alzheimer's disease.

Researchers at the University of Sydney in New South Wales, Australia, have found that anhedonia may be the first and most significant symptom of a type of early-onset dementia called frontotemporal dementia (FTD).

Anhedonia Differs from Apathy

FTD is different from Alzheimer's disease and other dementias. It develops earlier, usually between the ages of 40 and 65. Patients with other dementias and depression often feel apathetic toward things they usually enjoy, but apathy is not the same as anhedonia. Apathy is the loss of interest and motivation. Anhedonia is the loss of the ability to seek and feel pleasure.

Study details: The researchers compared symptoms and brain scans of 87 people diagnosed with FTD, 34 with Alzheimer's disease and 51 healthy older people. Using symptom scales that measure pleasure, apathy and depression, the researchers were able to show that loss of the ability to experience pleasure was only severe in patients with FTD. In these patients, anhedonia was a stand-out, early symptom of FTD and a major change from their former ability to experience pleasure. Their research study is published in the journal *Brain*.

Discovery May Help Avoid Misdiagnosis

When comparing brain scans, the researchers found that anhedonia causes the loss of brain cells (atrophy) in gray matter in the *frontostriatal* region of the brain. This area is responsible for sensing and seeking pleasure.

The researchers hope their findings will lead to an earlier diagnosis of FTD, which is often misdiagnosed as depression. Future studies will focus on how to manage the impact of anhedonia in patients with FTD and may lead to the development of specific treatments that will improve the quality of life for people who have lost the ability to seek out the joys of living.

For more information: Visit DailyCaring. com/elderly-losing-interest-in-life-ways-to-help-with-anhedonia for ways to assist a loved one experiencing anhedonia. See also the Alzheimer's Association website, Alz.org, for additional information on dementia and resources for help.

Disorders of the Gut-Brain Axis

Douglas A. Drossman, MD, president, Center for Education and Practice of Biopsychosocial Care (DrossmanCare) and Drossman Gastroenterology; and Johannah Ruddy, MEd, executive director of the Rome Foundation and secretary-treasurer of DrossmanCare. Dr. Drossman and Ms. Ruddy are coauthors of *Gut Feelings: Disorders of Gut-Brain Interaction and the Patient-Doctor Relationship.*

Your brain and gut are hardwired to work together. It doesn't always go smoothly.

If you've ever gotten diarrhea from being nervous or felt excessively anxious after a stomach bug, you've experienced a gut-brain interaction.

The brain and gut are hardwired to maintain constant communication with each other. That means that when things go awry, they can each wreak havoc on the other, causing what's called disorders of gut-brain interaction (DGBI).

Symptom Diversity

DGBIs, formerly called functional gastrointestinal (GI) disorders, can cause anything from difficulty swallowing to lack of control over bowel movements (see box on next page). The most well-known DGBI is irritable bowel syndrome, which causes pain, bloating, diarrhea or constipation, and a high risk of depression or anxiety.

These disorders don't come from structural diseases: They're not visible on an X-ray or endoscopy or identifiable in a blood test. *Rather, they relate to abnormal functioning of the GI system caused by one or more of five elements...*

• **Abnormal movement inside the bowels (motility disturbance)**

• **More intense abdominal pain than usual in response to stimuli (visceral hypersensitivity)**

• **Changes to the bowel's mucous membrane and immune response**

• **Changes to the normal microbes found in a healthy gut (gut dysbiosis)**

• **Changes in how the brain processes pain and other GI symptoms.**

Because of the communication along the gut-brain axis, the pain, nausea, or vomiting that can come from these dysfunctions can directly cause anxiety or depression. In turn, emotional distress can affect motility, causing diarrhea or nausea, and even change the way we perceive pain.

Pain and the Brain

To understand how stress and emotions affect pain, envision a walkway with a gate. Pain signals from the gut have to pass through the gate on their way to the brain. At the same time, the brain acts as a gatekeeper, sending signals that determine how far the gate will open—and how much pain you will feel. For example, if you're running a race and sprain your ankle, the brain could send norepinephrine (similar to adrenaline) to slam the gate shut and block the pain signals. Emotional distress has the opposite effect: It causes the brain to throw the gate wide open, allowing a flood of pain signals to rush through.

When you experience gut pain, nerves in the spinal cord amplify the signals, making the same pain feel worse. That produces emotional distress, which further lowers the pain threshold, creating a vicious circle that creates hypersensitivity in both the gut and the brain, sometimes transforming acute pain into a chronic condition.

Disorders of Gut-Brain Interaction

Doctors and scientists at the Rome Foundation identified 33 disorders of gut-brain interaction. A partial list is included here. The Rome Foundation's symptom-based criteria are the gold standard for identifying, defining, and classifying DGBIs.

Esophageal disorders

- Functional chest pain
- Functional heartburn
- Reflux hypersensitivity
- Globus (sensation of having a lump in the throat)
- Functional dysphagia (sensation of foods passing abnormally through the esophagus)

Bowel disorders

- Irritable bowel syndrome
- Functional constipation
- Functional diarrhea
- Functional abdominal bloating/distension
- Unspecified functional bowel disorder
- Opioid-induced constipation

Gastroduodenal disorder

- Functional dyspepsia (sensation of food staying in the stomach after a meal)
- Postprandial distress syndrome (feeling full too soon after eating a meal)
- Epigastric pain syndrome (pain or burning under the ribs)
- Belching disorders
- Chronic nausea
- Cyclic vomiting syndrome
- Rumination syndrome (repetitive, effortless regurgitation)

Gallbladder and sphincter of Oddi (SO) disorder

- Biliary pain
- Functional gallbladder disorder
- Biliary pain with pancreatitis

Centrally mediated disorders of gastrointestinal pain

- Centrally mediated abdominal pain syndrome (continuous or frequently recurrent abdominal pain)
- Narcotic bowel syndrome/opioid-induced abdominal pain

Anoretal disorders

- Fecal incontinence
- Levator ani syndrome (ache or pressure high in the rectum)
- Proctalgia fugax (pain in the rectal area)
- Functional defecation disorders (frequent excessive straining, feeling of incomplete evacuation with defecation)
- Inadequate defecatory propulsion
- Dyssynergic defecation

For more information on diagnostic criteria and treatment recommendations, visit http://therome foundation.org.

Brain scans show that chronic pain and chronic and severe stress can cause the deterioration of brain cells (neurodegeneration) in the brain's pain center, the anterior cingulate cortex. Fewer cells in that area make it harder to control pain. Fortunately, this process is reversible. Physical and mental activity, yoga, meditation, and medications called neuromodulators can promote regrowth of those cells (neurogenesis) and reduce GI pain.

Treatment Approaches

DGBI can be harder to diagnose than illnesses that show up on diagnostic tests, so if you suspect you may have one (see sidebar above), do a little homework before seeing your physician. Keep a diary of your symptoms. Record the time, severity, and presence of associated factors. If you identify triggers, such as specific foods—alcohol, caffeine, lactose, and fatty foods are common culprits—eliminate them from your diet. Share the diary with your doctor to help guide a treatment plan.

He or she may recommend medications that address specific symptoms, such as diarrhea or pain, and may prescribe neuromodulators like *amitriptyline* (Elavil), *nortriptyline* (Pamelor), *desipramine* (Norpramin), and *duloxetine* (Cymbalta). You might recognize some of these drugs as antidepressants, but that doesn't mean that DGBIs are in your head. Just like aspirin can prevent a heart attack and tackle pain, neuromodulators have more than one function: They can treat pain, lessen emotional distress, and promote nerve-cell growth. When it comes to DGBIs, that's a particularly powerful combination. Brain-gut behavioral treatments, such as cognitive behavioral therapy, relaxation, hypnosis, and mindfulness can reduce anxiety levels, encourage health-promoting behaviors, and potentially improve pain tolerance.

Patient-Doctor Communication Required

The cornerstone of all of this, however, is the patient-doctor relationship. Disorders of gut-brain interaction are complicated and often chronic illnesses, so it's important to have a doctor who will be a trusted partner. You'll be working together to customize a treatment plan that works best for you. That means you need to know how each treatment works, what side effects are expected, how effective it's expected to be, and how long it will take. Be honest with your physician about any questions or concerns that you have. A doctor who is a good partner will answer your questions and pay attention to your experiences.

You might not have that experience with the first doctor that you see. DGBI can be frustrating for doctors who like to deal with concrete test results and clear answers.

If you feel like your doctor doesn't understand your illness, refer him or her to the Rome Foundation and the book *Gut Feelings* (by Douglas Drossman, MD, and Johannah Ruddy, MEd), to learn the diagnostic criteria for DGBIs and best practices for medical treatment and patient-doctor communication.

The Stress Factor

If you meet a doctor who tries to dismiss your symptoms as stress, dig a little deeper into his or her thought process. Stress can indeed worsen GI symptoms because of the gut-brain axis, but what comes next is essential. A doctor who puts that information

---

Alzheimer's Disease Protein Travels in Blood

Investigators report that beta-amyloid, a protein that forms plaques in the brains of people with Alzheimer's disease (AD), appears to leak into the brain from fat-carrying particles in blood called lipoproteins. The discovery suggests that dietary changes and drugs that alter how lipoproteins interact with beta-amyloid could prevent or slow AD.

Curtin Health Innovation Research Institute, Curtin University, Bentley, Australia.

---

into context and includes stress management as part of an overall management strategy understands the condition. But if the doctor suggests that stress is entirely the problem and that you need to live with it or see a psychologist instead of a medical doctor, you may need to move on to a physician with a better understanding of DGBIs.

A neurogastroenterology pain treatment center can provide a multidisciplinary approach that addresses pain management, coping skills, and overall well-being. A comprehensive listing can be found in *Gut Feelings* at https://romedross.video/GutFeelings.

Preparing for the Stages of Alzheimer's

Monica Moreno, senior director for care and support at the Alzheimer's Association in Chicago, where she works with families after an Alzheimer's disease diagnosis. Alz.org

Alzheimer's disease is life-altering and frightening not just for the person receiving the diagnosis but also for his/her family. When you or a loved one hear this diagnosis, you likely will think of the end—or final—stages of this disease. However, diagnosed individuals can continue to live meaningful and productive lives in the early stages.

The first step is to understand and accept the diagnosis. That starts with getting educated about the stages…how the disease will progress…and what treatments and services are available today and in the future so that you can be prepared. There is a lot of information available…in fact, so much that it can be overwhelming. Take your time and go at your own pace. Alzheimer's is a journey, not a sprint.

Most important: You do not have to go through this alone. Once you reach out and get support, you will feel some relief and less isolated.

Each person's progression is different, but there are changes that characterize each stage and things you can do to prepare for the next stage…

Early-Stage or Mild Alzheimer's

What to expect: In the early stage, people often still are independent and able to drive and can continue to enjoy being social, though they might have a hard time planning and organizing tasks.

Symptoms: Mild memory issues, including struggling to find the right word when speaking…forgetting words or something you just read or heard, perhaps the name of someone you just met. You may start to lose things. Loved ones may notice these problems, but they might not be obvious to the outside world.

Steps to take…

•**Take care of yourself.** Many people who are newly diagnosed take the opportunity to look at their lifestyle and make changes that will enable them to live their healthiest life. Adopting lifestyle changes, including controlling blood pressure, healthy eating, exercising and staying socially and intellectually engaged, may help slow cognitive decline and preserve existing cognitive function longer.

•**Discuss medications.** Early detection gives you the chance to start taking medications that might help now. It also provides an opportunity to enroll in a clinical trial exploring new medications and treatments. Talk to your doctor.

•**Prioritize what matters to you.** In the wake of a diagnosis, many people choose to spend time doing meaningful activities and spending more time with the most important people in their lives.

•**Build your support team.** This is a good time to start building the right support team so that you'll have people to rely on as the disease progresses. This also is important for the spouse or care partner, whose support needs will grow as well.

One option: Connect with others who are living with Alzheimer's or other caregivers by joining an Alzheimer's Association support group (see page 40 for suggestions). Being able to share your experiences with others living your journey can be helpful.

•**Take practical steps to prepare.** Put legal and financial documents and end-of-life plans in place. Doing so now allows the person with Alzheimer's to be part of the conversation and share his/her wishes with family and friends. Later on, family members will have peace of mind knowing that they're following their loved one's wishes.

•**Put safety measures in place.** Most people want to stay in their home as long as possible, so creating a safe environment is critical. Remove tripping hazards such as throw rugs, and secure bookshelves and other heavy furniture to prevent them from tipping over. Other steps become more important when Alzheimer's worsens and affects judgment—securing hazardous items, such as medication, liquor, sharp objects and cleaning products, from easy access…putting stickers on glass doors to prevent walking into them…and securing exterior doors or installing motion detectors to prevent wandering from the home. Remove locks on bathrooms and bedrooms so the person cannot lock himself in accidently. When to take these actions will depend on Alzheimer's progression.

•**Consider when to stop driving.** This is a very difficult and complicated decision. The Alzheimer's Association offers online tools to help families discuss this sensitive topic, including signs of unsafe driving and transportation alternatives.

Middle-Stage or Moderate Alzheimer's

What to expect: This often is the longest stage—it can last for many years, and the person living with dementia can require more and more care as damage to nerve cells in the brain increases. Dementia symptoms become more pronounced, and loved ones may see clear personality and behavior changes.

Symptoms: Worsening language and cognitive problems, forgetting basic personal information and not knowing what day it is…difficulty doing—or even refusing to do—everyday activities such as bathing or needing help with those tasks…and emotional issues that manifest as anger and frustration and refusal to participate in social situations. Wandering and getting lost—either on foot, by car or on public transportation—may become a problem and pose a threat to safety.

Also: The person may become increasingly suspicious, have delusions or engage in repetitive compulsive behaviors. Physical changes can include sleep problems, such as nighttime restlessness and daytime sleepiness, and difficulty with continence.

Steps to take…

•**Consider additional help.** As care needs increase, families may consider adult-day-care centers, aides and other outside support. These resources not only provide additional assistance but also offer caregivers a break to attend to their personal care and well-being.

•**Adapt your communication.** As the disease progresses, and communication becomes more challenging, adapt your communication. This may include slowing down and making eye contact with the person as you speak…and using short, simple sentences.

More from Monica Moreno…

Help When You Need It

General help: The Alzheimer's Association has a 24/7 helpline at 800-272-3900 with masters-level counselors available to guide you. There also are chat boxes throughout the website. Alz.org

Online community: The website AlzConnected.org connects you to people who have walked in your shoes and will provide support by sharing their experiences, tips and strategies.

Action plans: At AlzheimersNavigator.org, you can create your own action plan for any of 10 of the most common concerns facing caregivers, such as care options and legal planning. For each topic, you'll answer a group of questions and, based on your answers, receive back an action plan along with resources to help you apply it. Over time as your needs change, you can go back and answer the questions again.

E-learning: At the Alzheimer's Association Education Center, you'll find many Alzheimer's and dementia learning programs available online. Alz.org/education

---

Ask one question at a time, rather than overwhelming the patient with a series of questions. Give him time to process and respond before continuing the conversation.

Late-Stage or Severe Alzheimer's

What to expect: This is the most difficult stage, with profound changes, such as loss of speech and movement and the inability to walk and swallow. General health worsens with an increased risk for infection, especially pneumonia. Significant personality changes may take place, and there may be little awareness of recent experiences or one's surroundings. But the person living with Alzheimer's still can benefit from some types of interaction and may be soothed by relaxing music or a gentle touch.

Talking Two Languages Fights Cognitive Decline

Dementia rates are 50 percent lower in countries where more than one language is regularly spoken than in countries whose populations speak only one language.

Study by researchers at Open University of Catalonia and Pompeu Fabra University, Barcelona, Spain, published in Neuropsychologia.

Steps to take: Around-the-clock assistance for daily personal care usually is needed. Families may consider nursing homes or other long-term-care options. Hospice care may be available for individuals nearing the end of life. See the box on the previous page for resources that can provide help.

Keeping Your Brain Sharp

Henry Mahncke, PhD, CEO of Posit Science, San Francisco, which created the BrainHQ brain-training program. Previously, he served as a science and technology advisor to the British government. Dr. Mahncke earned his PhD in neuroscience at the University of California, San Francisco, where he studied brain plasticity.

Brain fog. Senior moments. Alzheimer's disease. At nearly every stage of adult life, memory and cognition top the list of health concerns for Americans. Indeed, scientists have found that cognitive function, speed, and memory start to slowly decline at age 30.

Fortunately, researchers have good news, too: We can harness the power of neuroplasticity—the brain's ability to build new neural connections throughout the entire life span—to regain and even improve upon the mental sharpness of youth. Just as a muscle grows stronger with exercise, the brain grows stronger when challenged.

Try these three simple strategies to boost your brainpower at any age…

Try New Things

Your brain isn't just designed to think: It's designed to learn. To fulfill its potential, it needs to encounter new challenges and novel experiences. Novelty can come in the form of taking a different route to work, or in trying a different role once you're there. It can mean learning a musical instrument or studying a new language. The idea is to do something that doesn't come easily so your brain will grow and develop new neural connections to meet the additional cognitive demand.

Play New Games

Crossword puzzles, Sudoku, and games like poker, bridge, and chess all keep your mind busy, but it's really only when you're learning them that they change your brain. Once they become easy, you can add more challenge by seeking out more advanced puzzles or opponents or start learning a new game to add to your repertoire.

Train Your Brain

There are countless apps and computer programs that offer what's called brain games that are designed to challenge your memory and skill, but it's important to differentiate these from brain-training programs. Brain games are fun and stimulating, and you may become more adept at them the more you play, but they don't necessarily help you develop skills that translate to other tasks.

Brain-training programs can look a lot like brain games, but there's a key difference. Legitimate programs are developed by neuroscientists to improve on the building blocks of cognition in a way that yields real-world benefits. Brain-training has been used in neurorehabilitation programs to help people with brain injuries regain lost skills, but it's now also available to anyone with a phone or computer and a desire to improve daily cognitive abilities.

When scientists study cognitive function, they break it down into different domains that brain-training exercises can then target…

•**Processing speed refers to how quickly your brain can make sense of information.** For example, how quickly can you decipher a simple code?

•**Attention refers to your ability to zero in on what you want to notice while also suppressing what you don't.** Can you read this article while the radio is on in the background?

•**Executive function is your ability to plan and organize.**

•**Memory refers to several things.** Your working memory is the ability to keep information in mind in the moment, while short-term and long-term memory refer to storage and retrieval. In healthy people, these domains are all related—and all trainable.

If you practice a skill in a brain-training program and then see improvement in a similar cognitive task, it's called *near transfer.* For example, if you train with an exercise in which you have to remember a growing list of words and can then remember more words when your doctor tests your memory, your performance on the test represents "near transfer" from the brain-training program.

Unexpected Benefits

The more desirable—and more elusive—goal is called "far transfer." That means that the skill you learned in the game can lead to improvements in unrelated or real-world tasks.

•**Peripheral vision and driving.** As we get older and our processing speed slows, our peripheral vision diminishes. This isn't a problem in the eyes: It's a change in how quickly and accurately the brain is processing information coming from the periphery. Because this is a processing issue, it's a trainable skill.

To improve it, neuroscientists at Brain-HQ developed a game in which one image briefly appears in the center of the computer or phone screen while a second appears in the periphery. The player must answer questions about both of the items. Each time the player answers correctly, the exercise speeds up slightly, gently nudging the

Choosing a Brain-Training Program

The brain-games industry has come under fire for making unsubstantiated claims about the value of their products. At the root of the problem is the falsehood that all brain games work the same way. That is as false as suggesting that all pills work the same way.

To help consumers choose legitimate brain-training companies, the National Academy of Medicine (formerly called the Institute of Medicine) included a five-point checklist in its 2015 report *Cognitive Aging: Progress in Understanding and Opportunities for Action. When evaluating potential programs, look for the following information…*

•**Has the product demonstrated transfer of training to other laboratory tasks that measure the same cognitive construct as the training task?** For example, if some aspect of memory is being targeted in the product, is transfer demonstrated to other memory tasks?

•**Has the product demonstrated transfer of training to relevant real-world tasks?**

•**Has the product performance been evaluated using an active control group whose members have the same expectations of cognitive benefits as do members of the experimental group?**

•**How long are the trained skills retained?**

•**Have the purported benefits of the training product been replicated by research groups other than those selling the product?**

Once you find a program that you like, check with your insurance company and local library to see if the program you are interested in is available at a discount or for free before you make the final purchase.

—Dr. Henry Mahncke

brain toward faster processing speeds. If it gets too fast and the player begins to make errors, the game slows down so the player can catch up.

Over time, the training rewires how the brain processes information and provides real-world benefits: In a study of 2,800 adults, an independent team of researchers reported that people who trained with the exercise experienced a 48 percent reduction in at-fault car crashes.

●**Balance.** That same slowed visual system is one of the reasons for the higher risk of falls in older people. The briefest delay in transmitting visual data to the brain can mean the difference between quickly steadying oneself or experiencing an injurious tumble. After studying the effects of brain training on balance and walking in seniors, researchers from Chicago's Northwestern University and the University of Illinois Chicago suggested that improving visual speed and attention appear to improve walking speed and steadiness.

●**Hearing.** Slowed processing speed can affect hearing as well. While physical causes of hearing loss are common as we age, they're not always what's causing you to struggle to hear in a noisy restaurant or to need to turn up the television. In many cases, the brain's auditory system no longer has the speed and accuracy needed to hear fast speech amidst noise. Furthermore, a large study at the Mayo Clinic found that using brain training to rewire the brain to make the auditory system faster and more accurate improved memory, too.

Multifaceted Approach

Brain training has been shown to improve cognitive performance in a growing body of research, but there's more you can do to enjoy a brain-healthy lifestyle. Exercising, eating a healthy diet, managing chronic health conditions, and maintaining social connections are all strongly linked to cognitive benefits.

Can Vitamin B-12 Reverse Poor Cognitive Function?

Mira Ilic, MS, RDN, LD, registered dietitian nutritionist in the department of gastroenterology, hepatology and nutrition at Cleveland Clinic. ClevelandClinic.org

Replacing B-12 in people who are deficient may improve their cognitive function, according to a recent study in *Cureus Journal of Medical Science.* Of the 202 participants, 84 percent reported that having their B-12 deficiency treated first with infusions and then with daily oral supplements for three months led to a significant improvement in their energy, concentration, memory loss and disorientation...and 78 percent had improved scores on the Mini-Mental State Exam (MMSE), which evaluates memory, attention, and language. Even among those who said their symptoms didn't improve, more than half did better on the MMSE.

Brain function is just one of B-12's roles, along with helping red blood cell production and DNA synthesis. A B-12 deficiency can cause demyelination, loss of the outer sheath of neurons, which helps explain the tingling and numbness in the hands, feet, and legs. These symptoms may not show up for a few years and may be accompanied by concentration problems, memory loss, disorientation and, over time, confusion, and depression.

●**Causes of B-12 deficiency.** Some medical conditions put you at risk for B-12 deficiency—the autoimmune disease pernicious anemia...diseases that affect the small intestine (where B-12 is absorbed), such as Crohn's and celiac disease...long-term use of PPIs for acid reflux...taking *metformin* for diabetes and *colchicine* for gout...resectioning of the stomach or terminal part of the small intestine...and weight-loss surgery. Because foods highest in B-12 are animal-based, being vegan or vegetarian can cause a deficiency.

Simply getting older also can increase incidence of the naturally occurring condition atrophic gastritis, when the stomach fails to produce enough of the acids needed to extract B-12 from food before it reaches the intestines. This condition may affect about 30 percent of people over age 50, and the likelihood increases with age.

• **B-12 to the rescue.** Problems caused by a deficiency may be reversed by restoring B-12 levels through diet, supplements and/or injec-

tions. Treatment is most effective when the deficiency is caught early. People at risk should have their B-12 levels checked regularly.

• **To prevent a B-12 deficiency.** Adults generally need 2.4 micrograms of B-12 daily. Top sources include beef liver, clams, bluefin tuna, Atlantic salmon, milk, yogurt and eggs, fortified cereals, and other enriched foods.

Food, Drink, and Fun Ways to Stop Cognitive Decline

Apples Keep Your Brain Healthy

Apple nutrients injected into mice increased the gray matter in their brains—similarly to the brain-function boost from exercise. Antioxidants stimulated generation of new neurons in the mice's hippocampus, which controls memory, learning and navigation. No benefit to brain health was seen when the mice received only apple juice. One key nutrient was quercetin, found particularly in apple skins—so don't peel your apples.

Study by researchers at German Center for Neurodegenerative Diseases, Bonn, Germany, published in *Stem Cell Reports*.

Strawberries May Reduce Alzheimer's Risk

Older adults who regularly ate at least one serving of strawberries per week were 34 percent less likely to develop Alzheimer's disease than those who ate strawberries once a month or less. The association does not prove causation—but strawberries are known to contain compounds that have antioxidative and anti-inflammatory properties, which could account for the findings.

Study of 925 people, ages 58 to 98, who were dementia-free at the start of the study by researchers at Rush University's Memory and Aging Project, Chicago, published in *Nutrients*.

Drinking Two Cups of Coffee Staves Off Alzheimer's

An 18-month-long study found that coffee consumption slowed the accumulation of amyloid (a protein associated with AD) in the brain and

increased study participants' executive function, which is responsible for planning, self-control, and attention.

Edith Cowan University

Afternoon Naps May Boost Cognitive Ability

People over age 60 who regularly napped for five minutes to two hours after lunch scored significantly higher on tests of working memory, attention span, problem solving, verbal fluency, and other cognitive measures than people who did not nap. It is possible that napping helps regulate the body's immune response, reducing the generalized inflammation that relates both to sleep disorders and cognitive decline.

Study of 2,214 residents of several large cities in China, all of whom averaged 6.5 hours of nighttime sleep, by researchers in Shanghai and elsewhere in China, published in *General Psychiatry*.

Choir Singing Has Cognitive Benefits

In a Finnish study, researchers found that elderly choir singers had better verbal and cognitive flexibility than their non-singing peers in a control group. Choir singing involves complex information processing. It combines learning and memorizing lyrics and melodies; processing sensory stimuli, motor function related to voice production and control, and linguistic output; and it stirs emotions. Choir singers in the study also reported greater happiness.

Emmi Pentikäinen, PhD, doctoral student, University of Helsinki, Finland.

Synthetic supplements are effective for people who can't absorb the B-12 in food.

Work with your doctor to determine what's best for you based on your bloodwork, health, and medications you're taking. You also may need the B vitamin folate, which works in tandem with B-12.

Three Life Stages When Alcohol Is Most Toxic to the Brain

Editorial titled "Lifetime Perspective on Alcohol and Brain Health," by researchers at University of New South Wales and University of Sydney in Australia and King's College, London, published in *The BMJ*.

It's a well-known fact that heavy alcohol use is toxic to brain cells. But at certain stages of human development, according to recent studies, alcohol should be avoided completely.

Recent development: In an editorial, published in *The BMJ*, researchers in Australia and Britain warn that during three critical periods of life, the brain is more sensitive to alcohol toxicity and at greatest risk for damage. *When you should avoid alcohol…*

• **While pregnant.** During the prenatal period, the developing brain is most vulnerable. Heavy drinking during pregnancy can cause *fetal alcohol syndrome*, a condition in which the fetal brain does not grow and many types of brain function do not develop. Despite this risk, about 10 percent of pregnant women continue to drink. Even low to moderate use of alcohol during pregnancy may cause significant behavioral and psychosocial problems in children.

• **During adolescence.** More than 20 percent of adolescents ages 15 to 19 admit to binge drinking (about four to five drinks in two hours). During this time of life, the brain is establishing connectivity between brain cells and developing the protective covering of nerve fibers. Alcohol toxicity in adolescence can decrease brain volume and cause loss of mental ability (cognition).

• **Older age.** After age 65, the brain starts to lose some brain cells due to aging (atrophy). During this time, even low to moderate use of alcohol may increase the risk of dementia. Alcohol is a strong risk factor for dementia along with smoking and high blood pressure.

The researchers warn that current trends in alcohol use are worrisome. Imbibing is predicted to continue on its uphill climb in coming years. Women are now as likely to abuse alcohol as men. In developed countries, more individuals over age 65 are drinking. In past periods of health crisis, use of alcohol has increased, and this may also be the case with the recent COVID pandemic.

Bottom line: The researchers conclude that guidelines are needed to encourage low-risk drinking, as well as increased training for treatment of alcohol use disorder. They suggest actions such as regulating the price of alcohol and deceasing legal alcohol limits for driving. An integrated approach that involves both health-care and social-services professionals is needed to reduce alcohol intake and abuse across all life stages to increase healthful longevity.

Some Blood Pressure Meds Preserve Memory

Daniel Nation, PhD, associate professor of psychological science at University of California, Irvine, and lead author of a meta-analysis of 14 studies, published in *Hypertension*.

Angiotensin-converting-enzyme (ACE) inhibitors and angiotensin II receptor blockers (ARBs) that cross the blood/brain barrier do more than control blood pressure—they also slow memory loss. Memory-preserving ACE inhibitors include *captopril* (Capoten), *fosinopril* (Monopril), *lisinopril* (Qbrelis), *perindopril* (Aceon), *ramipril* (Altace) and *trandolapril* (Mavik). ARBs include *telmisartan* (Micardis) and *candesartan* (Atacand).

Eat a Mediterranean-Style Diet to Stay Mentally Sharp

Janie Corley, PhD, research associate, Centre for Cognitive Ageing and Cognitive Epidemiology, University of Edinburgh, Scotland, United Kingdom.

In this study, people in their late 70s who most closely adhered to a Mediterranean diet had the highest scores on a range of memory and thinking tests, even when accounting for childhood IQ, smoking, physical activity, and health factors. The most significant dietary factors were high consumption of leafy green vegetables and a lower red meat intake.

Taking Breaks Improves Learning

Study titled "Spaced Training Enhances Memory and Prefrontal Ensemble Stability in Mice," by researchers at the Max Planck Institute for Biological Intelligence, Martinsried, Germany, published in *Current Biology*.

Have you ever crammed for an exam and struggled to remember what you learned the next day? Learning more slowly over several days is almost always better. Retaining new information in smaller bites with pauses between sessions is called "the spacing effect." This effect was discovered by neurobiologists more than 100 years ago and it applies to almost all animals.

A new study from neurobiological researchers at the Max Planck Institute for Biological Intelligence may be the first study to explain why slower is better when it comes to learning and memory. When you store new information in your brain, neurons in the complex-thinking region—called the prefrontal cortex—are activated. They make connections with other neurons to retrieve the information when you want it.

Why Breaks Are Better: Of Mice and Neurons

The research team taught mice to find hidden pieces of chocolate in a maze. One group of mice had training sessions without any rest. Other groups had breaks of up to 60 minutes between sessions. All the mice had neuron activity recorded during the research experiments. The results are published in the journal *Current Biology*.

Right after the session, the mice that had the crammed sessions remembered where to find the chocolate more quickly. The spaced-learning mice found the chocolate also, but more slowly. However, the next day, the mice that took breaks during the training did better at finding the chocolate than the crammed-learning mice. The longer the breaks, the better the memory.

The neuron activity of the mice showed that the crammed-learning mice had to activate more neurons than the spaced-learning mice. It may be that more neurons are needed to absorb quick learning. The spaced-learning mice activated the same group of neurons during each session. The breaks strengthened the connections between the neurons and made retrieving the information easier. The study confirms what human experience shows. Taking breaks between learning takes longer, but the knowledge you acquire will remain longer in your memory.

Space Out Learning

If there's a test on your horizon, space out your study. If you're outside the traditional classroom and learning something new, such as a language or a musical instrument, practice consistently...but give yourself time to retain and process the material.

Salami May Be Bad for Your Brain

Scientists examined data from 500,000 people and discovered that eating 25 grams (0.88 ounces) of processed meat a day is associated with a 44 percent increased risk of developing dementia.

University of Leeds

Artificial Intelligence Can Improve Brain Function

Alik Widge, MD, PhD, assistant professor of psychiatry, University of Minnesota Medical School, Twin Cities, Minnesota.

Artificial intelligence plus targeted electrical brain stimulation can improve mental function. Stimulating the part of the brain that is responsible for cognitive control can make it easier for a person to shift from one thought pattern or behavior to another, an ability that is impaired in most mental illnesses. This method could be used to treat patients with severe and medication-resistant anxiety, depression, or other disorders.

Nitrate-Rich Foods Promote Healthier Brain Function

Anni Vanhatalo, PhD, professor of human physiology, University of Exeter, United Kingdom.

Older people often have lower nitric oxide production, which is associated with poorer blood-vessel and brain health. In this study, drinking nitrate-rich beetroot juice for 10 days increased levels of specific oral bacteria that help convert nitrate to nitric oxide. As a result, the study participants experienced lower blood pressure, higher nitric oxide levels in the blood, and better performance on attention tests.

Young-Onset Dementia May Be More Prevalent Than Previously Thought

JAMA Neurology

A systematic review showed that there are approximately 119 causes of dementia per 100,000 people under age 65, more than double previous estimates. The most common cause is Alzheimer's disease, followed by vascular dementia and frontotemporal dementia.

New Brain Imaging Study Predicts Deadly Brain Aneurysms

Study titled "Relationship Between Cerebral Aneurysms and Variations in Cerebral Basal Arterial Network: A Morphometric Cross-Sectional Study in Computed Tomography Angiograms from a Neurointerventional Unit," led by researchers at University of South Australia, published in *BMJ Open*.

Arteries that carry oxygen to your brain keep it alive. Sometimes the wall of an artery inside the brain weakens and blows up like a small balloon. This is called a cerebral aneurysm. Every year, about eight to 10 people out of 100,000 have a rupture of a cerebral aneurysm that causes deadly bleeding inside the brain.

Fifty percent of people with a ruptured aneurysm will die, and most people who survive will be disabled. A test that could predict an aneurysm before it ruptures would be an enormous boon. It would help doctors monitor individuals at risk. It would enable early treatment to reduce the risk, and repeated imaging studies to find small aneurysms before they rupture.

A Test to Measure Arteries

Researchers at the University of South Australia may have found the test. The test is not new—it is a brain imaging study done after injecting a dye into the blood stream, called cerebral CT angiography (CCTA). What is new is that the research team took measurements of arteries in the base of the brain and used their measurements to determine standard sizes for these arteries. This had never been done before.

Four arteries come up through the neck to supply the brain. As they enter the brain, they branch out into a network of arteries called the cerebral basal arterial network (CBAN). Because the blood supply from the four main arteries comes in at different rates, CBAN not only distributes blood to the brain, it dampens the flow and smooths out blood delivery, so small arteries inside the brain do not get stressed. The investigators wanted to find out if blood flow abnormalities in a person's CBAN might be a risk factor for a cerebral aneurysm. Their study is published in the British Medical Association journal *BMJ Open*.

The research team used 145 CCTA images to standardize the sizes of arteries in CBANs. Patients in the study were men and women from ages 18 to 100 who had a CCTA for various reasons. All the patients had been seen in the neurology department of a university hospital between 2011 and 2019. Along with standardizing the size of CBAN arteries, the researchers found one or more aneurysms in 83 of the 145 patients.

Asymmetrical Arteries Provide a Clue

The key finding was that patients who had arteries in their CBAN that were significantly asymmetrical had a significantly higher percentage of aneurysms in their brains. For example, people who had a ratio deference between their right and left anterior cerebral arteries in their CBANs of more than 1.4 had about an 80 percent risk of aneurysm. A ratio below 1.4 only had a 7.8 percent risk.

Based on their study, the investigators say that the size of arteries in the CBAN should be measured when a patient has an arterial brain study. Patients with asymmetry should be followed closely and checked for the beginning of a cerebral aneurysm. Early discovery of a brain aneurysm could save lives.

Insomnia May Be a Risk Factor for a Brain Aneurysm

Susanna C. Larsson, PhD, associate professor in the unit of cardiovascular and nutritional epidemiology at the Karolinska Institutet in Stockholm, Sweden.

Researchers studied data on 6,300 cases of intracranial aneurysm and nearly 4,200

High-Risk Factors for Memory Loss

Air Pollution Is Linked to Alzheimer's Disease

Duke University researchers report that people living in zip codes with more than 10 micrograms of particulate matter per cubic meter (mcg/m3) of air have a 35 percent higher risk of death from Alzheimer's disease than people living with cleaner air. The Environmental Protection Agency sets the limit for particulate matter at a substantially higher level of 35 mcg/m3.

Duke University

Alzheimer's Link to Early-Onset Diabetes

Type 2 diabetes at any age is associated with increased risk for Alzheimer's disease.

Recent finding: The earlier the onset, the greater the risk. For each five years earlier onset, risk for dementia increases by 24 percent. While association does not mean either condition causes the other, it is likely that an underlying condition is responsible for both…and new research reinforces the importance of diagnosing and treating type 2 diabetes as early as possible.

Study of more than 10,000 people, ages 35 to 55 at the start of the study, by researchers at Inserm, the French national health institute, published in *JAMA*.

Highly Processed Food Is Linked to Memory Loss in Rodents

Rats fed highly processed food for four weeks experienced a strong inflammatory response and behavioral signs of memory loss. Adding the omega-3 fatty acid docosahexaenoic acid (DHA) to their diets reversed the effects.

Ohio State University

cases of aneurysmal subarachnoid hemorrhage and found that a genetic predisposition for insomnia was associated with a 24 percent increased risk for intracranial aneurysm and aneurysmal subarachnoid hemorrhage. The risk for intracranial aneurysm was three times higher for each 10 mmHg increase in diastolic blood pressure, and three times higher for smokers.

Light Stimulation May Treat Neurodegenerative Diseases (NDs)

Study by researchers at Soochow University, Suzhou, Jiangsu, China, published in *Chinese Medical Journal*.

Controlled exposure to daylight or specific wavelengths of artificial light may alleviate ND symptoms that disrupt circadian rhythms, causing Alzheimer's sleep disturbances and Parkinson's insomnia, depression, and fatigue.

Inflammation-Blocking Nasal Drug May Help Stop Multiple Sclerosis

Study titled "Intranasal Anti-caspase-1 Therapy Preserves Myelin and Glucose Metabolism in a Model of Progressive Multiple Sclerosis," by researchers at University of Alberta Faculty of Medicine and Dentistry, Canada, published in *Glia*.

Multiple sclerosis (MS) is a debilitating disease of the central nervous system (spinal cord and brain) that damages the protective lining covering nerves and eventually the nerves themselves. The damage is caused by an inflammatory attack from a patient's own immune system.

Recent development: A new anti-inflammatory medication and a novel way of delivering the medication may be in the future, according to a study from researchers at the

University of Alberta Faculty of Medicine and Dentistry.

Background: The lining covering nerves, called myelin, acts like insulation on an electric wire. MS inflammation causes damage known as demyelination, which creates early MS symptoms. Blocking the MS inflammation attack is the key to preventing MS progression.

The Canadian researchers have identified a new drug called VX-765, which they focused on in their study, published in *Glia*. This drug blocks an integral step in the inflammation process that relies on inflammasomes. These are molecules that promote inflammation in the body. VX-765 blocks a component of inflammasomes called caspase-1.

Study details: Studying brains from people who died with MS, the researchers were able to show that caspase-1 entered the brain as a pivotal part of MS inflammation. They then created a model of MS by giving mice cuprizone, a drug that causes progressive nerve damage similar to that found in MS. After creating MS in mice, they gave them VX-765 through a nasal injection.

Brain imaging and brain sampling of the mice showed that mice given VX-765 did not develop MS demyelination or nerve damage. MS mice not given VX-765 developed progressive nerve damage.

Takeaway: The researchers say the study's outcome is very promising, although the research is in its early (preclinical) stages. An intranasal drug that blocks central nervous system inflammation would be valuable for people with MS because it provides a more precise and targeted treatment for a disease that still has no cure.

Faith Lives in a Specific Region of the Brain

Study by researchers at Brigham and Women's Hospital, Boston, published in *Biological Psychiatry*.

Researchers have found that an evolutionarily ancient area of the brain that is associated with fear conditioning, pain modulation, altruistic behaviors and unconditional love also is associated with religious feelings. And in case studies, patients have become hyper-religious after brain trauma in that region.

Antidepressants May Increase Stroke Risk

Allison Gaffey, PhD, a psychologist at Yale School of Medicine, New Haven, and VA Connecticut Healthcare System, West Haven, Connecticut, and leader of a study published in *Stroke*.

When researchers studied one million veterans with posttraumatic stress disorder, those who took a selective serotonin reuptake inhibitor (SSRI) were 45 percent more likely to suffer a hemorrhagic stroke. Interestingly, SSRIs were previously shown to reduce risk for ischemic stroke. Since this study concludes that serotonin-norepinephrine reuptake inhibitors (SNRIs) don't seem to carry the stroke risk, they may be a safer treatment.

A Simple Surgery Reduces the Risk of Stroke

A simple surgery reduces the risk of stroke in people with atrial fibrillation. Removing the left atrial appendage, a heart structure that traps blood in the heart chamber and increases the risk of clots, can reduce the risk of stroke from 7 percent to 5 percent. Surgeons have removed appendage during previously planned cardiopulmonary bypass surgery but noted that the procedure could also be done through less invasive methods for patients not having heart surgery.

Richard Whitlock, MD, professor of surgery, McMaster University, Hamilton, Ontario, Canada.

Clue That a Stroke Is Imminent

Alis Heshmatollah, MD, PhD candidate, neurology resident of Erasmus MC University Medical Center, Rotterdam, the Netherlands, and first author of a study published in *Journal of Neurology, Neurosurgery & Psychiatry.*

Cognitive function declines as much as 10 years before a stroke.

Recent finding: Compared with people who had not had strokes, stroke patients showed greater and faster decline in cognitive function and ability to handle activities of daily living over the previous 10 years. These may be early signs of the physiological changes that lead to stroke. Standard cognition tests may help identify those at higher stroke risk.

Stroke: Act Fast from Onset to Rehab

Mark Tornero, MD, medical director of vascular rehabilitation at The Ohio State University Wexner Medical Center in Columbus, Ohio.

From the moment a stroke hits, the clock starts ticking, and there isn't a second to waste. Whether blood flow needs to be restored by dissolving a clot in an ischemic stroke, or a brain bleed from a hemorrhagic stroke needs to be halted, speed is the key to limiting the damage and providing the best long-term recovery.

If you recognize—or even suspect—signs of stroke in yourself or a loved one (see graphic on page 52), the most important thing you can do is immediately call an ambulance. People who take an ambulance get better care faster than those who have a family member drive them to the hospital. That care includes access to tissue plasminogen activator (tPA), a lifesaving drug that can immediately break up a clot, but only if administered within three hours of the onset of

An Anti-Stroke Vaccine

Researchers reviewed more than one million medical records and found that people who received the first-generation shingles vaccine, zoster vaccine live (Zostavax), had a 10 to 20 percent lower risk of stroke. A newer vaccine, *zoster vaccine recombinant, adjuvanted* (Shingrix), may provide better stroke protection, as it's more effective against shingles (90 percent vs 50 percent). It's recommended for anyone over age 50, even those who have already had the Zostavax shot (which provides five years of protection) or who have already had shingles.

—Dr. Mark Tornero

symptoms. As few as 15 percent of patients with ischemic stroke arrive at the hospital in time for this treatment—but those who do experience fewer poststroke impairments and better recoveries.

A growing number of cities have mobile stroke units—enhanced ambulances that are equipped to provide stroke diagnosis and care as soon as they arrive at the patient's home—saving even more precious time.

Quick tip: If you call for an ambulance from a cell phone, your address might not be available to the dispatcher like it would if you called from a landline. To make it available, register your cellphone now at Smart911.com.

A Whirlwind of Activity

Once you arrive at the hospital, you'll be medically stabilized, but the race against time continues. Whether your stroke is minor or significant, the rehabilitation process will begin within just 24 to 48 hours. You may go to a rehabilitation unit in the hospital you are already in, a unit in a different hospital, a freestanding inpatient rehabilitation facility, or a skilled nursing facility. If you can care for yourself or have enough help to safely return home, you can take part in outpatient rehabilitation programs or, in

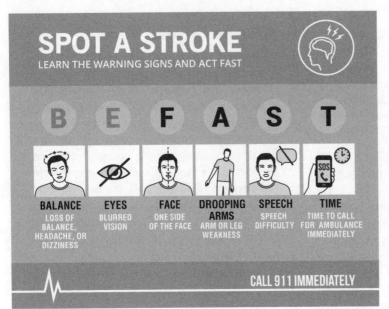

SPOT A STROKE
LEARN THE WARNING SIGNS AND ACT FAST

B E F A S T

BALANCE
LOSS OF BALANCE, HEADACHE, OR DIZZINESS

EYES
BLURRED VISION

FACE
ONE SIDE OF THE FACE

DROOPING ARMS
ARM OR LEG WEAKNESS

SPEECH
SPEECH DIFFICULTY

TIME
TIME TO CALL FOR AMBULANCE IMMEDIATELY

CALL 911 IMMEDIATELY

Getty Images

some cases, receive your rehabilitation in your own home.

The setting you choose will depend upon your needs, your doctor's recommendations, your insurance, and your preferences. Carefully consider the technology available at different facilities. Generally, academic hospital programs will have the most up-to-date treatments and access to innovative technologies. The Ohio State University Wexner Medical Center, for example, has specialized walking and electrical stimulation equipment that smaller programs or community facilities may not be able to house or afford.

What to Expect

When you begin stroke rehabilitation, you'll first undergo a battery of evaluations and assessments by a variety of specialists to identify what you'll need to work on. Stroke can have wide-ranging effects on everything from memory to movement, so it's not uncommon to have a large team of health-care providers that includes a physical medicine and rehabilitation physician, a neurologist, a neurosurgeon, a neuropsychologist, a certified rehabilitation nurse, a physical therapist, an occupational therapist, a speech-language pathologist, a recreational therapist, a respiratory therapist, a dietitian, a social worker, a case manager, and a rehabilitation engineer. Your team will create an individualized rehabilitation plan designed to address any deficits that impair your ability to function normally. Different team members will work on specific tasks.

For instance, if you have difficulty swallowing and cannot safely eat without the risk of choking, you'll work with a speech therapist to strengthen the muscles you use to swallow. If you're having trouble with things like bathing and grooming, an occupational therapist will teach you strategies to increase your independence while you rebuild your skills. Your team will also assess external factors such as your home environment, transportation concerns, social interactions, emotions, and coping skills.

You're an active part of this process: Be sure to tell them about anything that you specifically want to focus on so they can include it in your care plan. Once you go home, you can expect several weekly sessions with different therapists, and exercises to do on your off days, too.

Enjoyable Activities

Though stroke rehab involves lots of hard work and traditional exercise, you may be pleasantly surprised at how enjoyable some therapies can be. Activities involving art, video games, and virtual reality bring together multiple areas of the brain to perform complex activities, which can help augment core rehabilitative services.

Horseback riding has gotten a lot of attention for its healing benefits and can help with posture, muscle strengthening, and balance, but it requires a certain level of functioning, so if you're interested in that activity, ask your therapy team if it's appropriate for you.

Setting Goals

With difficult tasks, you can motivate yourself by setting small, achievable goals that you can build on as your skills grow. For instance, if leg paralysis is hindering your ability to walk, don't make running a 5K your first goal. Start with smaller goals, such as getting in and out of bed or mastering the use of mobility equipment. As you meet each mini-goal, set the next one to work toward your larger goal, and keep track of your accomplishments.

Your Recovery Timeline

The complexity of the brain and the amount of damage you sustain during a stroke will factor into how well you recover and how long it takes.

The first three months after a stroke form the core foundation of your stroke rehabilitation program. That's when you'll see the quickest and most dramatic improvements. You might even experience spontaneous recovery of a lost skill or ability as your brain finds new ways to perform tasks.

After that, your recovery may slow, but you will continue to augment and expand your rehabilitation strategies to continue working on any lingering problems. You may continue to see improvements for up to a year or two after your stroke.

Some people recover fully after a stroke, but others may have lingering impairments. Even if the rehabilitation process can't eliminate all impairments, it can help you learn ways to cope and adapt to them. Even after your official rehabilitation program is finished, it's important to continue to do physical and cognitive exercises to enhance and sustain your functional levels.

Future Stroke Prevention

Furthermore, the exercises and lifestyle strategies that you learn during rehab help lower the risk of having another stroke. (About 23 percent of stroke survivors have another.) Exercising, managing your blood pressure and cholesterol, eating a healthy diet, not smoking, and managing diabetes can all help lower your risk.

Walking Faster May Improve Stroke Recovery

Study titled "Dual-Task Walking and Automaticity After Stroke: Insights from a Secondary Analysis and Imaging Sub-Study of a Randomized Controlled Trial," by researchers at Oxford Brookes University, UK, published in *Clinical Rehabilitation.*

Being able to walk is one of the foremost abilities to recover after a stroke. Many stroke victims can walk on a treadmill but have trouble in their everyday lives, which entails walking while also watching your step and thinking about where you're going (among other things). Walking about in one's community is known as *dual-task walking* by medical researchers and rehabilitators and is something usually done automatically. Walking happens without too much focus on the movement, which frees up the brain to look, hear, maneuver and plan while walking. Stroke victims can have limited cognitive ability to achieve this basic task that most people take for granted.

Plain Treadmill versus Treadmill and Planning

In a previous study, researchers at Oxford Brookes University in the UK compared two types of rehabilitation methods for recovery of both walking speed and community walking at six weeks after a stroke. One group walked on a treadmill without any other intervention, tagged as single-task walking. Another group walked on a treadmill and were also asked to perform thinking, listening, and planning tasks while walking. This was the dual-task group. After 20 sessions of 30-minute training over 10 weeks, both groups improved walking speed. However, the researchers were surprised to find that the dual-task walkers were no better at dual-task walking than the single-task walkers.

A Theory About Walking Speed

The researchers suspected that patients who were able to walk faster at the beginning of their rehabilitation were more likely to be walking automatically and would be better at dual-task walking. They did a secondary analysis of the first study. The new findings are published in the journal *Clinical Rehabilitation*. The second analysis confirmed their hypothesis. Patients who were able to walk fastest at the beginning of the study were significantly more likely to regain dual-task walking by the end of the study, compared to the slower walkers.

The researchers further confirmed their hypothesis by looking at brain scans done while the study participants walked. When you have to think about what you're doing, you use part of your brain called the prefrontal cortex. When you're doing something automatically, the prefrontal cortex is quiet. The scans confirmed that the slower walkers were not walking automatically. They had to concentrate on walking and had little brain availability for community distractions. They had more prefrontal cortex activity.

The researchers conclude that for people who have limited walking capacity after a stroke, increasing walking speed should be a priority in rehabilitation. Before a person can learn to walk in a community setting, they need to regain the ability to walk automatically.

One of Your Carotid Arteries Is Blocked...

One of your carotid arteries is blocked, but your doctor says surgery to clear it is too risky. What should you do?

When a carotid artery is blocked and is discovered while testing for another health condition, typically no procedure is recommended. If the blockage has not already caused a stroke, it is unlikely to do so in the future, and if other arteries are clear, they can continue supplying blood to the brain. Surgery can be risky because there's a chance that a small clot or piece of plaque could break loose and travel to the brain, causing a stroke. In lieu of surgery, your doctor may recommend medication, such as aspirin or *clopidogrel* (Plavix), and lifestyle changes.

If you begin having symptoms such as dizziness, blurred vision, weakness, and/or numbness, it might make sense to have a procedure such as surgical removal of plaque or the insertion of a stent to hold the artery open. All these options should be discussed with your doctor.

Deepak L. Bhatt, MD, MPH, executive director of interventional cardiovascular programs, Brigham and Women's Hospital, Boston.

Chapter 3

CANCER BREAKTHROUGHS

Natural Breakthroughs in Breast Cancer Prevention

T*he statistics are well-known but still shocking:* Every year, more than 330,000 women are diagnosed with breast cancer, and more than 43,000 die from it.

Those frightening numbers are a relatively recent development: Breast cancer rates have more than doubled over the last few decades.

Modern Lifestyle, Rising Cases

During my more than 20 years as a practicing gynecologist, I've seen a growing number of cases among my patients. *I think there are several reasons for this steady rise...*

• **There is an increasing level of exposure to chemicals** such as bisphenol A (BPA) found in many water bottles, and phthalates, found in soaps and shampoos, that interfere with our hormones (the body's endocrine system). Exposure to these endocrine disruptors can upset the balance of the female sex hormone estrogen—a leading trigger of breast cancer.

• **Our highly processed diets alter the gut microbiome**—the trillions of friendly and unfriendly bacteria in the gastrointesti-

nal tract. When there are more "unfriendly" bacteria, there are higher levels of the enzyme beta-glucuronidase, which prevents the intestinal breakdown of estrogen, resulting in the reactivation of estrogen and an increase in the risk of breast cancer.

• **Non-stop stress generates excess cortisol,** a hormone that interferes with the breakdown of estrogen and increases inflammation (another risk factor for cancer).

• **A sedentary lifestyle has been linked to an increased risk of breast cancer,** perhaps because of increased body fat, poor blood sugar regulation, and inflammation.

• **There are several hormonally driven gynecological conditions that indicate a woman has excess levels of estrogen**—a leading risk factor for breast cancer, including endometriosis, uterine fibroids, heavy menstrual bleeding, and polycystic ovary syndrome (PCOS). If you have any of these

Tara Scott, MD, chief medical officer at Revitalize Medical Group in Akron, Ohio, clinical assistant professor at Northeast Ohio Medical University in Rootstown, Ohio, and Medical Director of Integrative Medicine at Summa Health in Akron, Ohio. Dr. Scott is board certified in obstetrics/gynecology, functional medicine, and integrative medicine, and is a passionate advocate for breast cancer prevention. RevitalizeMed.com

The Limitations of Early Detection

Most of the emphasis on controlling breast cancer is on early detection with mammography, but early detection should go hand-in-hand with prevention.

● **In a recent 23-year study published in the *International Journal of Cancer,*** researchers analyzed health data from the entire population of Norwegian women ages 30 to 89. They found that regular mammograms did not reduce the incidence of death from breast cancer compared to women who didn't get mammograms. In other words, mammography provided no benefit in terms of longer life.

That doesn't mean they're not important: They're the only tool we currently have for screening. Women between ages 45 and 54 should be screened once per year. After 55, screening can be performed annually or once every other year, according to the American Cancer Society.

● **If a mammogram detects cancer,** consider getting a second opinion to explore what treatment is best for your specific case. According to a recent study published in the *Annals of Internal Medicine,* one in three women with breast cancer detected by a mammogram is treated unnecessarily because the detected tumor is so slow-growing that it's essentially harmless. Experts call this overtreatment, meaning that it provides no benefit but can cause harm. There are many short- and long-term side effects from the treatment of breast cancer with chemotherapy, radiation, and surgery. Further, the hormone-blocking treatment common in breast cancer increases the risk of heart disease and osteoporosis.

The best strategy for dealing with breast cancer is to prevent the disease in the first place. You should also learn and perform breast self-exams once a month—statistically, this is the way most cancers are found.

—Dr. Tara Scott

conditions (or a family history of breast cancer), prevention is extra important for you.

These and other lifestyle factors, such as being overweight or having more than one alcoholic drink a day, can nearly double your risk of breast cancer, according to a new study published in *JAMA Network Open*. But that means that healthy lifestyle factors can do the opposite. Recent scientific studies show that the following steps can help you prevent breast cancer and, if you've already had it, keep it from coming back.

Eat More Fiber

Researchers at Harvard Medical School analyzed data from 20 studies on fiber and breast cancer and found that people who ate the most fiber lowered their risk of breast cancer by 18 percent.

Why it works: Higher fiber intake feeds the friendly bacteria in your gut, crowding out unfriendly bacteria. It also bulks up your stool and helps counter constipation, both of which help with estrogen detoxification.

What to do: Increase your intake of high-fiber fruits, vegetables, and whole grains. To ensure maximum fiber intake, consider taking a fiber supplement, too. Psyllium husk works great.

Spice with Onion and Garlic

In a study published in the journal *Nutrition and Cancer*, women who ate a dish spiced with onion and garlic more than once a day had a 67 percent lower risk of breast cancer than women who never ate onions or garlic.

Why it works: Onions and garlic are loaded with prebiotics, a type of fiber that feeds probiotics, allowing them to flourish in your gut. Probiotics may help increase levels of estrobolome, a type of bacteria that specifically metabolizes estrogen.

What to do: Make sure you eat a dish containing onion or garlic at least five days a week.

Eat Less Red Meat and More Poultry

In a seven-year study published in the *International Journal of Cancer*, researchers analyzed health data from more than 40,000 women. They found that women who ate the most red meat had a 23 percent higher risk of breast cancer than those who ate the least. However, those who ate the most poultry had a 15 percent lower risk of breast cancer compared with those who ate the least. Women who substituted poultry for red meat had a 28 percent lower risk of breast cancer.

Why it works: Red meat typically delivers high levels of fat and growth hormones, both of which have been linked to breast cancer.

What to do: Eat red meat no more than a few times a month. Increase your intake of organic poultry. You might also want to eat more wild-caught fatty fish like salmon and sardines. They are rich in omega-3 fatty acids, and studies link a higher intake of omega-3s with a lower risk of breast cancer.

Exercise Regularly

Many studies link regular exercise to a lower risk of breast cancer. Now, a new study published in the *Journal of the National Cancer Institute* shows the unique power of exercise for secondary prevention, too. Looking at more than 1,300 women diagnosed with breast cancer, the study found that women who exercised at a moderate intensity for at least 2.5 hours per week before and *after* their cancer diagnosis were 55 percent less likely to have their cancer return and 68 percent less likely to die of the disease. Even women who started exercising after the diagnosis were 46 percent less likely to have a recurrence and 43 percent less likely to die of the disease.

Why it works: Regular exercise helps improve and regulate nearly every cell, tissue, system, and organ—including strengthening your immune system, your main defense against cancer. Regular exercise also reduces circulating estrogen.

Menopausal Hormonal Therapy: It's Not What You Think

Researchers recently conducted a meta-analysis of 58 studies involving more than 100,000 women on menopausal hormonal therapy.

They confirmed what previous studies have found: Conventional menopausal hormonal therapy with estrogen and progestagen doubles the risk of breast cancer, they reported in *The Lancet*. (Topical vaginal estrogen did not increase risk.)

It's important to note that these studies looked at the use of synthetic hormones. Menopausal hormonal therapy with bioidentical estrogen and progesterone—medications that are chemically and structurally similar to the hormones manufactured by your body—have been shown in several large studies to actually lower the risk of breast cancer. If you're interested in menopausal hormonal therapy, find a physician who offers bioidentical hormones, measures your hormone levels before therapy, and prescribes an individualized rather than a standardized dose.

—Dr. Tara Scott

What to do: Aim for a weekly minimum of 2.5 hours of moderate aerobic exercise like brisk walking, biking, water aerobics, dancing, doubles tennis, or hiking.

Lose Weight

A study of more than 180,000 women published in the *Journal of the National Cancer Institute* found that women who lost weight after the age of 50 and kept it off had a lower risk of breast cancer. And the more weight they lost, the lower the risk. Women who lost 20 pounds or more decreased risk by 26 percent. But even women who lost 5 to 10 pounds decreased their risk by 13 percent.

Why it works: Fat cells generate *estrone*, the type of estrogen generated after menopause. It is even a more stimulatory hormone than *estradiol*, which is generated by the ovaries, and can cause growth in breast tissue that leads to cancer.

What to do: Look at the main cause of your overweight. It's different for each person. Are you eating too much? Are you an emotional eater? Are you not exercising enough? Is your thyroid out of whack? Is your stress too high?

Explore and address the causes of your weight gain—ideally, with the help of a physician, health coach, or weight loss program.

Skip Hair Dyes and Straighteners

An eight-year study published in the *International Journal of Cancer* looked at more than 46,000 women and their use of permanent hair dyes and straighteners. *The researchers found a consistent pattern of increased risk for breast cancer in women who used the products in the year before the study began...*

• **African American women who used permanent hair dye every five to eight weeks or more had a 60 percent increased risk.** (In general, the higher the frequency of use, the higher the risk, said the researchers.)

• **Caucasian women who used permanent hair dye every five to eight weeks or more had an 8 percent increased risk.**

• **Women who used chemical hair straighteners every five to eight weeks had a 30 percent increased risk.**

• **Women who used semipermanent or temporary hair dye had very little increase in risk.**

What happens: Hair dye and straighteners contain endocrine disruptors, and the latter also contains formaldehyde, a carcinogen.

What to do: It's best to just avoid these products.

Many Older Patients With Breast Cancer Can Safely Ease Up On Treatment

Priscilla McAuliffe, MD, PhD, surgical oncologist at UPMC Hillman Cancer Center and University of Pittsburgh School of Medicine and leader of a study of 3,000 women, published in *JAMA Network Open*.

Recent finding: Among women aged 70 and older who were diagnosed with and had surgery for early-stage breast cancer, the recurrence and survival rates were the same for women who did not have their lymph nodes removed and/or radiotherapy as for those who did. Treatment side effects, such as nerve pain and lymphedema, can be especially hard on older women.

Increased Genetic Risk Does Not Decrease Breast Cancer Survival

Study titled "Association of Genetic Testing Results With Mortality Among Women With Breast Cancer or Ovarian Cancer," by researchers at Stanford University, University of Michigan, et al., published in the *Journal of the National Cancer Institute*.

Usually, the focus of gene mutations BRCA1 and BRCA2 is on increased risk for cancer, so women who test positive with these specific mutations can work toward deterring eventual cancer development. Yet according to a new study, women with these mutations who develop breast or ovarian cancer survive just as long as women with these cancers who don't possess *BRCA1* and *BRCA2*.

How Cancer Genes Work

Mutations of breast or ovarian cancer genes can increase the risk of breast and ovarian cancer because healthy genes are responsible for making proteins that repair cell DNA. When mutated cells can't repair DNA, they are more likely to become cancerous.

BRCA1 and BRCA2 are passed down through families in both men and women. In men they may increase the risk of male breast cancer and possibly prostate cancer. For all women, the average risk of developing breast cancer is about 13 percent, but having a BRCA1 mutation raises the risk to between 55 and 72 percent. Having the BRCA2 mutation increases the risk to 45 to 69 percent.

Ovarian cancer is less common than breast cancer. It affects just over one percent of women but having the BRCA1 mutation increases the risk to 39 to 44 percent, and the BRCA2 mutation to 11 to 17 percent.

Does BRCA1 and BRCA2 Affect Cancer Survival?

The risk for cancer associated with BRCA1 and BRCA2 is known, but little has been discovered about the effect these genes have on cancer survival. A study out of Stanford University is good news for women with breast or ovarian cancer who have these gene mutations. Although BRCA1 and BRCA2 increase risk, they do not decrease survival; in fact, in some cases, they may increase chances of survival.

Using the Georgia and California Surveillance Epidemiology and End Results (SEER) database, the records of 22,495 women with breast cancer and 4,320 women with ovarian cancer were analyzed over 41 months. All the women had stages I through IV breast or ovarian cancer, and all were treated with chemotherapy. The study is published in the *Journal of the National Cancer Institute*.

Breast cancers have receptors that doctors can use to treat cancer, so these receptors were considered along with survival. The receptors are the female hormones estrogen (ER), progesterone (PR), and the protein human epidermal growth factor (HER2). *These were the key findings…*

- **Women with triple negative breast cancer (no ER, PR or HER2 receptors)** who

had a BRCA1 or BRCA2 mutation had better survival rates than women without genetic mutations.

- **Women with triple negative breast cancer who had a genetic mutation** other than BRCA1 or BRCA2 had the same survival rates as women without any genetic mutation.

- **Women with ovarian cancer who had a BRCA2 mutation** or a mutation other than BRCA1 or BRCA2 had better survival rates than women without a genetic mutation.

BRCA1 and BRCA2 Make Chemo More Effective

The researchers suspect that because BRCA1 and BRCA2 mutations make it hard for cells to repair DNA damage, chemotherapies that damage DNA in cancer cells may become more effective. Damaged DNA cannot regenerate. If you have breast cancer and the gene mutations associated with increased risk, be sure to discuss with your doctor chemotherapy options that enhance long-term survival.

For additional help: For more information on BRCA gene mutations, cancer risk, testing and treatment, visit Cancer.gov/about-cancer/causes-prevention/genetics/brca-fact-sheet.

Exercise Reduces Chemotherapy Brain Fog in Breast Cancer Patients

Study titled "Physical Activity Patterns and Relationships With Cognitive Function in Patients With Breast Cancer Before, During, and After Chemotherapy in a Prospective, Nationwide Study," by researchers at Washington University School of Medicine, St. Louis, published in *Journal of Clinical Oncology*.

"Chemo brain" is a real threat for women with breast cancer treated with chemotherapy. The medical term for this foggy chemical reaction is *cognitive dysfunction*. Symptoms include lapses in memory, difficulty finishing sentences and poor concentration. Some studies suggest that physical activity can help, but research on the effects of physical activity before, during and after chemotherapy are scarce.

More Exercise Relieves Chemo Brain

A new study led by researchers at Washington University School of Medicine in St. Louis suggests that increasing physical activity to the levels recommended by the U.S. Department of Health and Human Services (DHHS) may help prevent cognitive decline related to chemotherapy. DHHS guidelines are a minimum of 150 minutes of moderate to vigorous physical activity per week.

The research team analyzed physical activity levels using a self-reporting questionnaire before, right after, and six months after chemotherapy in 580 women with breast cancer. At the same time, the women were tested for cognitive functions in visual memory and attention span. They were also asked to rate their own level of cognition. As a control, 363 age-matched women without cancer answered the same physical activity questions and had the same cognitive measurements at the same time points.

Their findings are published in the American Society of Clinical Oncology's *Journal of Clinical Oncology.*

Cancer Patients Should Exercise Despite the Stress of Chemotherapy

At the start of the study, 33 percent of the cancer patients met the DHHS physical activity guidelines. Right after chemotherapy, that number dropped to 21 percent, and at six months, the number had gone up to 37 percent. *Key findings also included…*

• **In the control group,** about 40 percent of the women met the DHHS physical activity guidelines at all the time points.

• **On all the cognitive tests,** the more-active cancer patients did better than the inactive cancer patients.

• **The women without cancer performed similarly on all the cognitive testing,** despite their physical activity level.

• **Breast cancer patients who met the physical activity levels before chemotherapy** performed similarly on cognitive function testing as the control group on the memory and attention span, but they rated their own cognition lower than it actually was. The researchers think this may be due to anxiety, fatigue or depression related to cancer diagnosis and treatment, not to actual cognitive decline.

The researchers conclude that maintaining adequate physical activity before and during chemotherapy results in better cognitive function immediately after chemotherapy and at six months after completion of chemo treatment.

For more information: For resources and assistance on exercise and breast cancer, including steps to exercise safely, visit Breast Cancer.org/tips/exercise.

Best Treatment for Metastatic Breast Cancer

Study titled "ASO Author Reflections: Surgery Offers Survival Advantage in Treatment-Responsive Metastatic Breast Cancer," by researchers at Penn State College of Medicine and Cancer Institute, Hershey, Pennsylvania, published in *Annals of Surgical Oncology.*

For patients with metastatic (or stage IV) breast cancer, the standard treatment approach has been drugs or what is known as *systemic therapy*—chemotherapy, hormone therapy, and immunotherapy. About 6 percent of newly diagnosed breast cancers are metastatic (which means that the cancer has spread to other parts of the body).

Review of Combined Therapy

A team of researchers from Penn State College of Medicine and Cancer Institute have recently investigated surgery as a viable treatment option for patients with metastatic breast cancer. They reviewed the records of close to 13,000 stage IV breast cancers treated between 2010 and 2015 from the National Cancer Database.

Their findings suggest that surgery improves survival when it's combined with systemic therapy. The study was published in the *Annals of Surgical Oncology*. They excluded patients who died within six months of diagnosis, as these patients did not respond to systemic therapy.

Study details: The researchers identified whether the breast cancer patients had HER2, estrogen (ER), and progesterone (PR) tumor status. HER2 is a protein that promotes tumor growth. ER and PR are hormone receptors. They investigated how these receptors or the HER2 protein responded to different treatments and timing of drug intake, such as chemotherapy. *They compared systemic therapies without surgery to treatments with surgery…*

• **The addition of surgery to systemic therapies** regardless of ER, PR, and HER2 status improved survival.

• **The best survival benefit was giving systemic therapies before surgery,** rather than after surgery, in patients who were ER, PR, and HER2 positive.

Several clinical studies have concluded that surgery did not add a survival benefit to systemic therapies in stage IV breast cancer. However, studies that have looked back at medical records (retrospective studies) have found that surgery reduced death rates (mortality) by 35 percent to 50 percent. This new retrospective study supports these findings.

Surgery for Stage IV Breast Cancer

Although additional clinical studies could be helpful, it is difficult to recruit enough patients to make these studies reliable, and trials can take a long time. The research team believes their real-world data offers a timely guide for clinicians who treat breast cancer. Surgery has been shown to benefit other stage IV cancers, such as colon cancer. The researchers urge clinicians to consider surgery for patients with metastatic breast cancer who respond to systemic therapies. This combined therapy could make a significant impact on how long a patient survives.

Combining Chemotherapy and Gene Therapy for Metastatic Melanoma

Study titled "Combination of Chemotherapy with BRAF Inhibitors Results in Effective Eradication of Malignant Melanoma by Preventing ATM-dependent DNA Repair," by researchers at Stem Cells and Cancer Research Laboratory-IMIM, et al., Barcelona, Spain, published in *Oncogene*.

Metastatic malignant melanoma is the most advanced form of melanoma and the leading cause of death from skin cancer. There currently is no cure. According to a new study published in the journal *Oncogene*, combining low-dose chemotherapy along with gene therapy, called BRAF inhibition, may offer new hope for patients with this deadliest type of skin cancer.

BRAF Gene Therapy Defined

About half of patients with melanoma skin cancer have an abnormal gene (gene mutation) called a BRAF mutation. This mutation allows melanoma cancer cells to grow and spread. Drugs have been developed to block the BRAF mutation, called BRAF inhibitors. Using this type of treatment is called a targeted cancer therapy.

Chemotherapy drugs are not effective against metastatic melanoma. BRAF inhibitors are the best treatment, but BRAF inhibitors only stop the cancer cells from growing—they do not destroy and eliminate them. Over time, the cells become resistant to

Unexposed Skin Still Can Be Damaged By the Sun

Genetic mutations to the skin can be caused by the body's own processes over time, as well as by exposure to UV light. When researchers compared the roles of those different causes of skin changes in 21 adults, they took samples from the volunteers' hips, reasoning that skin in that area was unlikely to have been exposed to much direct sunlight. Still, they found that UV-related changes to skin cells were common even in sun-shielded tissue.

Study by researchers at National Institute of Environmental Health Sciences, Research Triangle Park, North Carolina, published in *PLOS Genetics*.

BRAF inhibitors and start to develop again, triggering a relapse.

Combination Therapy Stops Cancer Cells

In previous studies, researchers from the IMIM Stem Cell and Cancer Research Group showed that BRAF inhibitors could prevent colon cancer cells damaged by chemotherapy from revitalizing themselves by blocking DNA-damage repair. The researchers decided to try a combination of chemotherapy along with a BRAF inhibitor to see if it could work against metastatic melanoma.

In animal models as well as in human cancer cells, the combination of the chemotherapy and the BRAF inhibitor not only stopped the cancer cells from growing, but it also destroyed them completely. The combination approach provided the best results in all trials after one week of treatment.

The researchers hope that the combination therapy could eliminate metastatic melanoma treatment resistance and relapse. They believe that it may even be effective on types of untreatable malignant melanoma that do not have the BRAF mutation. Future developments include cancer-treatment trials of

the combination therapy in human patients with metastatic melanoma.

A Fiber-Rich Diet Improves the Response to Melanoma Treatment

Giorgio Trinchieri, MD, chief of the laboratory of integrative cancer immunology in the National Cancer Institute's Center for Cancer Research, Bethesda, Maryland.

Researchers looked at hundreds of melanoma patients and reported that higher dietary fiber intake was associated with disease non-progression among patients on immune checkpoint blockade (ICB) treatment. The most pronounced benefits were found in patients with high fiber intake and no probiotic use. The findings suggest that some commercially available probiotics may be harmful for patients on ICB.

Why People with Parkinson's Get More Melanoma Cancers

Study titled "An Amyloid Link Between Parkinson's Disease and Melanoma," by researchers at the National Heart, Lung, and Blood Institute, presented at the American Chemical Society Spring Meeting 2021.

Individuals with Parkinson's disease are two to six times more likely to develop a melanoma skin cancer. The medical community has known about this risk for nearly 50 years. But what has remained a mystery is how a progressive brain disease can make you more likely to get a serious skin cancer. A new study from researchers at the National Heart, Lung, and Blood Institute (NHLBI) (part of the National Institutes of Health) may have found the link—a type of protein called *amyloid*. Their research was presented at the 2021 meeting of the American Chemical Society.

The Amyloid Connection

With Parkinson's disease, an abnormal amyloid protein called α-*synuclein* forms deposits that destroy brain cells needed to make the brain chemical dopamine. Low levels of *dopamine* cause the common symptoms of the disease, such as slowed movement and tremors. But this protein is not only found in the brain. Research shows that α-synuclein can be found in the cells that produce melanin. Called melanocytes, these are the cells that become cancerous in melanoma.

Melanin's Risk

Melanocytes make the skin pigment melanin. Melanin makes your skin darker, and it also protects skin from the ultraviolet rays of the sun that cause skin cancer. Researchers at NHLBI had previously studied another amyloid protein found in healthy melanocytes called *premelanosomal protein* or Pmel. Pmel is an integral part of skin structure because it stores melanin.

In the NHLBI study, the research team combined α-synuclein with Pmel in the laboratory. They found that α-synuclein could cause Pmel to lose its ability to store mela-

nin. The loss of melanin may decrease skin protection from the sun, and it may be the reason people with Parkinson's disease and the abnormal protein α-synuclein are at risk for melanoma skin cancer.

More Parkinson's-Melanoma Research to Follow

The researchers describe their finding as just the tip of the iceberg, and plan future experiments to learn more about the interaction of α-synuclein and Pmel.

Is That Spot Dangerous?

Carolyn I. Jacob, MD, a board-certified dermatologist and associate clinical instructor at Northwestern University Feinberg School of Medicine. She is the founder and medical director of Chicago Cosmetic Surgery and Dermatology.

Skin irregularities can be harmless or a sign of something serious. Here's how to know the difference.

Some of us age with subtle, gradual, changes in our complexions, while others show dramatic effects from a lifetime of sun exposure and other influences. But, at some point, most of us encounter unexpected bumps and spots.

So how do you know which skin spots are harmless and which should concern you enough to check in with a doctor? *Here's a quick guide to help you know…*

Urgent Issues

The most important reason to pay attention to the marks on your skin is to detect the earliest signs of melanoma, a cancer that can develop in the cells that give skin its color. Melanoma is less common than other types of skin cancer, but more likely to spread to other parts of the body. Risk factors include having many moles, many unusual moles (large or oddly shaped), a family history of melanoma, or fair skin, though darker-skinned people can get it too. Exposure

---

Vitamin B-3 (Niacin) Protects Against UV Exposure

In the lab, treating skin cells with vitamin B-3 before exposing them to ultraviolet light protected them from DNA damage caused by direct sunlight, the main risk factor for non-melanoma skin cancers. Niacin from food is not protective. Take a supplement (500 mg to 1 g) prior to sun exposure. People with a history of non-melanoma skin cancer should take B-3 daily.

Lara Camillo, PhD, and Paola Savoia, MD, PhD, University of Eastern Piedmont, Novara, Italy, leaders of a study presented at the European Academy of Dermatology and Venereology Congress.

to the sun and tanning beds raises the risk, but melanomas can also grow on skin that doesn't get much exposure, such as the soles of the feet. Some melanomas develop from existing moles, while others arise as new growths.

Here are the signs that should prompt an immediate visit to a dermatologist...

• **Asymmetry.** If you draw an imaginary line down the middle of the spot, do the two sides look the same or different? Melanomas may look different on each side.

• **Border.** A melanoma may have an irregular, scalloped, or poorly defined border.

• **Color.** A melanoma may have a mixture of colors, such as tan, brown and black, or even red, white, and blue.

• **Diameter.** Typical melanomas are larger than a pencil eraser, about 6 millimeters, when diagnosed.

• **Evolving.** The most concerning sign may be if a spot on your skin is getting bigger, changing color or shape, rising up from the skin, or looking different from anything else on your skin.

A melanoma doesn't have to show all of these attributes. In some cases, it may show just one, such as rapid growth. If you have a new mole or even a bump that looks like a pimple that keeps growing, visit the dermatologist. When melanoma is caught early, the survival rates are excellent, but they drop precipitously if it spreads to other parts of the body.

Lower-Risk Spots

The most common forms of skin cancer are basal and squamous cell carcinomas. They are rarely life-threatening, but they can be disfiguring, so a doctor's visit is in order if you have a spot that sounds like those described below. Anyone can develop these cancers, but they are most common in people with fair skin who have spent a lot of time in the sun.

Basal cell carcinomas most often appear on the face, ears, and hands. They can look

like pearly, shiny bumps with tiny blood vessels. They can be the same color as your skin or a little reddish and may have a dip in the middle. They can look like a pimple, a minor injury, or a wound that won't heal. They can have a waxy, scar-like appearance. They may bleed, ooze, become scaly, or start to itch.

Squamous cell carcinomas most commonly appear on the face, scalp, lips, and hands, but they can also appear in the mouth, under a nail, or even inside the anus.

The earliest sign of what could become a squamous cell carcinoma is a lesion called an actinic keratosis. Usually appearing in people ages 40 or older, these are often dry, scaly pink or red patches, but they also can be brown or white. They may feel rough, sensitive, painful, itchy, prickly, and burning. They may look and feel inflamed, and they may come and go in the same location. Left untreated, these lesions can progress to squamous cell carcinoma. They may then become a raised, red bump, or even stick out like a small horn. These skin spots are highly treatable, but shouldn't be ignored.

Benign Spots

There are many benign causes of spots, lumps, and bumps that can appear—especially as we get older...

• **Acrochordons (skin tags)** tend to grow in areas where there are skin folds. They are harmless and do not require removal, but your dermatologist can take them off if they are bothersome.

• **Warts are caused by the human papilloma virus,** and they can take many forms. They may be flat, cauliflower-shaped, or have finger-like projections. You can treat them at home with over-the-counter salicylic acid. If that fails, see your dermatologist for other options, such as laser therapy or cryotherapy.

• **Cherry angiomas.** These are small, bright red spots that are flat or slightly raised and typically appear on the trunk and extremities. They can be as small as a pinpoint and as large as a quarter inch in diameter.

They most often grow on the arms, legs, or trunk, and are considered harmless.

•**Age spots (also known as lentigines).** These flat, oval spots are tan to dark brown. You are most likely to notice them on skin that has had heavy sun exposure, such as the back of your hands, shoulders and face. They can be lightened with creams and lotions or treated with lasers or chemical peels.

While these are all examples of benign conditions, it's wise to always remember the adage: When in doubt, check it out.

Minimize Your Risk of Lung Cancer

Jamie Garfield, MD, associate professor of thoracic medicine and surgery, and an interventional pulmonologist, Temple Lung Center at Temple University Hospital, Philadelphia.

When you think of lung cancer, you likely think of cigarettes, and for good reason. Cigarette smoking is linked to 80 to 90 percent of all lung cancer deaths in the United States.

But every year, nonsmokers get lung cancer too. *Here's what you need to do to protect your lungs…*

If You Smoke, Quit

If you smoke, talk to your physician or a trained smoking cessation expert to get help with quitting. The process may be eased with medications and behavioral counseling. Even smokers who are diagnosed with cancer benefit from quitting. It improves the response to treatment and healing, and it can reduce the risk of death.

Despite lingering misconceptions that e-cigarettes and vapes are a comparatively harmless alternative to the real thing, the U.S. Centers for Disease Control and Prevention has determined that they are still unsafe. They often contain nicotine and a variety of chemicals with unknown safety profiles.

The risk of lung cancer isn't limited to the smoker: Secondhand exposure to smoke is the No. 1 risk factor for the development of lung cancer in nonsmokers. Even thirdhand smoke—residual chemicals and nicotine left on clothes and surfaces by tobacco smoke—can increase the risk of asthma, ear infections, pneumonia, and cancer of the bladder, cervix, kidney, mouth, throat, and pancreas.

Eat for Your Lungs

A healthy diet high in fruits and vegetables has been shown to decrease the risk of cancer—even among smokers. It doesn't make smoking safe, but it can help protect your lungs while you work on quitting.

A 2017 study suggested that beta-cryptoxanthin (BCX), a carotenoid in yellow, orange, and red fruits and vegetables, reduces the number of receptors that nicotine binds to in the lungs. Researchers reported in *Cancer Prevention Research* that a daily dose of 870 micrograms of BCX (about two tangerines) could reduce the risk of lung cancer and cut lung tumor growth by 52 to 63 percent.

Another study reported that eating a wide variety of fruits and vegetables may be the best bet. Smokers who reported that they ate between 23 and 40 different types of fruits and vegetables during the prior two weeks were almost one-third less likely to get squamous cell lung cancer than people who ate 10 or fewer types, the researchers reported in *Cancer Epidemiology, Biomarkers & Prevention*.

Researchers postulate that compounds in fruits and vegetables may repair some smoking-induced DNA oxidative damage, regulate anti-tumor pathways, inhibit tumor cell proliferation, induce tumor cell death, and reduce the inflammatory reaction to nicotine.

Exercise

Regular exercise can improve lung and cardiovascular health, and it appears to reduce the risk of developing lung cancer by 20 to 30 percent for women and 20 to 50 percent for men. Researchers suggest that the protective effects may come from better pulmonary and immune function, improvements in DNA repair, lower inflammation, and reduced concentrations of carcinogenic agents in the lungs.

Aim for at least 150 minutes per week of moderate-intensity aerobic activity or 75 minutes per week of vigorous aerobic activity, but don't walk or jog along highways, where pollution levels are high.

Reduce Radon

Exposure to high levels of radon, a naturally forming radioactive gas that can rise to dangerous levels in the home, is the second-leading cause of lung cancer in the United States. Exposure to the combination of radon gas and cigarette smoke creates a greater risk of lung cancer than does exposure to either factor alone, but more than 10 percent of radon-related cancer deaths occur among nonsmokers.

You can purchase an inexpensive radon test kit in most hardware and home-improvement stores. If the radon levels in your home exceed 4 picocuries per liter, hire a radon remediation company to install a venting system.

Use Personal Protective Equipment

Occupational and recreational exposure to substances such as asbestos, silica, coal, wood dust, and mold can increase your risk for cancer and chronic lung diseases, such as chronic obstructive pulmonary disorder and asthma. Wearing personal protective equipment and working in well-ventilated areas can help reduce risk.

Reduce Environmental Exposure

Forest fires, cars, power plants and many other sources emit tiny particles—much smaller than a grain of sand—that can worsen lung disease and lead to cancer. Children, the elderly, and people with lung and heart disease and diabetes are at the highest risk. To lower risk, pay attention to the air quality forecast

Mushrooms Lower Cancer Risk

Eating 18 grams of mushrooms daily (less than one-quarter cup) was associated with a 45 percent lower risk for cancer. Mushrooms are high in cell-protecting vitamins and antioxidants, including the especially protective amino acid *ergothioneine*. All mushrooms are high in these antioxidants, but shiitake, oyster and maitake have the most.

John Richie, PhD, professor of public health sciences and pharmacology at Penn State Cancer Institute, Hershey, and coauthor of a review of 17 cancer studies and data from more than 19,500 cancer patients, published in *Advances in Nutrition*.

(find your local forecast at AirNow.com) and limit your outdoor activity when air quality is poor.

Cut Down on Recurrent Infections

Recurrent infections can put you at risk for acute and chronic lung disease and even lung cancer. Stay up-to-date on vaccinations that protect against respiratory infections, such as pneumococcal, influenza, and COVID vaccines.

Unravelling the Mystery of Lung Cancer in Nonsmokers

Study titled "Genomic and Evolutionary Classification of Lung Cancer in Never Smokers," by researchers at the National Cancer Institute, Bethesda, Maryland, et al., published in *Nature Genetics*.

When you hear about lung cancer, the leading cause of cancer deaths, the first cause-connection that comes to mind is "smoking." And that's a correct link…to a certain extent. Although smoking is the biggest risk factor for lung cancer, about 10 percent to 20 percent of individuals with lung cancer have never smoked tobacco. Researchers refer to these people as "never smokers." Lung cancer in never smokers is more common in women and tends to occur at an earlier age than the average diagnosis (which is 65 and older).

Why never smokers get lung cancer for the most part is a mystery. Now, a team of international investigators has begun to crack the genetic code of never smokers to unravel why some of these individuals develop this deadly disease.

Gene Mutations Tell a DNA Story

Led by the National Cancer Institute, part of the National Institutes of Health, the research team used whole-gene sequencing on tumor tissue from 232 never smokers with lung cancer and compared their genes to tissues from healthy never smokers. Whole-genome sequencing means identifying all the DNA in a person's cells. The researchers were looking for patterns of gene mutations called *mutational signatures.*

A mutational signature tells researchers how a tumor starts to grow. From prior research, mutational signatures have been cataloged for many types of cancer. There are mutational signatures that are caused by specific types of carcinogens, the substance that causes cancer. Cancer mutations may also start from the natural process of cell damage and repair not caused by a carcinogen, which also has a mutational signature. The results of the study are published in the journal *Nature Genetics.*

Three Cancer Subtypes Can Target Treatment

Based on the mutational signatures they found, the investigators created three subtypes for lung cancer in never smokers. *They gave the subtypes musical names based on the levels of genetic changes...*

• **Piano subtype is the most common.** It has the fewest mutations, and it grows slowly over years.

• **Mezzo-forte subtype has more mutations,** grows more quickly than piano type and has a known lung cancer mutation gene called EGFR.

• **Forte subtype grows most quickly,** and has a genomic signature called whole-genome doubling, which is also seen in smokers. Whole-genome doubling means that all the chromosomes in cancer cells have been doubled, giving cancer cells a high survival rate.

Knowing the subtype helps doctors determine how a cancer will behave and may lead to better treatments, called targeted therapies. Many targeted therapies are already being used. For example, the *EGFR* mutation helps cancer tumors increase their blood supply, and drugs that target this gene specifically curb this activity.

As researchers learn more about the genes of these cancers, strategies for prevention and treatment may follow. The research team would like to do genomic testing on more patients and focus on possible risk factors such as race and geographic location.

For more information on lung cancer in nonsmokers: Visit the Centers for Disease Control and Prevention website at CDC. gov/cancer/lung/nonsmokers.

Breakthrough Genetic Testing for Non-Small Cell Lung Cancer

Study titled "Real-World Utilization of Biomarker Testing for Patients with Advanced Non-Small-Cell Lung Cancer in a Tertiary Referral Center and Referring Hospitals," by researchers at University of Twente, Enschede, the Netherlands and University of Melbourne Centre for Cancer Research, Australia, published in *The Journal of Molecular Diagnostics.*

Advanced non-small-cell lung cancer (NSCLC) is difficult to treat. Targeted remedies and immunotherapy require genetic testing to find out if the patient's cancer cells have genes that can respond to treatment. These genes are called *biomarkers*. There are many possible biomarker genes. Biomarkers are also used to measure response to treatment.

Whole-Genome Sequencing Tests All Genes

Biomarkers with the highest prevalence are usually tested first. These include the cancer genes *EGFR, ALK, BRAF V600E* and *ROS1*. However, new biomarkers are being discovered, as well as new tests to find them. Some biomarker testing looks for a few genes, and some only test for single genes. There is a wide variation in both testing and treatment selection. One possibility is to do a complete genetic test of all genes, called whole-genome sequencing, which can be an expensive process and used less often than selective gene testing.

Study details: To learn more about how genetic testing is done at a cancer center treating advanced NSCLC, researchers from University of Twente, the Netherlands and University of Melbourne Center for Cancer Research, Australia, reviewed testing for 102 patients referred to a comprehensive cancer center in the Netherlands between 2017 and 2018. The results are published in *The Journal of Molecular Diagnostics*.

Extensive test combinations: The study found 99 different test combinations. Common biomarkers were usually tested first, but many new and emerging biomarkers were also tested. There was a wide variety in the number of tests and the timing of tests. The researchers found that the mean testing cost per patient was more than $2,000, the most expensive test being the whole-genome sequencing.

Benefits of Whole-Genome Sequencing

Despite the expense, the researchers concluded that whole-genome sequencing would be less time consuming overall and would find some biomarkers that would not have been found by current testing options. Other studies have found that delays in testing can lead to delays in NSCLC treatments and decreased treatment response. The researchers conclude that replacing current testing with whole-gene sequencing could be an exciting avenue for future studies and yield better results for individuals with this difficult-to-treat cancer.

Antacids Might Limit Lung Cancer Treatment

Study titled "Efficacy of First-line Atezolizumab Combination Therapy in Patients with Non-small Cell Lung Cancer Receiving Proton Pump Inhibitors: Post Hoc Analysis of IMpower150," by researchers at Flinders University, Adelaide, Australia, published in *British Journal of Cancer*.

It is estimated that about 30 percent of cancer patients frequently use a PPI to relieve heartburn symptoms. Could these PPIs possibly block the effectiveness of immune checkpoint inhibitors?

Study Presents Evidence That PPIs Block Immunotherapy

A new study from researchers at Flinders University in Australia has found that patients with non-small cell lung cancer had a lower overall survival and a shorter progression-free survival when they were taking a checkpoint inhibitor and a PPI. The study is published in the *British Journal of Cancer*.

In this trial of 1,202 patients with advanced non-small cell lung cancer who were having their first chemotherapy treatment, 441 patients (37 percent) were taking a PPI in the 30 days before and after chemotherapy. The researchers compared survival between the PPI patients who took a checkpoint inhibitor along with traditional chemotherapy to PPI patients who took chemotherapy drugs without a checkpoint inhibitor.

The key finding was that PPI users taking a checkpoint inhibitor and traditional chemotherapy had worse survival than patients taking just chemotherapy. PPI use did not affect survival in patients who were taking chemotherapy without a checkpoint inhibitor. The researchers conclude that PPI use decreases survival in patients who are taking a checkpoint inhibitor. They suggest that doctors who treat cancer (oncologists) need to monitor PPI use in their patients.

Why PPIs and Immunotherapy Are a Bad Mix

The reason that PPIs may interfere with checkpoint immunotherapy is that these antacids change the microbe balance in the intestines, called the gut microbiome. The microbiome plays an important role in regulating the immune system. Checkpoint inhibitors work by turning off proteins in immune system cells that slow down an immune response, called checkpoints. Opening up checkpoints allows the immune system to go into overdrive and attack cancer cells. PPIs seem to interfere with the ability to open the checkpoints.

This is not the first study to find a link between PPIs and checkpoint inhibitors. Checkpoint immunotherapy is used for other cancers also. According to the American Association for Cancer Research (AACR), PPIs have been shown to reduce the effects of checkpoint inhibitors on bladder cancer. In a study reported by AACR, PPIs reduced the response of advanced bladder cancer to checkpoint inhibitors by about 50 percent. Patients taking PPIs had about a 50 percent higher risk of their cancer getting worse during treatment.

If you are being treated with a checkpoint inhibitor for cancer, it makes sense to check with your oncologist before taking a PPI.

New Cell-Phone Health Risks

Devra Lee Davis, PhD, MPH, founder and president of Environmental Health Trust in Teton Village, Wyoming. She is author of Disconnect: The Truth About Cell Phone Radiation, What the Industry Is Doing to Hide It, and How to Protect Your Family. EHTrust.org

While 5G cellular service sounds exciting, the health risks of this fifth-generation wireless technology and the radiation it emits are concerning. Cell-phone companies warn shareholders that they may be sued for cancer and other health impacts from 5G and other wireless devices, while at the same time aggressively marketing these same devices to consumers.

Talking about the risks of cell-phone radiation is not new—Environmental Health Trust has been warning about it for many years. But 5G and wireless dramatically increase the risk. These new networks rely on 4G connections and use the same wireless frequencies we have now but with new, higher frequencies. More than a million new "short" cell towers are being built, bringing microwave-radiating antennas closer than ever before and more than tripling exposure. You have no say at all about antenna location—one could be right outside your bedroom wall! And you're at risk of exposure whether or not you have a 5G phone.

One of the most ironic things about 5G is that it actually doesn't improve reception for voice calls. What it does do is create a new, faster way for wireless devices to communicate with one another, such as in a smart home. It also boosts download speeds for data, movies and video games.

How to Reduce Your Exposure

To protect yourself and your family from radiation associated with 5G—as well as from 4G and 3G—follow these guidelines. *These steps are more important than ever…*

• **Don't carry your cell-phone in your pocket, bra or against your body** unless it is turned off.

• **When you are not using the phone, power it off or set it to Airplane/Flight mode.** Also turn off Wi-Fi and Bluetooth.

• **When talking on the cell phone, use speaker mode or a plug-in earpiece** to keep your the phone away from your brain and body. Or, even better, send texts rather than make voice calls.

• **Don't use your cell phone when you have only one or two bars or when you are between cell towers.** A cell phone sends signals to a tower up to 900 times a minute, and each time, some of that radiation is absorbed into your body.

• **Don't sleep with your cell phone nearby.** If you use your phone as an alarm, set it to Airplane/Flight mode and turn off Wi-Fi and Bluetooth before putting it on your nightstand.

Better: Purchase a battery-powered alarm clock (plug-in digital clocks can emit EMF radiation).

• **Keep your corded-phone landline,** which is free of wireless radiation and works in an emergency. Cordless home phones emit the same type of radiation as cell towers.

• **Use a wired mouse, keyboard and printer** to avoid unnecessary radiation, and don't buy smart-home wireless devices.

• **Get engaged in your community and at the state and federal levels** to prevent cell-phone towers from being built near your home and schools.

• **Hang onto your non-5G phone as long as possible.** Newer phones usually have more antennas, and you can't always turn them off.

Daily Aspirin Fights Inherited Bowel Cancer

Five-year study of 861 Lynch syndrome patients in 16 countries by researchers at Newcastle University, UK, published in *The Lancet*.

People with a hereditary condition called Lynch syndrome are at high risk for colon cancer.

Recent finding: Lynch syndrome patients who took two full-strength aspirin a day for two years were 50 percent less likely to develop colon cancer over a decade than those who did not take aspirin. Lynch syndrome affects about one out of 200 people. Talk to your doctor if you have Lynch syndrome or any strong family history of cancer—the benefits of aspirin may outweigh the known risks for stomach ulcers and bleeding.

WHO Study Links Moderate Alcohol Use to Cancer

Study titled "Global Burden of Cancer in 2020 Attributable to Alcohol Consumption: A Population-Based Study," by researchers at the World Health Organization's International Agency for Research on Cancer, et al., published in *Lancet Oncology*.

For decades, those who imbibe a daily glass of wine have toasted to a healthy heart. And several studies do say that moderate alcohol consumption is linked to lower risk of death from heart disease. Other studies say that alcohol intake for heart health is open for debate. More recently, an international team of researchers from the World Health Organization has published a global population study finding a strong link between alcohol consumption and cancer risk. Their findings were published in the journal *Lancet Oncology*.

Female Breast Cancer Is Now the Most Diagnosed Cancer Worldwide

In 2020, there were an estimated 2.3 million new cases of cancer, with 11.7 percent being female breast cancer…11.4 percent lung cancer…10 percent colorectal cancer…7.3 percent prostate cancer…and 5.6 percent stomach cancer.

Study by researchers from the American Cancer Society, Atlanta, and International Agency for Research on Cancer, Lyon, France, published in *CA: A Cancer Journal for Clinicians*.

Alcohol Intake and Risk for Cancer

The research team looked at cancers diagnosed in 2020. They reviewed cancers that are known to have an increased risk from alcohol, which includes cancers of the mouth, throat, esophagus, breast, colon, rectum, and liver. Alcohol consumption was broken down into moderate, risky, and heavy use. Moderate use is one to two alcoholic drinks per day. *Some key findings included…*

- **Alcohol-related cancers were highest in men** (about 77 percent of the cancers).
- **The most common cancers linked to alcohol use were esophageal, liver, and breast cancers.**
- **Although most cancers were found in risky or heavy drinkers,** one in seven cancers were linked to just one to two drinks per day.
- **The research team estimates that drinking one to two alcoholic drinks per day caused more than 100,000 cancers in 2020.**
- **About one in four breast cancers may be linked to alcohol use.**

The researchers expressed concern that the impact of alcohol on cancer risk is unknown or overlooked. In fact, current policy tells people that if they choose to drink alcohol, drink in moderation (one drink per day for women and two drinks per day for men), which implies a level of safety. In fact, say the researchers, all drinking involves risk. For women, each six-ounce glass of wine per day increases the risk of breast cancer by 6 percent.

How Alcohol Is Linked to Cancer

Alcohol is known to cause cancer by inhibiting DNA repair in cells and altering proteins and lipids. In the liver, alcohol turns into *acetaldehyde*, which is a cancer-producing substance (carcinogen). In mouth and throat cancers, alcohol acts as a solvent making it easier for carcinogens in tobacco to reach cells. That is why these cancers occur most in people who smoke and drink alcohol.

What's in a Drink?

In the United States, one alcoholic drink is any beverage containing 0.6 fluid ounces or 14 grams of pure alcohol, according to the National Institute on Alcohol Abuse and Alcoholism. That translates into 12 ounces of regular beer (at five percent alcohol), five ounces of wine (at about 12 percent alcohol) and 1.5 ounces of distilled spirits, which includes gin, rum, tequila, vodka, etc. (at about 40 percent alcohol). Note that alcohol content (or ABV, alcohol by volume) can range extensively— for example, some craft beers can contain as much as 12 percent alcohol and some dessert wines run as high as 20 percent.

WHO researchers conclude that public policy needs to catch up to the research. The cancer risk for alcohol is an addition to the known risks of alcohol addiction and liver failure (cirrhosis). The researchers suggest policy changes that include higher taxes on alcohol, bans on advertising and cancer warnings on alcohol labels.

For more on alcohol and alcohol abuse: Visit Rethinking Drinking online at RethinkingDrinking.niaaa.nih.gov.

New CAR T-Cell Therapy Triples Remission Rates for Refractory Multiple Myeloma

Larry D. Anderson Jr., MD, PhD, director of the myeloma, Waldenström's, and amyloidosis program, UT Southwestern Medical Center, Dallas, Texas.

The therapy, called *idecabtagene vicleucel* (ide-cel) or bb2121, engineers patients' T-cells to target a molecule called B-cell maturation antigen, which is found only in plasma cells and myeloma cells. Nearly three-quarters of the patients in the study had at least a partial response to the therapy, and one-third achieved complete remission. Most participants experienced low-level side effects. The U.S. Food and Drug Administration has granted the drug priority review status.

Cutting Down Chemotherapy Side Effects

Keith Block, MD, the medical and scientific director of the Block Center for Integrative Cancer Treatment in Skokie, Illinois, editor-in-chief of the medical journal *Integrative Cancer Therapies*, and author of *Life Over Cancer*. BlockMD.com

Chemotherapy saves countless lives, but it comes with a high cost of side effects, such as fatigue, nausea, diarrhea, mouth sores, nerve pain, increased susceptibility to infections, hair loss, mouth ulcers, brain fog, and muscle damage. The side effects can be so severe that about 30 percent of patients abandon the treatment prematurely.

Research links this type of incomplete treatment to significantly shorter survival times. In one study of more than 400 people with colon cancer, the patients who didn't complete the prescribed three rounds of che-

---

Appetite-Boosting Tips

- **Consider when your appetite is best**—which for many people is at breakfast—and try to get most of your nutrients and calories for the day then.
- **Exercising shortly before mealtime can also stimulate appetite.**
- **Pain and pain medications can interfere with appetite,** so schedule your meal or snack at least 30 minutes after you take the medication.
- **Rather than eat regular-size meals,** have a healthy snack every two to four hours.
- **If family members or friends offer to help cook, take them up on it**—nothing increases appetite like someone else doing the cooking.
- **Make every bite count** by choosing whole, nutrient-rich foods that provide plenty of calories and protein.
- **During meals,** limit the amount of liquid you drink, since drinking may make you feel full.
- **Herbal teas such as fennel or anise,** mixed with verbena or mint, may stimulate your appetite.

—Dr. Keith Block

---

motherapy were more than twice as likely to die during a 10-year follow-up.

The good news is that there are protocols that can reduce toxicity and side effects, improve quality of life, and allow patients to complete their chemotherapy treatment. An integrative oncologist who is open to a cancer protocol that uses both conventional treatments and natural therapeutics makes an excellent resource in this pursuit.

Couplers

Clinical trials show that several natural therapies can mitigate the toxicity of specific chemotherapy drugs.

The Antioxidant Controversy

Using antioxidant supplements such as co-enzyme Q10 or vitamin E during chemo has been controversial because of concerns that they might interfere with the oxidizing free radicals generated by chemotherapy drugs to kill cancer cells. But two major studies show that this controversy has no basis in science.

My colleagues and I conducted an exhaustive review of every randomized controlled trial in which antioxidants were administered during chemotherapy. Not a single study showed evidence of a decrease in efficacy from antioxidant supplementation during chemotherapy. In fact, many of the studies showed that antioxidant supplements increased tumor responses to chemo, reduced toxicity, and increased survival times. These findings were published in *Cancer Treatment Reviews*.

Bottom line: When implemented under the supervision of an experienced integrative cancer specialist, you can take carefully selected antioxidants during chemotherapy without concern that they are interfering with your treatment.

—Dr. Keith Block

•*Cisplatin* (**Platin**). Vitamin E appears to reduce the risk of nerve, kidney, and inner-ear damage that can come from taking this drug. One clinical trial found that taking 300 milligrams (mg) of vitamin E twice a day cut the risk of developing neurotoxic symptoms from 68 to 21 percent.

•*5-fluorouracil* (**5-FU**). Glutamine can reduce intestinal toxicity and diarrhea from 5-FU. *Common dosage:* 10 to 20 grams (g) daily, sipping, swishing and swallowing throughout the day. Sucking on ice chips for five minutes before, during, and after drug infusion can reduce intestinal toxicity and inflammation of mucous membranes inside the mouth and/or gut.

•*Paclitaxel* (**Taxol**). Alpha-lipoic acid (300 to 600 mg, once or twice daily) has been reported to minimize the neuropathy associated with paclitaxel. Glutamine (5 to 10 g) and vitamin B6 (50 mg twice daily) also may counter the weakness and numbness occurring from Taxol-induced peripheral neuropathy.

•*Doxorubicin* (**Adriamycin**). Coenzyme Q10 may help protect the heart against damage from this medication. *Common dosage:* 200 to 600 mg per day. An extract of the herb hawthorn (300 mg to 600 mg, twice daily) may also help protect the heart.

•*Oxaliplatin* (**Eloxatin**). Pre-treatment with intravenous calcium and magnesium may reduce the risk of neurotoxicity from oxaliplatin. Alpha-lipoic acid, glutamine, vitamin B6 and acetyl-L-carnitine may also help.

•*Silymarin.* An extract from milk thistle, given at a dose of 250 to 500 mg, two to three times daily, may help prevent liver damage from a large number of chemotherapies.

Controlling Side Effects

Several nutritional and herbal protocols can help control and reverse specific chemotherapy side effects.

•*Fatigue.* Try Siberian ginseng (Eleutherococcus senticosus), 2 to 4 g per day or rhodiola rosea, 300 mg per day. Engaging in 10 to 15 minutes of gentle aerobic exercise (such as walking or stationary bicycling) right before a session of chemotherapy can cut acute toxicity by 50 percent.

•*Nausea.* Try ginger as a tea or supplement (500 mg, every four hours).

Caution: You should not take ginger when your platelet count falls below 50,000 due to marrow suppression from chemotherapy, since it may have anticoagulant effects.

Aromatherapy with peppermint oil also may tame nausea: Carry a small bottle of peppermint oil with you throughout the day and sniff it occasionally.

•*Urinary symptoms.* Drink cranberry juice (blended with other natural juices instead of sugar to improve taste) or take concentrated cranberry tablets to prevent urinary tract infections.

• **Joint or muscle pain (myalgia).** Tart cherry juice concentrate may relieve muscle pain and improve sleep. Glutamine (10 to 20 g per day) may help with muscle pain due to treatment with paclitaxel.

• **Upper respiratory tract infections.** Chemotherapy patients may find that they are prone to colds because of a compromised immune system. Herbs that are commonly taken at the first sign of a cold include kan jang (*Andrographis paniculata*); echinacea or a combination of echinacea, wild indigo, and baptisia; *Pelargonium graveolens* (a South African herb called umcka); and *Sambucus nigra* (elderberry).

• **Congestion.** Soups containing garlic and hot pepper can help relieve congestion, and gargling with salt water helps relieve a sore throat.

Supportive Diet

To prepare your body for chemotherapy, base your diet on unrefined and minimally processed foods with plenty of plants (which are anti-inflammatory) and minimal amounts of meat and dairy products (which are pro-inflammatory).

• **Eat a rainbow of vegetables,** emphasizing brightly colored ones (pigments contain cancer-fighting phytochemicals), leafy greens, cruciferous vegetables (like broccoli, cauliflower, and kale), onions, and garlic.

• **Consume plenty of whole grains,** the richest source of complex carbohydrates and fiber, which provide a slow, sustained supply of fuel for your daily activities while reducing fuel for cancer.

• **Avoid cancer-promoting foods,** including excess dietary fat (particularly saturated fats in meat and dairy, and trans fats found in many processed foods), and refined carbohydrates.

• **Consume plenty of legumes (lentils, chickpeas, beans), soy foods, fish, and occasional omega-3 eggs.** These choices have cancer-fighting properties, contain many of the nutrients found in meat, and are an excellent source of complex carbohydrates and digestion-regulating soluble fiber.

• **To satisfy meat cravings,** try grilling, barbecuing, or baking salmon, halibut, tuna, or haddock steaks. Try tofu hot dogs, veggie burgers, vegetarian bacon, and vegetarian cold cuts.

• **To satisfy cravings for sweets,** eat fruit (no more than two to three servings per day, because the high amount of natural sugar can make you gain weight and cause your blood sugar to fluctuate). You can also use small amounts of unrefined, healthful sweeteners, such as monk fruit, rice syrup, barley malt, agave, kiwi sweetener, stevia, or maple syrup.

• **Every day, drink eight cups of water,** three to five cups of green tea, plus other fluids such as vegetable juices and herbal teas. Green tea is even better for rehydrating than water. It contains many antioxidants and anti-cancer phytochemicals.

Reduce Stress

When dealing with cancer, you need a way to calm yourself to curb and counteract the stress hormones coursing through your body, which contribute to cancer's ability to multiply and spread and are linked to poor outcomes. One excellent way to relax is to use relaxed abdominal breathing.

Another Reason to Give Up Sugary Soda

Yin Cao, ScD, MPH, associate professor of surgery at Washington University in St. Louis, Missouri, and senior author of a study of more than 95,000 women published in *Gut*.

Drinking two or more sweetened drinks per day more than doubles risk for early-onset colorectal cancer (EO-CRC). Each additional drink adds another 16 percent increase in risk.

Good news: Replacing sugary drinks with artificially sweetened beverages, coffee and especially milk was associated with up to 36 percent lower EO-CRC risk.

Cancer Is More Prevalent in Night Shift Workers

Washington State University

Researchers now suspect that disruption of the body's natural 24-hour rhythms throw off the timing of the expression of cancer-related genes in a way that reduces the effectiveness of the body's DNA repair processes when they are most needed.

CT Scan Is Best for Non-Invasive Colorectal Cancer Screening

Perry J. Pickhardt, MD, is professor of radiology at University of Wisconsin School of Medicine & Public Health, Madison, and leader of a study published in *American Journal of Roentgenology.*

In a comparison of stool DNA, fecal immunochemical test (FIT) and CT colonography (CTC, a type of X-ray), CTC proved best for finding polyps 10 mm or larger. (Smaller polyps are benign and need no immediate action.) Colonoscopy would be used if significant findings appear on the CTC, but using CTC first reduces unnecessary colonoscopies.

Bonus: CTC bowel preparation is simpler than typical colonoscopy preparation.

Dangerous Chemicals in Your Clothes and Furniture

Results of chemical tests run on 60 products by research company Toxic-Free Future, Seattle. ToxicFree Future.org

Stain- and water-resistant materials, such as used for rain jackets, hiking clothes, mattress pads, comforters, napkins and tablecloths, have been found to contain *perfluo-roalkyl and polyfluoroalkyl* (PFAS) chemicals. PFAS are sometimes called "forever chemicals" because they do not degrade. They are linked to heart and liver damage as well as cancer and hormone disruption.

Self-defense: Don't purchase items marked "stain-resistant" and "water-resistant"…and choose rainwear that repels water with fabrics made of tighter weave or coated with paraffin wax.

Immunotherapy Could Improve Survival in Pancreatic Cancer

Study titled "T Cell Inflammation in the Tumor Microenvironment After Agonist CD40 Antibody: Clinical and Translational Results of a Neoadjuvant Clinical Trial," by researchers at the Abramson Cancer Center, University of Pennsylvania, Philadelphia, presented at the American Association for Cancer Research 2021 annual meeting.

Even in its early stage, pancreatic cancer is difficult to treat. A new study from cancer researchers at the University of Pennsylvania's Abramson Cancer Center may have found a way to increase treatment response by jump-starting a patient's own immune system. This type of treatment is known as immunotherapy.

Immune system cells, called T cells, attack and destroy some cancer tumors, but pancreatic cancer can be stubbornly resistant. The researchers used a drug called *selicrelumab* to trigger T cells to be more active against pancreatic tumor cells. Selicrelumab works by activating tumor cells in a way that helps T cells find them and strengthens the immune system attack. This type of drug is called a *CD40 agonist.*

First Trial to Use CD40 Agonist in Early-Stage Pancreatic Cancer

In the study, presented at the American Association for Cancer Research annual meeting, researchers gave selicrelumab before surgery, changing the environment around the tumor from T cell "poor" to T cell "rich." In previous studies, a CD40 agonist was used to treat advanced pancreatic cancer along with other treatments. This was the first trial of this drug in early-stage pancreatic cancer.

Promising Results with Immunotherapy

Fifteen patients had surgery after taking selicrelumab. Imaging of the tumor cells in these patients were compared to patients who did not receive selicrelumab before surgery. Eighty-two percent of the selicrelumab patients had high levels of T cells in their surgically removed tumor cells compared to 37 percent of the patients not treated with selicrelumab. This was a phase 1b clinical trial, which is an early trial to see if larger trials are warranted.

The researchers were encouraged by their findings and hope this study is the first step in strengthening treatment for pancreatic cancer with immunotherapy. They are now looking forward to the next set of trials.

For more information: For support, resources, and services concerning pancreatic cancer, visit the Pancreatic Cancer Action Network online at PanCan.org or call 877-272-6226.

Researchers Have Developed Microrobots That Can Be Guided Directly to Cancer Cells

American Chemical Society

In the laboratory, investigators prompted the fish-shaped microrobots to open their mouths and release chemotherapy drugs directly at the cells. If the microrobots can be made small enough to travel through human blood vessels, they could help reduce the systemic side effects of chemotherapy.

Chapter 4

DIABETES BREAKTHROUGHS

Women with Diabetes Are at Higher Risk of Heart Disease

When it comes to cardiovascular health, men are usually the focal point since they develop heart disease sooner than women and are at higher risk for certain fatal conditions. Yet according to the American Heart Association (AHA), studies show that women with type 2 diabetes have twice the risk of heart disease as men with type 2 diabetes. They are also at higher risk for early heart attacks and fatal heart attacks than men. Type 2 diabetes increases the risk of coronary heart disease (CHD) by narrowing the arteries that supply the heart. Women may have a greater risk than men due to female hormones, higher cholesterol, and a higher proportion of body fat.

Higher Risk of CHD... But Less Care

A new study published in the American Medical Association (AMA) journal *JAMA Cardiology* shows how dangerous type 2 diabetes is for a woman's heart. This study reviewed data from over 28,000 women over more than 20 years. It found that women who developed type 2 diabetes before age 55 had more than 10 times the risk for CHD over the next 20 years compared to women without type 2 diabetes. Younger age was associated with the greatest risk. Women diagnosed with diabetes at age 75 had a more than three-fold higher risk of CHD. The women were part of a long-term Women's Health Study from 1993 through 2020.

Although diabetes was the highest risk factor for CHD in these women, other risk factors also played a role. These included high blood pressure, obesity, and smoking, all of which increased CHD risk at least four-fold. These studies point to the importance of reducing type 2 diabetes risk factors for women. Obviously, prevention is the best medicine when it comes to these diseases. Yet one study found that women at risk were less likely than men to use drugs and procedures to protect against high cholesterol and heart disease.

Study titled "Association of Lipid, Inflammatory, and Metabolic Biomarkers With Age at Onset for Incident Coronary Heart Disease in Women," by researchers at Brigham and Women's Hospital, Harvard Medical School, Boston, et al., published in *JAMA Cardiology*.

Diabetes Brings Women to the Same Age Risk as Men

Heart disease usually starts in men about 10 years earlier than women. Women with diabetes have CHD at similar ages as men. They tend to develop cardiovascular risks between the ages of 40 and 50. Women also have risk factors for diabetes that men don't experience, such as polycystic ovary disease and weight gain from pregnancy.

Takeaway: Both the AHA and AMA conclude that doctors need to be more aware of the dangers of CHD in women with diabetes. Women should work with their healthcare providers to control the risk factors. Risk factors such as gender and family history cannot be changed, but controllable lifestyle habits can. Controllable risk factors for both diabetes and CHD include quitting smoking; controlling blood sugar, cholesterol, and blood pressure; and adopting a consistent exercise regimen along with a heart-healthy diet.

For more information: For resources and support concerning heart disease conditions specific to women, visit WomenHeart.org.

Natural Ways to Help Prevent Diabetes

Jamison Starbuck, ND, a naturopathic physician in family practice in Missoula, Montana, and producer of *Dr. Starbuck's Health Tips for Kids*, a weekly program on Montana Public Radio, MTPR.org.

Many *patients fear diabetes for good reason:* Like heart disease and cancer, diabetes is a leading cause of death. It's often the underlying cause of cardiovascular problems like stroke and high blood pressure, too. The good news is that action, rather than fear, can make type 2 diabetes a preventable disease.

Insulin, secreted from the pancreas, is a substance that moves glucose (blood sugar) from the blood into the cells. Glucose is necessary for many essential bodily activities as well as organ, muscle, brain, and nervous system function. While people with type 1 diabetes are deficient in insulin, those with type 2 usually make plenty of insulin, but due to obesity, problems with fat metabolism, a poor-quality diet, and an overabundance of sweets or alcohol, their cells have become resistant to it. The cells become so full of sugar they cannot take in more. When the blood is unable to dump sugar into the cells, blood-sugar levels rise and create diabetes.

You can prevent and even reverse diabetes with a few basic strategies...

●**Diet.** In addition to avoiding sugar, choose a high-fiber diet as often as possible. Plant fiber, such as that found in vegetables, whole grains, and legumes, slows the absorption of glucose into the blood from the intestines, keeping levels steady and reducing the possibility of developing insulin resistance. Legumes, rich in protein and fiber, are particularly good at regulating blood sugar absorption. Include beans, lentils, split peas, and garbanzo beans in your daily menu as a great diabetes prevention tactic.

●**Stress management.** Stress increases glucose levels through adrenal gland function. This is useful when glucose gives us energy, but when stress is prolonged and unrelenting, adrenal and pancreatic function become dysregulated and blood sugar levels rise. Thus, stress management strategies such as meditation, yoga, therapy, and supportive friendships are all good diabetes prevention medicines.

●**Exercise** burns glucose, helps maintain a healthy body weight, lifts mood, and can lessen sugar cravings. Timing your exercise can help prevent diabetes, too. Recent studies with men at high risk for diabetes, indicate that vigorous exercise between 3 and 6 p.m. is more helpful in stabilizing blood sugar levels than the same exercise done in the morning. Though this study was limited to males, I think it's likely that women would see the same benefit. For many years, I've prescribed late-afternoon exercise as an effective treatment to reduce nighttime sweet cravings in both male and female patients.

• **Sugar-busting supplements.** If you have prediabetes or have a genetic risk for diabetes, talk with your doctor about chromium picolinate and the botanical medicine Gymnema (*Gymnema sylvestre*). Both of these over-the-counter supplements help with blood sugar control by slowing the absorption of glucose from the digestive tract into the bloodstream. Gymnema has been used in India to treat diabetes for more than 2,000 years. I've used it with patients for over two decades. I typically prescribe 200 to 500 micrograms of chromium and 200 to 600 milligrams of Gymnema daily, both taken with meals.

Diabetes During Pregnancy Is on the Rise

Study titled "Trends in Gestational Diabetes at First Live Birth by Race and Ethnicity in the US, 2011–2019," by researchers at Northwestern University Feinberg School of Medicine, Chicago, published in *JAMA*.

Pregnant women have to keep an eye out for a lot of things, including blood sugar, because being diagnosed with diabetes during pregnancy is both common and dangerous. Diabetes while pregnant is called gestational diabetes. Although the condition usually causes no symptoms and goes away after pregnancy, women with gestational diabetes are as much as 10 times more likely to develop long-term diabetes or prediabetes and twice as likely to develop cardiovascular disease. Children born to mothers with gestational diabetes are at higher risk for childhood obesity and earlier adult cardiovascular disease.

Asian, Hispanic Women at Highest Risk

A new study from researchers at Northwestern University Feinberg School of Medicine warns that gestational diabetes is on the rise, especially for certain ethnic groups. Their findings are published in the *Journal of the American Medical Association*. Using data from the National Center for Health Statistics, the research team looked at first births in 12.6 million women between 2011 and 2019. *Key findings included…*

• **Women's ages ranged from 15 to 44.**

• **The rate of gestational diabetes increased from 47.6 to 63.5 per 1,000 births.**

• **The rate of gestational diabetes increased by 3.7 percent each year.**

• **Gestational diabetes increased in all ethnic groups,** but Asian and Hispanic women were at the highest risk.

More Obesity, More Gestational Diabetes

The researchers say the increase in gestational diabetes goes hand-in-hand with increases in obesity, lack of exercise and poor diet in pregnant women. Other factors that increase the risk for gestational diabetes are previous gestational diabetes or prediabetes, polycystic ovary syndrome, a family history of diabetes and previously delivering a baby weighing more than nine pounds. Identifying and treating gestational diabetes early in pregnancy is important because untreated gestational diabetes can cause pregnancy complications such as high blood pressure, larger babies and a higher risk for C-section birth, pre-term birth and breathing problems for newborns.

When to Screen and How to Live

Currently, pregnant women are screened for gestational diabetes with blood testing at 24 to 28 weeks. The researchers support a recommendation by the American College of Obstetricians and Gynecologists to start screening earlier in women at higher risk, such as women of Asian or Hispanic descent. Controllable risk factors need to be addressed before pregnancy, which include maintaining a healthy weight, regular physical activity and a healthy diet.

Although there is no sure way to prevent gestational diabetes, women can reduce their risk with healthy lifestyle choices during pregnancy that include…

●**Eating foods that are high in fiber, lower in calories and low in fat**…such as fruits, vegetables and whole grains.

●**Exercising before and during pregnancy for about 30 minutes on most days of the week.**

●**Starting pregnancy at a healthy weight.**

●**Not gaining more weight than recommended during pregnancy.**

A New Treatment for Diabetic Heart Disease

Study titled "Diabetes Induces Dysregulation of MicroRNAs Associated with Survival, Proliferation and Self-renewal in Cardiac Progenitor Cells," by researchers at University of Otago, Dunedin, New Zealand, published in *Diabetologia*.

About 50 percent of people with diabetes die from heart disease. One reason for this large percentage is the progressive loss of "functional efficacy" in heart muscle stem cells known as cardiac progenitor cells. Cardiac progenitor cells are responsible for the survival, growth, and replacement of heart muscle cells.

Other than a heart transplant, the only treatment for the loss of these stem cells has been heart muscle stem cell transplant. Attempts at this kind of transplantation have had mixed results. The procedure is also time consuming and expensive.

How to Regenerate Heart Muscle Stem Cells

Researchers at the University of Otago in New Zealand have found one reason that heart stem cells fail in people with diabetes. Their discovery may lead to a new way to regenerate the stem cells and to treat diabetic heart disease. Their research is published in the journal *Diabetologia*.

Using heart stem cells from diabetic mice and from heart tissue removed during heart surgery in human patients, the researchers were able to show that diabetes causes changes in the way a type of RNA acts in heart cells. This change is called *dysregulation* and the type of RNA is called microRNA. Dysregulation of microRNA plays a role in several diseases because microRNA helps control DNA of cells, called *gene expression*.

Four types of microRNA were identified. One of the microRNA molecules, called miR-30c-5p seemed to be particularly important. The researchers were able to increase the levels of miR-30c-5p (called *overexpression*) by injecting it into the human and mice heart cells. This significantly improved the survival and growth of the cardiac progenitor stem cells. If further studies in the lab are successful, and can be confirmed in human trials, injecting microRNA could be a quicker, cheaper and more effective way to curb diabetic heart disease than trying to transplant stem cells. The next stage of research will be to evaluate the three other microRNA candidates.

Best Way to Stop Diabetic Heart Disease

MicroRNA may be a future treatment for diabetic heart disease, but it will not take the place of healthy lifestyle choices for people with diabetes. The best way to not die from diabetic heart disease is to prevent it. *According to the American Diabetes Association, these include…*

●**Exercise for at least 150 minutes per week.**

●**Don't sit for more than 30 minutes.** Get up and walk around.

●**Maintain a healthy weight.**

●**Take your medications.**

There's No One-Size-Fits-All Lifestyle Approach for Diabetes

Recent finding: Intensive lifestyle intervention (diet and exercise) benefited most subgroups—but among those with poor glycemic control at the study start, intensive lifestyle intervention was associated with 85 percent higher risk for cardiovascular events. Ask your doctor about the best approach, which may include glucose-lowering drugs to improve cardiovascular risk factors and modest exercise when feasible.

Michael Bancks, PhD, is assistant professor of epidemiology and prevention at Wake Forest School of Medicine, Winston-Salem, North Carolina, and leader of a 10-year study of 5,145 adults, published in *Diabetes Care*.

• Follow your diabetes meal plan.

• Pay attention to stress and your mental health.

• Work with your diabetes care team.

• Learn about diabetes in a diabetes education program.

• Track your diabetes numbers such as your A1C, blood sugar and cholesterol.

• Get six to eight hours of sleep every night.

Tight Blood Sugar Control Reduces the Risk of Stroke and Heart Attack in People with Diabetes

Jun Young Chang, MD, PhD, clinical assistant professor, department of neurology, University of Ulsan College of Medicine, Seoul, Korea.

Researchers tested the hemoglobin A1C levels of 18,567 people with diabetes who had been admitted to the hospital for ischemic stroke and followed them for one year. People with initial A1C levels above 7.0 percent had a 28 percent greater risk of having a second stroke and a 27 percent greater risk of having a cardiovascular event compared with people whose A1C levels were below 6.5 percent. The ideal A1C range, the researchers concluded, is 6.8 to 7.0 percent.

If You Have Diabetes... Lowering Blood Sugar Improves Brain Health

Study titled "Long-term Change in Physiological Markers and Cognition Performance in Type 2 Diabetes: The Look AHEAD Study," by researchers at Pennington Biomedical Research Center in Baton Rouge, Louisiana, published in *The Journal of Clinical Endocrinology & Metabolism*.

You probably know that people with type 2 diabetes are at higher risk for heart disease and stroke. What you might not realize is that type 2 diabetes also increases risk for cognitive decline. The ability to think clearly, learn, and remember important details can simply slip away. In fact, having type 2 diabetes doubles the risk of developing dementia, including Alzheimer's disease.

Some promising research: A recent study has shown that lowering blood sugar through exercise and diet may be the best way to reduce the risk of cognitive decline in people with type 2 diabetes. The study is published in *The Journal of Clinical Endocrinology & Metabolism*.

Although previous studies have found that lowering blood sugar, losing weight and increasing physical activity all reduce the risk of cognitive decline in individuals with type 2 diabetes, there's been no long-term research that offered a clear understanding of how improving lifestyle habits actually benefits the brain.

Recent study: To gain greater perspective, researchers evaluated data collected from a long-term diabetes trial called the Look AHEAD (Action for Health in Diabetes) study. The Look AHEAD study included people diagnosed with type 2 diabetes ages 45 through 76.

Participants in the trial were offered three yearly sessions of education in physical activity and diet for diabetes or a more intensive lifestyle intervention for diet and activity designed to promote weight loss of more than 7 percent of body weight and the ability to maintain a healthy weight over several years.

More than 1,000 of the participants went through a series of cognitive tests during a span of about eight to 12 years to see how much losing weight and lowering blood sugar affected cognition. The participants were about equally divided between the two intervention groups.

Key results of the study included...

• **Any lowering of blood sugar led to improved cognition in all the patients.**

• **Weight loss improved short-term memory but not verbal learning or overall memory.**

• **People who were more overweight (obese) at the beginning of the study had less improvement in cognition.**

• **People who were overweight but not obese benefited most from physical activity.**

Takeaway: The researchers concluded that lowering blood sugar in people with type 2 diabetes reduced the risk of cognitive decline. Although weight loss may also help, it is not as effective as lowering blood sugar. People who are already obese may have less success in reversing the risk of cognitive decline, so it's important to maintain a healthy body weight throughout your life.

Experimental Drug Slows Progression of Diabetic Kidney Disease

Study titled "Effect of Finerenone on Chronic Kidney Disease Outcomes in Type 2 Diabetes," by researchers at University of Chicago Medicine, published in *The New England Journal of Medicine.*

Long-term (chronic) kidney disease affects one in four people with type 2 diabetes and may lead to kidney failure, requiring dialysis or organ transplant.

Recent finding: In the largest-ever clinical trial for chronic kidney failure in people with type 2 diabetes, an experimental drug was able to delay the onset of kidney failure and also reduce cardiovascular disease events, such as heart attack and stroke.

The new drug is called *finerenone.* It works by blocking the effects of a steroid hormone called a mineralocorticoid, which is generated by the body. Mineralocorticoids can cause inflammation and scarring in the kidneys and the heart. This was a Phase III study that may lead to approval of finerenone by the Food and Drug Administration. Other trials are currently being conducted to find out if finerenone can successfully treat heart disease.

Study details: Researchers led by University of Chicago Medicine studied finerenone in approximately 6,000 patients with type 2 diabetes and kidney disease, which was at a stage just short of kidney failure. The study, conducted at more than 1,000 sites in 48 countries, was sponsored by Bayer, the company that manufactures the new drug. The results of the study are published in *The New England Journal of Medicine* and were also presented at a meeting of the American Society of Nephology.

Patients were equally assigned to receive the new drug or a placebo. The primary goal (or endpoint) of the study was to find out if finerenone could reduce progression to chronic kidney disease by 40 percent. A secondary endpoint was to see if the drug could reduce cardiovascular events, including deaths, heart attack, stroke and hospital admission for heart failure. The treatment group had significantly less progression to kidney failure and significantly lower cardiovascular events than the placebo group. Bayer announced that the study's endpoints had been met.

According to the researchers, over a period of two to three years, patients taking finerenone reduced progression of kidney disease by 18 percent compared with standard care. The drug was considered safe. The only significant side effect was an elevation in blood potassium, which occurred in less than 3 percent of the patients.

Takeaway: The research team concluded that finerenone is a promising new treatment for patients with kidney disease resulting from type 2 diabetes and may delay the need for dialysis or a kidney transplant.

The Surprising Causes of Peripheral Neuropathy

Mary Vo, MD, an assistant professor of neurology and assistant attending neurologist at New York Presbyterian/Weill Cornell Medical College. Dr. Vo researches a form of peripheral neuropathy called chronic inflammatory demyelinating neuropathy at Weill Cornell Medicine's Peripheral Neuropathy Center and specializes in caring for patients with peripheral neuropathy, nerve injury, back and neck pain, muscle weakness, radiculopathy, and headache.

Diabetes isn't the only disease that can damage the nerves that lead to the hands and feet.

The pain arrives mainly at night: burning, tingling, or electric-shock stabbing that stymies sleep. Just covering your feet with a blanket can feel unbearable. If you get up in the dark, you may find yourself tripping or bumping into things, not because you can't see, but because you can't fully feel your feet. Creeping slowly from your toes upward over months or years, this pain and numbness, which can also affect your hands and arms, is perplexing and alarming.

The likely culprit? Peripheral neuropathy, which is damage to the peripheral nerves that reach throughout your body. While diabetes is the leading cause of this condition, peripheral neuropathy is surprising in both its origins and scope, with an extensive list of possible causes (see sidebar below).

The Many Causes of Peripheral Neuropathy

Peripheral neuropathy can be the result of an astonishing array of causes...

- **Diabetes,** usually because of poorly controlled blood sugar
- **Alcohol abuse**
- **Medications,** particularly chemotherapies
- **Thyroid disorders**
- **Degenerative disc disease and spinal stenosis**
- **Autoimmune conditions,** such as Sjogren's syndrome, lupus, and rheumatoid arthritis
- **Poisons,** including industrial chemicals and heavy metals such as lead or mercury
- **Infections,** including Lyme disease, shingles, Epstein-Barr virus, hepatitis, and HIV
- **Genetics**
- **Tumors**
- **Injury or surgery**
- **Vitamin deficiency or toxicity.** Pay close attention to the B vitamins, including B1, B6 and B12, but don't indiscriminately take supplements. Taking too much over months or years can build toxicity that leads to or worsens neuropathy. Ask your doctor how you can achieve the right balance.

The Root of the Problem

Peripheral nerves, which carry messages to and from the brain, contain large fibers that are covered with a type of fatty insulation and small, skinny, uninsulated fibers. The small fibers report sensory information such as pain, heat, or cold, while also controlling involuntary vital functions, such as heart rate and blood pressure. The most common form of peripheral neuropathy strikes the longest nerves in the body, those leading to the skin of the hands and feet, where it can cause pain or numbness. *Small-fiber nerve damage can also trigger problems in other parts of the body…*

• **Low blood pressure** can lead to symptoms that include fainting, dizziness, or lingering fatigue.

• **Bloating, nausea, indigestion, constipation, or diarrhea** are often misdiagnosed as irritable bowel syndrome.

• **Incontinence or sexual problems,** while rare, are unquestionably distressing when they occur.

• **Heat intolerance may lead to excessive sweating,** or sufferers may lose the ability to sweat.

Finding Answers

As with many conditions, early diagnosis and treatment offer the best chance for effective symptom and damage control. But by the time many people with peripheral neuropathy seek a diagnosis, doctors find that the condition is actually worse than a patient's symptoms may suggest, so don't delay. Even if your symptoms seem vague, see your primary care doctor as soon as possible.

Your physician will review your medications and supplements, screen you for diabetes, thyroid issues and vitamin levels, and may perform a variety of tests to pinpoint peripheral neuropathy and its causes. These may include nerve conduction and electromyography to measure large-fiber damage, a skin biopsy to count small-nerve fiber endings in the skin, or a sweat test to gauge the body's ability to regulate temperature.

Tailoring Treatment

If your doctor can pinpoint the cause of your neuropathy, your treatment options can be tailored to address the underlying issue. For example, patients with autoimmune disease will be referred to a rheumatologist, who may

---

Common Blood Pressure Drugs Are Linked to Diabetes

Lowering blood pressure is important for avoiding type 2 diabetes. Angiotensin-converting enzyme (ACE) inhibitors and angiotensin II receptor blockers (ARBs) lower diabetes risk, but diuretics and beta-blockers raise it. Individual risk for diabetes should be considered when prescribing a particular hypertension medication.

Barry R. Davis, MD, PhD, professor emeritus of biostatistics and data science at UTHealth School of Public Health in Houston and coauthor of a meta-analysis of 146,000 patients, published in *The Lancet.*

---

prescribe immune-modifying treatments that can actually reverse nerve damage and symptoms. Diabetes patients should work with an endocrinologist to improve blood sugar control and monitor medications.

Recovery can be more challenging when peripheral neuropathy has no traceable cause, which is true in up to half of all cases. Even then, a variety of approaches can provide meaningful relief, though full nerve repair is typically elusive.

• **Medication.** Over-the-counter pain medications, such as nonsteroidal anti-inflammatory drugs, can relieve mild symptoms, as can topical treatments such as capsaicin cream.

When these aren't sufficient, there are several types of drugs to try. Some patients find relief with anti-epilepsy drugs like *gabapentin* (Gralise, Neurontin, Horizant) and *pregabalin* (Lyrica) or antidepressants such as *duloxetine* (Cymbalta) and *venlafaxine* (Effexor XR). The antidepressants *amitriptyline* (Elavil), *doxepin* (Silenor, Zonalon) and *nortriptyline* (Pamelor) may also help.

• **Physical and occupational therapy** can help you cope with limitations in how you walk or use your hands.

Lifestyle Factors

Some simple lifestyle changes can also improve your symptoms…

- **Exercise regularly to improve blood flow to nerves.**
- **If you have diabetes, limit your sugar intake.**
- **Vitamin B12 protects nerves and may even enhance nerve regeneration.** Ensure that you get enough by eating foods like dairy, lean meat, poultry, and eggs. If you are vegetarian or vegan, talk to your doctor about taking a supplement.
- **Avoid eating fish that are high in mercury, a toxin that can worsen neuropathy.** The worst offenders are king mackerel, orange roughy, swordfish, tuna, and grouper.
- **Limit alcohol,** which is toxic to nerves and can make neuropathy symptoms worse.
- **Don't smoke.** Smoking narrows and damages peripheral blood vessels.
- **Review your medications regularly with your primary care doctor.** A variety of medications can cause reversible peripheral neuropathy—even long after you've been taking them with no problems.

Recent Study Nixes Dairy for Blood Sugar Control

Study titled "The Impact of Diets Rich in Low-Fat or Full-Fat Dairy on Glucose Tolerance and Its Determinants: A Randomized Controlled Trial," by researchers at Fred Hutchinson Cancer Research Center, Seattle, published in *The American Journal of Clinical Nutrition*.

For some time, research has suggested that eating yogurt and other dairy foods, such as milk and cheese, may reduce the risk of developing type 2 diabetes. However, this finding has been based on observational studies that may include inaccurate information from questionnaires completed by study subjects.

To get to the bottom of the hypothesis that dairy foods improve blood sugar regulation (glucose tolerance), researchers at Fred Hutchinson Cancer Research Center conducted a controlled trial of patients with metabolic syndrome, a combination of conditions that increases risk for diabetes, heart disease and stroke. The conditions include belly fat, high blood pressure, high blood sugar and/or high cholesterol.

The researchers included 72 people with metabolic syndrome in their study and divided them into three groups: Group 1 had no dairy foods other than three servings, at most, of skim milk per week; Group 2 had a low-fat diet with more than three servings of low-fat dairy per day; and Group 3 had a full-fat diet with more than three servings of whole milk and other full-fat dairy per day.

Study results: After 12 weeks, the participants were evaluated for glucose tolerance and weight gain or loss. Contrary to the observational research, dairy foods did not improve glucose tolerance in any group. In fact, in groups two and three, there was a decrease in insulin sensitivity, which refers to how the body's cells respond to insulin, and participants in the high-fat group gained an average of two pounds.

Although there was no effect on blood sugar in any of the groups, the decrease in insulin sensitivity is significant because this is a risk factor for type 2 diabetes. The study was published in *The American Journal of Clinical Nutrition*.

Conclusion: The researchers found that dairy foods do not improve glucose tolerance in people with metabolic syndrome. In fact, the study determined that more low-fat or high-fat dairy foods in the diet decreased insulin sensitivity, which may increase the risk of diabetes in people with metabolic syndrome.

A Diabetes Drug Boosts Weight Loss

Rachel Batterham, MD, head of the Centre for Obesity Research, Department of Medicine, University College London.

Adding 2.4 milligrams of weekly *semaglutide* (Ozempic, Rybelsus) to healthy lifestyle changes helped obese adults lose almost 15 percent of their body weight over 68 months, researchers discovered in a double-blind trial. Participants in the placebo group lost just 2.4 percent of their starting weight in the same timeframe. About 74 percent of people taking semaglutide reported at least one gastrointestinal side effect, such as nausea, diarrhea, vomiting, or constipation.

Get Up and Move to Reduce Risk of Chronic Disease

Study titled "Effects of reduced sedentary time on cardiometabolic health in adults with metabolic syndrome: A three-month randomized controlled trial," by researchers at Turku PET Centre, University of Turku and Turku University Hospital, Finland, published in *Journal of Science and Medicine in Sport*.

Many of us engage in a dangerous daily activity of sitting eight to nine hours, which increases risk for chronic diseases such as diabetes and heart disease. Experts advise at least 150 minutes of moderate to intense physical activity every week to remedy these risks. For many people who are overweight and physically inactive, this level of activity is difficult to start and even harder to maintain.

That's the bad news. The good news is that it may take less than 150 minutes intense exercise a week to make a big difference in your health.

Sitting Makes Us Sick

A new study from researchers at the University of Turku in Finland suggests that even a modest goal of sitting less can have health benefits. Their clinical trial included 64 middle-age sedentary individuals who were at risk for cardiometabolic disease. People in the trial were randomly selected to continue their usual activity level or to reduce their sitting time by one hour each day over a period of three months. The results of the study are published in the *Journal of Science and Medicine in Sport*.

People who qualified for the trial had metabolic syndrome and were physically inactive. They were not diagnosed specifically with heart disease or diabetes. Metabolic syndrome is a group of risk factors that include abdominal obesity, elevated fasting blood sugar, high triglycerides, low good cholesterol, and high blood pressure. Having three or more of these risk factors is what defines metabolic syndrome.

Before the trial started, all the participants had their physical activity and sitting times recorded for one month. They had body measurements and fat measured, blood pressure checked, and blood testing to measure liver health, insulin, and blood sugar. To measure how much sitting, standing, and exercise occurred during the day, the researchers had all the participants wear a movement-measuring device every day.

After three months, all the tests done before the trial were repeated. The group assigned to one hour less of sitting achieved an average of a 50-minute reduction in sedentary time. Most of their active time was used for mild to moderate physical activities instead of just standing. This group had significant improvement in insulin levels, blood sugar, triglycerides, liver health, and resting heart rate. There were no changes in the activity-as-usual group.

Just Sit Less

Based on the results of this trial, the research group concludes that replacing 50 minutes of daily sedentary time with low to moderate physical activity over three months reduces cardiometabolic risk. The next step for the research team is to study the effects of reducing sedentary time over six months on heart and diabetes risk as well as energy production and body composition.

Chapter 5

EMOTIONAL RESCUE

5 Surprising Causes of Hidden Stress...

We've all had nights when we collapse into bed after a stressful day of juggling work, family, caretaking and more. But even on days when we don't overtly feel "stressed," it's often there—impacting our health in hidden ways.

The way we treat our bodies—from how we move and eat...to the people, objects and energy surrounding us—has a direct impact on our stress response whether or not we realize it, promoting inflammation, accelerating aging, and hindering the body's anti-stress efforts.

If we know where stress hides in our lives, then we can combat it. *Headaches and digestive issues are common, but here are five hidden sources of stress—and how to overcome them...*

HIDDEN STRESSOR #1: **Poor foot biomechanics.** Feet are true taskmasters, keeping us moving while bearing the brunt of our weight. Poor foot biomechanics—the way the toes and feet function as they interact with our muscles and gravity—can reach up the body, making it hard for the other muscles and joints to work properly and leading to hip and back pain, poor balance and more. When feet are under stress, the whole body feels stress!

Ill-fitting shoes are a cause of stress in your feet, as are hard- or thick-soled shoes that prevent feet from receiving the stimulation they need—stimulation that forces them to work and keeps them strong and supple.

The fix: Walk barefoot. Feet are built to walk on varied terrain and need the stimulation that comes from that. Walking barefoot engages the bones, joints and dozens of muscles that work together to keep communications flowing through your body and improve your balance and feeling of stability.

Even better: Walk barefoot outside. The subtle negative electromagnetic charge from grass, moist soil and sand helps balance the positive electromagnetic charge that builds up in the body from the stress of daily living.

Also: Stimulate and massage bare feet by rolling them over a tennis ball for five min-

Integrative and functional medicine pioneer Frank Lipman, MD, founder of Eleven Eleven Wellness Center and chief medical officer at The Well, both in New York City. He is author of more than six books including, most recently, *The New Rules of Aging Well: A Simple Program for Immune Resilience, Strength, and Vitality* and *Better Sleep, Better You.* DrFrankLipman.com

utes a day. Strong, flexible feet translate into a strong, flexible body.

HIDDEN STRESSOR #2: Nighttime eating. We all know that eating at night is not good for digestion and metabolism. But research shows that late eating puts stress on the brain and the body, both of which interpret the incoming calories as *Food is coming in...time to start producing energizing hormones.* That, in turn, interferes with sleep.

The fix: Stop eating by 8 p.m. This will help lead your body toward restful sleep. If you crave the nightly ritual of snacking on the couch, try replacing food with a cup of herbal or decaffeinated tea. You may discover that the routine itself is what is enjoyable, not the food. And with less food in your belly, your sleep will improve.

Up for a challenge? Once or twice a week, try a 16-hour overnight fast. Finish dinner by 7 p.m. or 8 p.m. When you wake up the next morning, drink a large glass of water—this is always a healthy practice, even when you are not fasting. Don't eat your first meal before 11 a.m. or noon. Fasting for 16 hours kicks off a detoxification process called *autophagy* during which stress-induced cellular debris is cleared away. Does 16 hours feel too daunting? Begin with 14 or 12 hours.

HIDDEN STRESSOR #3: Clutter. In a study in *Personality and Social Psychology Bulletin,* women who described their homes as "cluttered" or "disorganized" (as opposed to "peaceful" or "comforting") experienced cortisol levels that indicated chronic stress. Our brains like structure and order. Piles of paper and overflowing closets can hinder concentration and are linked with procrastination, both of which further contribute to stress.

The fix: Purge, hide, and donate. Toss or donate unused clothing. Use decorative baskets and bins to store unfolded laundry, magazines, and other household items. Consider hiring a professional organizer to guide you through the process.

If you have time to tackle only one area: Focus on your bedside table. It often becomes cluttered with books, tissues, beauty products, and more. Seeing a big mess right before you go to sleep can cause your stress hormones to spike...precisely when you don't want them elevated.

HIDDEN STRESSOR #4: Out-of-whack light and dark cycles. Humans run on an internal 24-hour body clock that naturally syncs with the sun and moon. Morning light signals the brain to stop producing sleep-inducing melatonin and increase levels of energizing hormones. As darkness falls, melatonin production ramps up in preparation for sleep.

But modern life makes it easy to ignore these light and dark signals. Smartphone, tablet, and TV screens emit a blue light that is similar to the color and wavelength of daylight. Looking at these screens at night tells the brain to stay awake.

The fallout: Poor sleep, which is linked with a laundry list of bodily stressors—mood fluctuations...immune system suppression...system-wide inflammation...and impairment of the body's glymphatic system, which cleanses and clears the brain of toxins created throughout the day while you sleep. When these toxins accumulate, they can lead to cognitive decline and even Alzheimer's disease.

Important: Inadequate sleep also causes widespread stress and inflammation that shortens telomeres, the caps at the end of chromosomes that protect DNA. As telomere length shrinks, so does life span.

Recent finding: When researchers examined telomere changes in 239 postmenopausal women over a year-long period, they found that telomere shortening could be predicted by the number of stressful events the women experienced...except among women who engaged in higher levels of protective health behaviors such as getting quality sleep.

The fix: Expose yourself to bright light in the morning. Help reset your body clock by throwing open the curtains as soon as you wake up. Even better, step outside. As your eyes adjust to daylight, your hormones will program your internal clock to help energize you all day.

Quick Ways to Boost Your Mood

Compliment someone every day—find something sincere and positive to say to your partner, a friend, or a random stranger. *Look through old photos* to bring back positive memories from the past. *Write to someone you care about* to say what you like or admire about the person. *Play daily,* even in a small way, such as running, jumping, dancing, or doing crafts. *Practice gratitude* by writing down something you are grateful for every day. *Pause while doing an everyday activity*—notice a flower among weeds or make some other small observation to help ground yourself in the moment. *Engage your senses* by thinking about how specific things affect you—the smell and taste of a favorite meal, the sound of a child's laughter, the warmth of the sun. *Get some houseplants* and enjoy the way your care helps them flourish.

Roundup of experts on mood-boosting ideas, reported at BHG.com.

At night, power off screens by 10 p.m. and dedicate at least 30 minutes to a relaxing transition activity—take a warm bath, read a book, etc.

***HIDDEN STRESSOR #5:* Stressful texts and e-mails.** Junk e-mail…unnecessary texts…robocalls—we've come to accept these intrusions as normal parts of modern life. But anything that makes you feel annoyed, angry, or harassed triggers the same fight-or-flight hormonal stress response designed to propel you out of dangerous situations. The stress-inducing 24-hour news cycle is similarly toxic—levels of the stress hormone *cortisol* rise with every frightening or depressing story you hear or read. Following the 2016 election, a psychologist coined the term "Headline Stress Disorder" to describe this media-induced stress and anxiety.

Surprising: Even happy texts can create stress if announced with a *Ding!* on your phone—it diverts your attention and creates a sense of anxious anticipation that won't dissipate until you check the text.

The fix: Unsubscribe! Turn off your phone's notifications so that you don't hear that ding every time a message arrives. When you receive unwanted e-mails from companies and websites you've shopped at, scroll to the bottom and click "Unsubscribe." Reduce robocalls by enrolling in the Federal Trade Commission's National Do Not Call Registry at DoNotCall.gov. And limit your time reading or watching upsetting news… or at least try to balance things by purposefully seeking out feel-good news at sites such as GreaterGood.Berkeley.edu.

Head Games That Sabotage Your Health

Luana Colloca, MD, PhD, MS, MPower professor in the Pain and Translational Symptom Science Department at University of Maryland School of Nursing in Baltimore, physician-neuroscientist and a self-described "placebologist." Dr. Colloca is an international expert on placebos and nocebos. Nursing.UMaryland.edu

You swear the reason your headache won't go away is because you bought the generic pain reliever instead of the name brand…your spouse stops taking his newly prescribed statin because he is experiencing muscle pain, just as his pharmacist warned might happen…you receive a call from a member of your book club letting you know that she tested positive for COVID-19, and suddenly you notice you have a sore throat. If you can relate to any of these scenarios, you have experienced the power of the "nocebo effect," the opposite of the placebo effect.

Nocebos Defined

A nocebo is anything—a pill…a story in the news…a doctor's words…a list of side effects on a bottle of medication—that triggers medical side effects or adverse events. Unlike a placebo, which stimulates a positive response in a patient despite containing no active ingredients, a nocebo tricks you into thinking that you're ill when you're perfectly fine...or in more pain than you actually are...and it can slow recovery. ("Placebo" means "I shall please," and "nocebo" means "I shall harm" in Latin.) The nocebo effect is the direct result of personal expectations, past experiences and/or verbal suggestions. Both placebos and nocebos are rooted in the power of suggestion and brain chemicals being released, but only one is a threat to your well-being.

Nocebos are powerful and have been proven to exist in multiple studies exploring the mind-body connection in pain, chronic fatigue, depression and more. Consider a study published in *Journal of the American College of Cardiology* in which participants were assigned to take either *atorvastatin* (Lipitor), a placebo pill or no pill at all for one month at a time over a period of 12 months. During the months when participants were given pills, they did not know whether they were taking the drug or a placebo. They were asked to rate the severity of any negative effects on a scale of 0 to 100. Keep in mind that statin side effects often are mentioned in the media and discussed by doctors when prescribing, so most of the participants had heard statins could cause unpleasant symptoms.

Telling results: During the months when the participants did not take a pill, they reported an average score of 8/100. In months when they took a statin, 16.3/100 and 15.4 in the placebo months. The study authors determined that 90 percent of symptoms experienced by participants taking atorvastatin were also felt by those taking the placebo and thus could be blamed on the nocebo effect.

How Nocebos Work

The nocebo effect engages a complex set of mechanisms in the nervous system that can amplify how people perceive touch, pain, pressure, temperature and more.

Example: We know that when someone expects pain to occur, even nonpainful stimulations are perceived as painful and minimally painful stimulations as highly painful. At the molecular level, the body is releasing hormones called *cholecystokinins* that facilitate pain transmission, an evolutionary adaptation that primes the body to respond to a dangerous situation.

We also know from neuroimaging studies that certain parts of the brain become activated in anticipation of pain and other negative stimuli—enough so that they can override the effects of even the strongest pain medications.

Recent study: Patients who received morphine after a surgery felt relief. But when they were told that their morphine had been stopped, they reported an increase in pain—even if the medicine hadn't actually been stopped. (This phenomenon is called *nocebo hyperalgesia.*) On the flipside, when painkillers were stopped without notifying the patient, there were few complaints.

A third mechanism involves the autonomic nervous system (ANS), the branch of the nervous system that controls bodily functions that are not under conscious control, such as heartbeat, breathing, digestion, and more. The nocebo effect may be a result of the ANS responding to negative expectations, fear, or anxiety. This could explain how a 26-year-old showed up in the emergency room appearing drowsy and pale with dangerously low blood pressure and an elevated heart rate, saying, "Help me, I took all my pills," before collapsing...and yet lived to tell the tale. He had been enrolled in a clinical trial for depression and had a change of heart after attempting suicide by swallowing 29 capsules of what he believed to be antidepressants. ER staff began treating him for an overdose, but his symptoms wouldn't improve. A physician from the trial was contacted and revealed that the patient had been in the placebo group—the pills were inert. Within 15 minutes of being told this, the patient's blood pressure and heart rate returned to normal. The nocebo effect had caused his frightening symptoms.

Who Is Most at Risk?

Anyone can experience the nocebo effect, but people with a history of anxiety, depression or other psychiatric disorders are more prone, as are patients with negative expectations of or negative prior experiences with a treatment. Even though the nocebo effect might seem similar to hypochondriasis, the latter is an anxiety disorder. You don't need to have a mental health condition to be susceptible to nocebos. Women may be more sensitive to nocebos, but there are conflicting findings. (That said, women are more responsive to placebos compared with men.) Pessimists and people with type-A personalities also may be more nocebo-prone.

Living through a health outbreak, such as H1N1 influenza, Ebola, or COVID-19, heightens anxiety and can intensify the nocebo effect. Many people who have developed a headache, sore throat and more over the last two years convinced themselves that they were infected with COVID-19, thanks to the nocebo effect.

COVID-19 and nocebos: Researchers followed 74 people during the stay-at-home orders in Baltimore between May and June of 2020. Among the 72 participants not diagnosed with COVID during that time, 70 percent reported symptoms associated with the virus.

Moreover, a preregistered prospective longitudinal study conducted with a U.S. national sample of 551 individuals indicated that post-vaccine side effects are predicted by prevaccine expectations of side effects, worry about COVID-19, and depressive symptoms.

Outsmart the Nocebo Effect

Nocebos can thwart treatments and contribute to illness.

Examples: Many people who start taking cholesterol-lowering statin drugs discontinue them due to side effects. Widespread

discontinuation has led to an increase in fatal heart attacks and strokes. But how many of those side effects are just nocebos causing needless consequences? How many COVID tests will be run over the next few years, straining the health-care system, due to the nocebo effect?

Reading this article is the first step in breaking the pattern. Simply knowing that your brain can create new or worsening symptoms through the process of anticipation can help blunt the nocebo effect. *Other steps…*

•**Ask your doctor for help.** Health-care providers have the challenging job of striking a balance between being honest with patients about potential treatment side effects…but not being so open about every possible side effect under the sun that they spark anxiety.

Self-defense: If you tend to be anxious, ask your doctor to tell you only about the most common side effects…or request that he/she focus on how well-tolerated your treatment tends to be. Also, don't read the long list of possible side effects attached to your new medication if you tend toward anxiety. Many are relatively rare but can trigger a nocebo effect nonetheless.

•**Avoid negative stories and blogs.** Reading about another patient's negative experience with a treatment can act as a nocebo—simply knowing that she developed pain or nausea from a certain drug can contribute to an increase in your own pain or nausea. This may have to do with the fact that the areas of the brain involved in feeling empathy for others also are responsible for the way we interpret pain.

Self-defense: If you're starting a new drug and want reassurance from other people but know you are susceptible to the nocebo effect, Google strategically—search "chemotherapy + breast cancer + success story," not "chemotherapy + breast cancer + vomiting."

•**Try not to get caught up with labels and prices.** Consumers often think expensive and name-brand medications work better than cheaper or generic ones. In a study in *Neurology*, patients with Parkinson's disease (PD) were given one of two placebo injections and were told that it was a dopamine-agonist medication used to treat PD. One of the placebos was described as expensive…the other as cheap. Four hours later, those who received the "cheap" version then received the "expensive" version, and vice versa. Both placebos improved patients' motor function, but the benefit was larger among those who received the "pricier" drug first.

Self-defense: Don't fear that the price or brand name of your medication will make it less effective. If your doctor prescribes a generic drug, rest assured that it is pharmaceutically equal to its name-brand counterpart.

Stop Medicating "Normal"

Allen Frances, MD, professor emeritus and former chair of the department of psychiatry and behavioral science at Duke University School of Medicine, Durham, North Carolina. He chaired the DSM-IV Task Force. He is one of the experts featured in the documentary *Medicating Normal* and author of *Saving Normal* and *Essentials of Psychiatric Diagnosis.*

As a former practicing psychiatrist, Allen Frances, MD, is very concerned about how millions of people who are facing the unavoidable problems of everyday life and really are just the "worried well" are being overdiagnosed with psychiatric disorders and receiving unnecessary pharmaceutical treatment. Since the early 1980s, the number of Americans who meet the criteria for a mental disorder and who are being prescribed psychiatric drugs for depression, anxiety, sleep disorders and attention-deficit hyperactivity disorder (ADHD), among other conditions, has increased dramatically. So, too, are the diagnoses of autism and bipolar disorder in children. Some of these cases represent previously missed instances of mental illness, but more accurate diagnosis can't explain why so many people, especially children, suddenly seem to be mentally ill.

The Medicalization of Ordinary Life

Overtesting, overdiagnosing and overtreating are the hallmarks of our current health-care system, thanks to external forces that have put profit and expediency over appropriate care when it comes to mental and emotional issues.

One of the biggest drivers of this phenomenon is the *Diagnostic and Statistical Manual of Mental Disorders (DSM-5)*, published by the American Psychiatric Association. The current edition, updated in 2022, of the "psychiatric bible" converted millions of people into mental patients by arbitrarily broadening the definitions of existing disorders and adding new psychiatric illnesses.

Examples: Everyday overeating has become "binge-eating disorder." Normal concerns about physical symptoms now are considered to be "somatic symptom disorder." Normal grief now is easily mislabeled as "major depressive disorder."

Example: Sarah's 33-year-old son committed suicide, and she was inconsolable. She couldn't sleep or eat, cried all the time and was unable to focus or work. After two weeks, a friend suggested that she go to her primary care doctor, who diagnosed her as clinically depressed and put her on an antidepressant. Sarah took the medication for two weeks, but her symptoms grew so bad that she considered killing herself so she could join her son. Her doctor told her, incorrectly, that suicidal thoughts couldn't be a side effect of the drug. She decided to stop taking it and began attending counseling and grief group meetings and gradually improved. Two years later, she says she can experience joy and laughter again though she continues to live with her grief.

Another driver is the pharmaceutical industry, which earns billions of dollars by selling psychiatric drugs. Psychotropic drugs are among the top sellers for many drug companies. Pharmaceutical companies also are major supporters of continuing medical education today, which is more focused on prescription pads than healthy lifestyle and psychotherapy.

A third reason is the fact that there are no laboratory tests that can definitively say a person has a psychiatric illness. A diagnosis is made based on what a psychiatrist can glean from spending time with the patient during office visits and hearing about her symptoms, stressors, past history, family history, and supports. The diagnosis is subjective and sometimes differs widely from one psychiatrist to another.

What Is Normal?

Severe, classic mental disorders such as schizophrenia and major depression are unmistakable and can be reliably diagnosed. But mild cases are on a continuum with the normal ups and downs, stresses, disappointments, sorrows, and setbacks of living a typical life.

Examples: Temper tantrums can suggest bipolar disorder or, more simply, difficulty managing anger. Irritable, distancing behavior from veterans returning from tours of duty can indicate post-traumatic stress disorder or just a normal period of adjustment back to civilian life. Your grandson's precocious, obsessive interest in video games and science fiction can suggest autism or just the interests of a normal young man in today's world.

Consumer Self-Defense

Unfortunately, most psychiatric diagnoses and treatments now are handled by rushed primary care doctors, often after 10-minute visits with patients they don't know very well. General practitioners prescribe 90 percent of *benzodiazepines* (calming agents such as Valium, Xanax and Ativan)...80 percent of antidepressants...65 percent of ADHD drugs...and 50 percent of antipsychotics—even though primary care doctors

have little training in psychiatry or the medications they are prescribing. Writing a prescription is the fastest way to get the patient out of the office. On the flip side, patients have an inbred belief in the wisdom of doctors and have been trained through the last 50 years that taking a pill fixes things.

End result: The patient obediently follows the doctor's advice, and both the doctor and the patient feel satisfied that something has been done—whether or not the problem is accurately diagnosed and properly treated.

To protect yourself from being diagnosed with a psychiatric disorder when you don't have one...

•**Observe your symptoms for a few weeks.** Watchful waiting and several visits with your primary care doctor are the best first step for many people with mild issues. Symptoms often go away on their own with the passage of a few weeks, and what's often needed most is reassurance from a doctor that these feelings are normal—plus advice on how to cope and reduce stress without medication. Often, new symptoms result from increased life stress that is likely to be transient and better managed by problem-solving than pills. Psychotherapy also is often helpful. Be sure to rule out the possibility that symptoms may be due to a medication side effect or withdrawal...drug or alcohol use...or a medical illness.

Important: If your symptoms are severe, chronic, or worsening or if you fear that you might hurt yourself or others, seek immediate psychiatric assistance.

Serious challenges in our medical system: Insurance companies often refuse to pay for a mental health visit unless a DSM-5 diagnosis is made, forcing doctors to prematurely identify the so-called illness and treat it with medication. Another challenge is that many mental health clinicians do not accept insurance and patients must pay out-of-pocket. Fortunately, a number of lower-cost services now are available via teletherapy. Your primary care doctor also may be a good resource for a referral to a therapist. Often a brief series of therapy sessions with the right person will have a significant impact on your symptoms and your life.

• **Be skeptical and well-informed.** Don't passively accept a psychiatric diagnosis and drug treatment—especially from your primary care doctor—without doing some research on websites from reputable institutions such as a medical school like Harvard, Mayo Clinic and others, and the government website MedlinePlus.gov. Check whether your symptoms match the description of the disorder... have lasted long enough to meet the criteria...are causing you considerable distress... and/or are impairing your ability to work, take care of yourself and connect with others. Keep a diary of your symptoms to chart progress and share with your doctor.

• **Get more than one professional opinion and include your family in decision-making.** People usually come to their doctors' offices on one of the worst days of their lives with transient problems that often will improve on their own or with reduced stress and increased support.

If you're on a psychiatric drug currently: You may not need to take the medication for life, but don't stop taking it abruptly or on your own. Many meds cause withdrawal syndromes that can be disruptive and even dangerous. Going off psychiatric medications always should be done gradually over weeks or months and only under medical supervision.

When Depression Drugs Don't Work

Stephen S. Ilardi, PhD, an associate professor of clinical psychology at the University of Kansas, and the author of *The Depression Cure: The Six-Step Program to Beat Depression Without Drugs.*

Since World War II, the rate of clinical depression, also called *major depressive disorder*, has risen tenfold. It's not surprising, then, that about one in eight Americans takes a daily antidepressant.

For many of those people, though, antidepressants just aren't effective enough. In the largest "real-world" study of antidepressants—one that looked at more than 4,000 patients—fewer than 10 percent of those taking an antidepressant experienced complete remission that lasted longer than a year. Antidepressants can also deliver a slew of common side effects, like headaches, dry mouth, insomnia, digestive upset, sexual problems, weight gain, and fatigue.

Healing depression typically requires combating the disease from several different angles at once—and the following non-drug methods have particularly strong scientific support.

Exercise

This is the single most powerful tool we have for overcoming depression, probably because it affects so many systems in the body: It regulates neurotransmitters, improves sleep, and decreases brain inflammation, to name just a few. It's not an exaggeration to say that if all of the benefits of exercise could be packaged in one pill, it would instantly become the most useful overall medication in our psychiatric armamentarium.

Based on the best research, just 30 minutes of brisk, aerobic walking three times a week is usually effective. There is some evidence that boosting the exercise "dose" may carry even greater antidepressant benefits. If your depression makes it hard to exercise, a personal trainer, friend, or loved one who can walk with you regularly can help you start and keep up with this depression-busting habit.

Diet, Fish Oil, and Fiber

The Mediterranean diet, which emphasizes fish, vegetables, fruits, beans, whole grains, nuts, seeds, and olive oil, fights depression, likely because it controls inflammation. (The inflamed brain is usually a depressed brain.) You can also fight inflammation—and depression—with 1,000 to 2,000 daily milligrams of eicosapentaenoic acid (EPA), a powerful omega-3 molecule derived from fish oil. To avoid the dreaded "fishy burps," buy pharmaceutical grade, enteric-coated fish oil and store it in the freezer. Take your pill with a meal.

The Mediterranean diet also delivers high levels of plant fiber, which encourages the growth of healthy microbes in the gut, preventing or reversing dysbiosis, an imbalance of good and bad gut bacteria that has been linked to both depression and anxiety. To get even more fiber, take a soluble fiber supplement, such as psyllium husk or chicory root, at a dose of 5 to 7 grams each day. Cutting-edge research suggests we can also boost beneficial, depression-fighting gut microbes with probiotic supplements, especially those that feature *lacto* and *bifido* bacterial strains.

Caution: If you have a gastrointestinal problem such as irritable bowel syndrome or ulcerative colitis, talk to a gastroenterologist before taking fiber or a probiotic.

Acetyl-L-carnitine (ALC)

This brain-produced nutritional compound supplies energy to brain cells (neurons). ALC levels are often low in people with depression, particularly those over age 40. Several studies show that supplementing the diet with 2,000 mg of ALC can produce anti-depressive results comparable to medication, but with effects that kick in faster (about a week, as compared to four to six weeks for medications) and with minimal adverse side effects.

Bright Light

If your depression starts in the fall or winter, when the days are shorter, you may have

Symptoms of Depression

While symptoms vary from person to person, they often include the following...

- **Intense emotional pain** (similar to the agony of losing a loved one)
- **Loss of interest and pleasure in everyday activities**
- **Social withdrawal**
- **Fatigue**
- **Poor sleep**
- **Changes in weight or appetite**
- **Non-stop negative thinking**
- **Brain fog** accompanied by poor concentration, memory, and decision-making

seasonal affective disorder, which is best treated with bright light therapy. The eye is an outpost of the brain, and light works like a drug, resetting your body clock and normalizing the natural sleep-wake cycle (the circadian rhythm) for better mood, sleep, and appetite. Research also shows that light boxes are beneficial for anyone with depression, at any time of year.

To get the benefits of light therapy for depression, you need about 30 minutes of exposure to 10,000 lux, a unit of illumination, within an hour of waking up. It's important to read the manufacturer's instructions and use a measuring tape to make sure you're sitting at the correct distance to get the full brightness. Sitting too far away can reduce or eliminate the benefits of light therapy.

Spend Time with People

Social connection is a key component of overcoming depression, but when you're depressed, your brain tells you to stay away from people. It also says they don't want to be around you, anyway. That's the disease talking: Disregard the message and spend time with friends and family members in shared activities that you enjoy. For the 25 to 30 percent of depressed people who don't have supportive friends or family, a psychotherapist or therapy group can provide that type of support. You can also build connections by taking classes or participating in organized or informal group activities. Try Meetup.com to find groups of people who are interested in things that you are.

Hobbies Heal Your Mind

Hobbies Are a Form of Self-Care

If you've picked up a new hobby during the pandemic, you may want to resist the urge to commercialize it (unless you're truly desperate for money). The happiness and well-being that come from taking time to do something for the pure joy of it can vanish when you pressure yourself to compete in the marketplace.

Self.com

Relax with a Fun New Craft

Try dot mandala rock painting for a relaxing therapy. Water-based acrylic paint is used to create colorful, symmetrical patterns.

How to do it: Place a large dot of paint in the center of a smooth stone. Place four smaller dots evenly spaced around the center one. Then place four more dots, one between each of the first four dots, evenly spaced. Continue to add dots of different sizes using different colors of paint, spacing the dots evenly to keep the design symmetrical. Let dots dry between additions to keep the paint from flowing together.

Variations: Use a pin, toothpick, crochet hook or similar tool instead of a brush...use a pin or toothpick to drag the edge of still-wet dots in a curve. For inspirational examples and instructions, see *RockPainting 101's Dot Mandela* tutorial at bit.ly/3fuD2Or.

Miranda Pitrone, rock-painting artist, Lake Erie-Painesville, Ohio. MirandaPitroneArt.com

Stop Ruminating

Nonstop negative, anxious thinking about the past or the future creates a runaway stress response that worsens depression. To stop ruminating, you need to first notice that you are doing it, and then focus your attention elsewhere. Cognitive-behavioral therapy and mindfulness-based stress reduction are excellent tools in this process.

A rumination log can help, too. Every hour or so, note whether or not you've been ruminating. Over time, you'll develop a spontaneous "mental alarm" that will alert you any time your thoughts take a ruminative turn—and stop them.

Nitrous Oxide for Depression

Charles R. Conway, MD, professor of psychiatry, Washington University School of Medicine in St. Louis, Missouri.

In a small study, breathing the anesthetic drug, commonly called laughing gas, with oxygen for one hour significantly improved symptoms, and the benefits lasted for several weeks. The most common side effect was nausea. Nitrous oxide binds to N-methyl-D-aspartate glutamate receptors on neurons, as does ketamine, another anesthetic drug that is being widely studied for its antidepressant effects.

Loneliness Linked to Microbial Diversity of the Gut

UC San Diego School of Medicine

Researchers discovered that people with higher levels of wisdom, compassion, social support, and engagement have more diverse bacteria in their guts than people who report high levels of loneliness. That diversity may increase immunity and decrease systemic inflammation.

Stress Buster: It's Your Heart—Not Your Brain

Leah Lagos, PsyD, licensed clinical psychologist Board Certified in Biofeedback (BCB) who specializes in health and performance psychology in New York City. She is author of *Heart Breath Mind: Train Your Heart to Conquer Stress and Achieve Success.* DrLeahLagos.com

No matter how much stress you had in your life before 2020, the pandemic put everyone on edge. If you're like most people, you may have relied on one or more of the go-to approaches to tamping down that stress—mental imagery, journaling, knitting, reading a novel…you name it.

What you may not realize: The most widely used calming activities are based on the belief that stress lives in your brain, and if you can just think your way through it or distract yourself from it, it will improve.

But here's a secret that can revolutionize the way you deal with stress—it actually lives in your body, not in your brain. To tap into your body's hidden calming capacities, one of the most effective self-regulation approaches is to train your heart rate variability (HRV).

Here's what you need to know about training your heart to ease day-to-day stress…

What Is Heart Rate Variability?

Most people think that the heart beats with the regularity of a metronome. But the truth is, when you inhale, your heart rate naturally quickens…and when you exhale, it slows down. The result is a slight variation in the time between heartbeats—so slight that it's measured in milliseconds.

The degree to which the heart rate accelerates on inhalation and decelerates on exhalation varies from person to person. The more variation you have in those intervals—your HRV—the better. Too little variation suggests a condition called *sympathetic dominance,* meaning that the nervous system is essentially stuck in fight-or-flight mode. Sympathetic dominance is all too common today.

The goal is to balance the sympathetic nervous system and parasympathetic nervous system—the "rest and digest" or "tend and befriend" branch that handles day-to-day vitals such as digestion, along with helping the body relax and de-stress. When balanced, HRV is high, reflecting a strong ability to tolerate and bounce back from stress.

The Good News About HRV

Just as HRV responds to everyday life's stressors, it also can be significantly improved by strengthening your parasympathetic nervous system to assist your body in handling stress.

Result: Higher HRV…improved health and longevity…and a happier you.

In addition to mental and emotional resilience, high HRV is linked to a host of health benefits, including reduced blood pressure, improved cardiovascular health, lower rates of depression and more. In fact, research has shown that HRV is a more accurate predictor of future cardiac events in people who don't have heart disease than cholesterol, blood pressure or resting heart rate.

To track your HRV, you can use an HRV sensor, which usually comes as a chest-strap monitor…a fitness tracker, some of which have a wristband embedded with a sensor… or a fingerprint-scanning app.

Even though it can be interesting to have an exact measurement, most people can safely assume that they need to improve their HRV. The breath-pacing exercises below are easy and highly effective for most people.

Ways to Boost Your HRV

Increasing evidence shows that HRV can help anyone improve his/her physical and mental health—often by practicing for 20 minutes twice a day for four weeks. After 10 weeks of practicing at this frequency, you'll develop a reflex that kicks in during moments of stress to help you reset and recover. *Here's how…*

STEP 1: **Change your breathing.** Instead of breathing at a rate of 12 breaths per minute—as most adults do—slow it down. Breathing at a rate of approximately six breaths per minute triggers a systemwide relaxation response.

Inhale through your nose for four counts, filling your belly with air, and exhale for six counts through pursed lips, as if you're blowing on hot soup. Belly breathing stimulates the parasympathetic nerve receptors found in the lower lungs, helping to spread a sense of calm throughout the body and mind. When you breathe only into your chest, those lower-lung receptors go untouched.

Start with 10 minutes twice a day.

Helpful: Try a free app, such as *Awesome Breathing*. For maximum benefits, work your way up to 20 minutes twice a day. Don't try this while reading, watching TV, or listening to music. For best results, forgo other sources of stimulation and enjoy the feeling of your breath.

Fascinating research: Reciting the "Ave Maria" or a mantra can slow breathing to almost precisely six breath cycles per minute, according to a study published in *BMJ*. This may be one reason why people find the recitation of these words to be calming—it improves HRV.

STEP 2: Don't skimp on cardiovascular exercise. Cardiovascular fitness and HRV are strongly correlated—the fitter your heart, the higher your HRV. Follow the guidelines for physical activity—150 minutes per week of moderate-intensity aerobic exercise (challenging enough that you can carry on a conversation but not sing) or 75 minutes per week of vigorous-intensity aerobic activity (you can't say more than a few words without having to catch your breath).

Helpful: Try to incorporate some high-intensity interval training (HIIT) workouts, which alternate quick, intense bursts of cardio exercise with periods of low-intensity activity. Research shows that HIIT has even better potential for improving your body's response to stress because alternating the intensity of your workout challenges your nervous system. Start out with a 1:2 ratio—run for one minute then walk for two, and repeat...or go all-out on the elliptical for 30 seconds, then slow down for a minute,

and repeat. Most people can aim for a 10- to 20-minute HIIT session.

STEP 3: Practice "emotional pivoting." The next time you're feeling stressed—after a difficult conversation with a coworker, for example—try this mind-body strategy. Think back to a time in your life when you felt an incredible amount of love, gratitude, awe and/or safety. Take 10 breaths, focusing on the positive experience as you inhale for four counts through your nose. Really try to connect to the memory, almost as if you're reliving it. Exhale through your mouth for six seconds, releasing any anxiety, stress, or fear along with your breath. Do this for about five minutes after a stressful situation. With practice, this can help improve your HRV, allowing you to easily pivot away from negative emotional states.

STEP 4: Limit those cups of joe. Getting too much caffeine—for example, three or more cups of coffee a day—can reduce HRV. That's because excess caffeine stimulates the sympathetic nervous system.

Helpful: Consider swapping your coffee for green tea. It has less caffeine than coffee, so it's energizing without feeling overly stimulating. Green tea also contains an active compound called *L-theanine*, which can boost your HRV by increasing production of various calming neurochemicals while lowering levels of stress-producing brain chemicals.

STEP 5: Try cold therapy. Exposure to a cold temperature can increase HRV. Though no one knows exactly why, it's often attributed to a physiological survival mechanism called the "diving reflex," which kicks in when a person dives into cold water. The body responds to this sudden underwater immersion by conserving oxygen (via decreased heart rate) and prioritizing blood flow to the heart and brain. Don't worry—you don't need to sign up for a local polar bear plunge. You can trigger the diving reflex by splashing very cold water on your forehead, cheeks, and nose. Try this before your breathing practice to jump-start your HRV.

Keep a Crush from Ruining Your Marriage

Raffi Bilek, LCSW-C, director of the Baltimore Therapy Center, where he specializes in marriage counseling. BaltimoreTherapyCenter.com

Even women in good relationships can find themselves attracted to people other than their partners. And a crush is powerful—you feel giddy or melty when you're with the person, and that's a feeling you like.

Crushes and affairs are invariably more exciting than marriages. They are new and secretive and don't come with any of the challenges of a marriage. But in terms of your own feelings, the fact that you use the word "crush" is telling. A crush is just, well, a crush. You don't love this person. Remember in junior high when you had a huge crush on that cute girl or boy who sat next to you in class? Odds are that a few months later, you were over it. You won't have these feelings forever…but you may be prolonging them by keeping yourself in close proximity to the object of your crush.

There is no quick trick you can use to make a crush disappear. If you are committed to your marriage and want it to continue to flourish, you need to take deliberate precautions to avoid taking your crush too far.

Ask yourself how much time you really need to spend with this other person. The less time you spend together, the easier it'll be to shake off that crush.

Example: If it's a workmate, you don't have to have lunch together.

If you suspect that the other person shares your feelings, and thus this crush is an imminent threat to your marriage, the best course of action is to change the circumstances entirely. See whether you can be assigned to another work project. Or if this crush comes from a social or volunteer environment, spend less time with the associated group.

How to De-Stress Your Smile

High stress can lead to increased dental problems, including tooth grinding, jaw clenching, chipped and cracked teeth, and jaw pain.

Relieve jaw pain/spasms: Lightly hold (but don't bite) a pencil horizontally in your front teeth for about 20 minutes to loosen jaw muscles.

Prevent pain/strengthen jaw muscles: Place a thumb under your chin, and open your mouth, pushing against the thumb for five seconds…then try to close your mouth while pushing your chin down to keep it from closing.

Relax your jaw at bedtime/reduce nighttime clenching: Close your eyes, press your tongue against the roof of your mouth, and breathe deeply through your nose for several minutes.

Helpful: An ergonomic desk chair supports your back and encourages good posture, reducing muscle stress in your shoulders, head, and neck, which will relieve stress in the jaw.

Real Simple. RealSimple.com

Let Go of Envy…and Feel Happier

Mark Goulston, MD, Los Angeles–based psychiatrist, author of *Get Out of Your Own Way: Overcoming Self-Defeating Behavior*, host of the "My Wakeup Call" podcast and creator of the "Defeating Self-Defeat" audio course at Himalaya.com. MarkGoulston.com

Susan Krauss Whitbourne, PhD, adjunct professor of gerontology at University of Massachusetts Boston, and author of PsychologyToday.com's "Fulfillment at Any Age" blog.

Ramani Durvasula, PhD, professor of psychology at California State University, Los Angeles, and author of *"Don't You Know Who I Am?": How to Stay Sane in an Era of Narcissism, Entitlement, and Incivility.* Doctor-Ramani.com

Envy may be considered one of the seven deadly sins, but it's actually a perfectly normal, universal emotion. With envy, you see someone with a coveted attribute that you don't have—money, looks, professional success—and experience negative feelings as a result. You equate that person's gain with your loss.

Sadly, envy is a ubiquitous human emotion that doesn't feel good. A 2020 Cognitive Therapy and Research study confirmed that envy is associated with anger, anxiety, rumination, even depression.

Rather than allow envy to become self-destructive, why not take a fresh approach to this toxic and tricky emotion? *We asked three leading experts for their best advice…*

Mark Goulston, MD

Tame envy by using gratitude to move from a scarcity mindset to an abundance mindset. How people view life tends to fall into one of two categories—those with a scarcity mindset and those with an abundance mindset. Those with a scarcity mindset view life as a pie with a fixed number of slices, so if one person takes a big slice, then there is less for everyone else to enjoy. These folks see other people succeed and think, *I don't have that. They have it better than me, and now there's not enough for me.* Those with an abundance mindset see the world as a limitless pie, bursting with opportunity and potential for growth. They see others thrive and think, *Great work. Maybe I can aim for that kind of success, too.*

These terms, developed by Stephen Covey in *The 7 Habits of Highly Effective People*, can make an enormous difference in how you experience envy. A scarcity mindset can bring out the worst in a person, causing him/her to constantly thirst for more while robbing him of the optimism or motivation needed to go out and get it. Many people inherit a scarcity mindset from their parents who, rather than being grateful for what they had, walked around in a state of continuous disappointment. Poor self-esteem also is linked with feelings of scarcity. These people may leave their house one day wearing their favorite sneakers…see a friend wearing great new sneakers…and instantly wish

they had those sneakers, not the ones they are wearing. Their scarcity mindset triggers envy, making them feel as if they're somehow lacking simply because their attire isn't as high-end or eye-catching.

Now imagine a person with an abundance mindset in the same situation. She sees someone in an outfit that's a bit more fabulous than what she's wearing and thinks, *Wow, what a classy, elegant ensemble. Maybe I'll try something that color/material/style the next time I go shopping.* Rather than focus on what she's lacking, she finds inspiration in others' success. And because she's not coming from a glass-half-empty place, when she sees someone with a new car, great job success, high-achieving children, or abundant grandchildren, she isn't envious…she thinks, *I feel good about life, and maybe it could be even better.*

If you see yourself in this description of a scarcity mindset, one way to shift is to tap into the power of gratitude. When you wake up in the morning or before going to bed at night, write down three things you're grateful for. Ideas can be big and small—relationships…a great meeting at work…your home…doing more sit-ups than the day before…a recent feel-good experience. If you're religious, you could try a prayer of gratitude. You even could send a quick text or e-mail telling someone why you are thankful for him/her. Taking time every day to focus on all that you have takes power away from envious feelings.

Susan Krauss Whitbourne, PhD

Tame envy by mining it for inspiration. When we feel envious of someone, the natural tendency is to avoid him. We do this not only because we want to distance ourselves from what we consider to be the source of our resentment, but the envy itself tends to make people feel bad about themselves. (*If I were successful like he is, I wouldn't feel this way.*)

Let's say you have a friend or acquaintance who received an award for his community service. You've always wanted to get involved with volunteering but never had enough time to make the commitment, and now you're envious of the accolades he is receiving. Instead of distancing yourself from him, do the opposite—get closer. Ask him how he discovered the right cause to get involved with, how he found the time to do it and what are some of his favorite aspects of volunteering. The goal is to reframe your envy as a longing to better yourself and use that as motivation to grow and make positive changes in your own life. Researchers call this benign envy. Use it as a jumping-off point for your own success.

Dwelling on your envy will only make you more depressed. The healthier choice is to acknowledge your feelings and make the best of them.

Added bonus: By connecting with the source of your envy, you have the opportunity to spend time with a potentially remarkable person who is doing great things in the world.

Ramani Durvasula, PhD

Tame envy by figuring out what it's trying to tell you. We all have childhood experiences that shape who we are today, the emotions we feel and the way we react to the world around us. Those experiences—particularly the negative ones—can predispose adults to feelings of envy, triggered by seeing other people succeed in the same areas where we feel we have failed.

Maybe you were constantly critiqued by a parent for not being smart enough…felt like you never fit in at school…never excelled at sports, despite your best efforts…struggled with your weight…or didn't have your material needs met due to financial struggles in your household. These types of hurt and suffering can manifest in adulthood as something called a "core wound," and it usually is behind feelings of envy. Someone prone to envying people with large, luxurious homes may have grown up in a modest or even rundown house or apartment, and that envy represents the shame you felt as a child. If you and your sibling grew up arguing all the time, leaving you feeling disconnected, then you might now feel envious of a friend who has a rock-solid relationship with her brother and his family.

The key is identifying your core wound, which often requires the deeper dive of therapy. The depth of these experiences—and the defenses we develop over a lifetime—can make it difficult to identify these vulnerabilities. However, taking time on your own through journaling, reflecting on uncomfortable triggers in your life and trying to link them to origins earlier in life can be useful. What hurt you the most in childhood? Chances are, you'll quickly see the link between the core wound and your current feelings of envy. Treat yourself with compassion when you identify a core wound—imagine talking to yourself as a child—and remind yourself that these emotions you now feel don't make you a bad person…they're simply an activation of your own vulnerabilities. Now, instead of beating yourself up for coveting your neighbor's seemingly perfect marriage, you can dig deeper and realize how difficult it was for you to grow up as a child of divorce, and that pain is now materializing as envy.

Core wounds may never completely fade but are likely to remain "tender" areas. Be gentle with yourself, and you may be able to coexist with them peacefully and mindfully.

The same principle applies if you suspect that you are the object of someone else's envy. Something about you or your life may be triggering one of his core wounds. In this situation, the envious person may be prickly or even rude to you.

Your initial response may be to defend yourself or engage in an argument in response to a snide comment. Instead, remember that the other person is feeling insecure and treat him with compassion, humility, and grace—three things that the world is severely lacking right now.

Envy vs. Jealousy

Envy almost always involves just two people, with you wanting what he/she has. Jealousy typically involves three people—you, someone you care about and a third person whom you believe threatens that significant relationship.

Why We Constantly Want More

Daniel Z. Lieberman, MD, professor and vice chair for clinical affairs in the Department of Psychiatry and Behavioral Sciences at George Washington University, Washington, D.C. He is author of *The Molecule of More*.

Anyone who has made a large purchase, fallen in love, or overeaten at a party knows that humans face a perpetual pull between what we want and how we feel once we have it. While this is rich fodder for philosophical pondering, this dilemma has a simple cause: the competing interests of two types of neurotransmitters—chemicals in your brain that transmit messages between neurons. Neurotransmitters have a wide variety of mundane roles, such as affecting movement, heart rate, and sleep, but they also play a key role in how we feel about the present and the future.

Battling Brain Chemicals

Your feelings about the present are controlled by serotonin, oxytocin, endorphins (your brain's version of morphine), and a class of chemicals called endocannabinoids (your brain's version of marijuana). When they're working correctly, these "here-and-now" chemicals tell your brain to be happy and satisfied with what you have.

And then there is dopamine. Not interested in the present, dopamine is focused on maximizing the resources that will be available in the future. It can be a powerful positive force, motivating you to work hard, to learn, to earn money, and to grow. When it was first discovered, scientists thought it was a pleasure-inducing chemical, but when they dug deeper, they learned that it's not so simple. Dopamine induces pleasure when

you are *pursuing* things, but it offers no such benefits once you have them. In fact, part of its role is to make you dissatisfied with the present so you'll be motivated to work harder to improve the future.

Let's take a closer look at this lesser-understood chemical.

Dopamine Wants More

The dopamine desire circuit is a system in your brain that constantly scans the environment for new resources that will improve your chances of surviving and keeping your DNA replicating. As such, its primary focus is food, sex, and the ability to win competitions.

When the circuit finds something potentially valuable, dopamine floods the brain and creates feelings of pleasure, desire, and excitement to convey the message, "You desperately need this!" Whether you actually need something in the moment is irrelevant because dopamine is entirely focused on stockpiling resources for the future.

It's like a person at the beginning of the pandemic who stockpiled toilet paper. No one needed or enjoyed having 200 rolls of TP, but dopamine insisted that it was important to have just in case. Dopamine does the same thing with all sorts of resources. It can make your perfectly good house seem inadequate. It can make a new acquaintance seem more interesting and desirable than a current partner. It can make space for a third piece of cake even though you feel uncomfortably full.

The cruelty of the dopamine desire circuit is that as soon as you get what it told you that you wanted, its job is done and dopamine levels plummet—along with those feelings of desire and excitement. Buyer's remorse, the sinking feeling of regret that occurs after making a big purchase, is a perfect example of a dopamine drop.

Wanting and liking are produced by two different systems in the brain, so enjoying things once we have them requires finding balance between dopamine and the here-and-now chemicals. (More on that shortly.)

Overactive Dopamine Circuits

Some people have more active dopaminergic circuits than others, which can make finding that balance more difficult. People with elevated activity in the dopamine desire circuit can become trapped in an endless cycle of chasing the buzz and fall prey to compulsive spending, hypersexuality, gambling, or even becoming addicted to drugs, which provide an intense dopamine rush. (One in six people who take *levodopa* [L-Dopa], a Parkinson's disease drug that replaces missing dopamine, has a similar response.)

Others have too much activity in the dopamine control circuit. The dopamine *desire* circuit gives us urges, while the dopamine *control* circuit, when working properly, gives us the ability to manage those urges and guide them toward profitable ends. The latter lets us imagine the future to see the potential consequences of decisions we might make right now, and it gives us the ability to plan how to make that imaginary future a reality.

But when people have an overactive dopamine control circuit, they can become addicted to achievement. For them, life is about the future, improvement, and innovation—at the expense of being able to experience the joys of the present. This can cause people to neglect their emotions, abandon empathy, and miss out on enjoying the present. If you ignore your emotions, they become less sophisticated over time and may devolve into anger, greed, and resentment. If you neglect empathy, you lose the ability to make others feel happy. Living for the future can also rob you of the pleasure of the sensory world around you. Instead of enjoying the beauty of a flower, you can imagine only how it would look in a vase.

Finding Harmony

Dopamine naturally decreases as we age, so part of successful aging is transitioning to the here-and-now chemicals. Just as too much dopamine is detrimental, too little is problematic as well. Without adequate dopamine, you lose motivation and drive, and no

How Slot Machines and the Internet Hijack Your Brain

If you've ever played slot machines—the top moneymakers for casino owners—you've felt the exhilarating rush of believing that you might win big if you keep playing. Your dopamine will keep your excitement high for a while, but if you lose too often, the reward circuit loses interest, dopamine levels drop, and the game is no longer fun.

That's why the people who design slot machines provide random wins. Just before you lose interest, you'll make a little money that keeps the dopamine desire circuit guessing—and pumping out excitement.

The people who design social media sites and phone apps use the same principles to keep you coming back for more—and it's contributing to an epidemic of endless dopamine stimulation.

Short, snappy headlines that make you want to learn more, quick hits of social interactions, Facebook likes, and phone notifications all excite your dopamine with their promises that something rewarding might be a click away. Advertisers and media companies make money when you click, so they are working with highly skilled experts to manipulate your dopamine response and keep you coming back.

Of course, not everything online is positive, but that doesn't decrease your dopamine response. Because it wants to maximize your chances of survival, dopamine rewards you with a buzz of excitement and pleasure when you read about all of the terrible things it thinks it needs to prepare you for, leading to what's called doomscrolling.

To fight back, use the Internet and social media judiciously and be aware of the manipulation happening behind the scenes. Turn off notifications. Make your screen black and white. Embrace the materials world: Think atoms and molecules instead of zeros and ones.

—Dr. Daniel Z. Lieberman

longer experience excitement at the prospect of a brighter future. There are many ways to balance dopamine with the here-and-now neurotransmitters.

• **Master a skill.** Mastery is the ability to extract the maximum reward from a particular set of circumstances. That satisfies dopamine and causes it to pause for a little bit and let the here-and-now neurotransmitters shine. You can gain mastery over a game, a sport, an art, a musical instrument, or anything else that you enjoy.

• **Pay attention to what you are doing in the moment.** By spending time in the present, we take in sensory information about the reality we live in, which allows the dopamine system to use that information to develop plans that maximize rewards. That's dopamine and the here-and-now neurotransmitters working together. Further, when something interesting activates the dopamine system, if you shift your focus outward, the increased level of attention makes the sensory experience more intense. Being in nature is particularly beneficial because it's complex, has unexpected patterns, and there is a virtually limitless amount of detail to explore.

• **Download a meditation app.** You can strengthen your ability to be in the present with practice. It's like lifting weights. In fact, brain scans show that parts of the brain are thicker in people who meditate.

• **Create.** Because it is always new, creation is one of the best dopaminergic pleasures. Satisfy both your dopamine and you're here-and-now chemicals with activities like woodworking, knitting, painting, decorating, sewing, and using adult coloring books.

• **Fix things.** Solving problems by fixing things is a dopaminergic activity, but it also leads to a satisfying solution in the present. Plus, learning to fix your own broken appliances or other objects boosts your sense of self-efficacy and saves money.

Ditch the Baggage from Your First Marriage

Terry Gaspard, MSW, LICSW, therapist in private practice in Rhode Island and author of *The Remarriage Manual: How to Make Everything Work Better the Second Time Around.* MovingPastDivorce.com

"Love is better the second time around." That's what the song says, but remarriage is far from easy.

Fact: Although more than 40 percent of first marriages end in divorce, the divorce rate for second, third and fourth marriages is 60 percent or higher.

After interviewing more than 100 remarried couples, I've found that it's common for one or both partners to assume that a second union will automatically be better than the first because they think they've learned from past mistakes. In reality, many people haven't taken the time to examine their prior relationships for clues to why they failed, potentially dooming them to repeat self-sabotaging relationship patterns.

Second marriages also come with complicated relationships when kids are involved. Children can be a big factor in second-marriage failures if you and your spouse are not communicating well.

Whether you are newly remarried or you've been remarried for a while, here is advice for ditching unresolved baggage and putting your remarriage on the right path…

Rules for a Happy Remarriage

• **Cultivate realistic expectations.** In second marriages, couples typically get to know each other more quickly than first-time couples, have more baggage and have more complicated lives—especially if they have children from prior marriages.

Don't make assumptions about how your remarriage should work. That can lead only to misunderstandings and disappointment. No matter how much you love someone, you are going to have different ways of doing things when it comes to managing conflict around money, parenting, dealing with in-laws and ex-partners, and other issues. In many cases, new partners haven't yet learned successful ways to manage conflict. It usually takes a few years for family members to adjust to a remarriage or living in a stepfamily.

If you are widowed: If you had a happy first marriage, don't expect your second marriage to be exactly like the prior relationship and don't try to replace your first spouse. You will have to develop a unique relationship based on the person you're currently with.

• **Give the benefit of the doubt.** Many second-time spouses have less tolerance toward what they perceive as disrespect if they came out of an oppressive relationship and, over time, learned to be both defensive and offensive in communicating with a partner. In the heat of the moment, they may criticize and issue ultimatums, which only pushes the two parties farther apart.

Research by leading marriage counselor John Gottman, PhD, shows that successful couples perform five positive interactions for every negative one during conflict. Be positive by using statements that focus on your needs rather than your partner's negative behavior.

Example: If you are in the middle of a phone call and your spouse starts talking to you, instead of saying, "You are so selfish and unaware of your surroundings," say, "I would really appreciate if you would not talk to me when I'm on the phone."

• **Abandon the power struggle.** The need to be right is prominent in second marriages because partners have typically lived on their own for some time and figured out what they think is the best way to do things.

Example: Samantha and John, both of whom were left by their previous spouses, bicker a lot as they try to get the other to do things his/her way. They have trouble finding the middle ground without feeling as if one of them is losing.

Better: They need to learn to trust that they can be open with each other about what they really want in a given situation without feeling rejected or weak.

Many couples have hidden issues with control, and this usually means that they need to feel cared for and loved. Rather than digging their heels in and getting into a power struggle, they can ask for what they need in a positive way. Partners who learn to say "Yes" more often and see things from their partner's point of view are happier. And they need to learn how to compromise so that both feel like they are satisfied with the outcome. Those who can accept each other's influence are open to their partner's point of view even when they disagree. You can learn to do this by being more self-aware of your control issues and listening with curiosity to your partner's perspective.

Know Your Triggers

We all have basic needs and desires for acceptance, attention, safety, love, respect, being in control and being needed. In remarriages, each partner's unmet needs and desires may come to the surface and bump into the other spouse's vulnerabilities. Some of us may have trust issues or a fear of abandonment, while others have anxiety about being stifled or controlled.

Example: Kelly would go into a tailspin when her second husband, Mark, came home a little late from work without texting to let her know. She started micromanaging him and asking questions about where he was and why he was late. Once she realized that she was mistrusting Mark because her ex-husband had been unfaithful, she knew she was overreacting. She explained to Mark what she was feeling and asked if he could text or call her if he was going to be more than 15 minutes late. Mark was happy to oblige.

To gain self-awareness about your triggers when interacting with your new spouse, notice situations when your muscles tense up… your heart rate increases…you have hot or cold flushes or tingling…and/or you are having repetitive or intense thoughts such as *I can never win* or *This is so unfair.* Notice

105

what is going on when you have these physical responses or thoughts. Is your partner speaking very loudly? Are your children arguing? Did you have a stressful day at work?

Important: The more intense your reaction to your partner's behavior or words, the more likely it is your own issue that is causing the problem.

5 Ways Not to React Badly in the Moment

Once you become aware of the kinds of behaviors and situations that trigger you, you need to learn ways of coping with them so that you can remain calm and reflective rather than act out of fear and anger.

Example: My second and current husband, Craig, and I were at a wedding, and he was group dancing with other women while I sat on the sidelines fuming. I don't dance because I believe that I'm not a good dancer. Once I reflected on my feelings, I was able to realize that Craig's outgoing behavior was triggering my fear of abandonment. We talked it out and came to an agreement that he could dance with others at weddings but needed to check in with me on breaks so that I didn't feel ignored.

To avoid overreacting…

1. Remove your attention from the situation or person, and put it on your breath. Inhale slowly through your nose and exhale through your mouth, as you silently count to 10. Repeat until you feel calm.

2. Excuse yourself and walk away for five minutes. Go to the bathroom, get a glass of water or pace in the yard. Return when you've cooled down enough to speak rationally with your partner.

3. Ask yourself, *Why am I feeling so fearful or angry?* This often will lead to a litany of worst-case scenarios running through your head. In my case, I had to think, *Does Craig want to dance with someone else because there is something wrong with me? No. He just likes to dance more than I do.* Once I stopped taking his dancing at

parties as a personal affront, I was able to stop catastrophizing that it meant our relationship was over.

4. Find the upside or fun in the situation.

Example: Once I realized my husband wasn't participating in dance circles to be with other women, I could enjoy watching him dance and it made me want to invite him for a slow dance.

5. Delay your emotional reaction. Don't repress your feelings, but also don't explode in public or in the car. Talk about the situation that occurred once you've calmed down.

Tip: If you feel like you're ready to explode, release your negative feelings by exercising or going into a private room and screaming, or taking time alone with the breathing exercises above or a bit of journaling.

Remarriages often take more effort than first marriages because you are dealing with more baggage and more family members. But they also can be stronger and more resilient because both partners typically have some experience with marriage. Critical to success is that both partners need to be open and vulnerable when communicating with each other, as well as kind and forgiving when misunderstandings occur.

Choose Your Thoughts

Michael Anderson, PhD, professor of cognitive neuroscience, University of Cambridge, UK, quoted in *The New York Times.*

When you want to forget something, for instance, a fight with a friend—consciously flood your mind with positive memories of her so those pop up instead of the argument…or picture yourself putting up a "mental hand" and saying, "Nope, I don't want to think about that."

The Upside of Regret

Daniel Pink, JD, author of several books including *The Power of Regret: How Looking Backward Moves Us Forward*. He previously was a contributing editor at *Fast Company* and *Wired* magazines and host and co-executive producer of "Crowd Control," a National Geographic Channel series about human behavior. DanPink.com

"Non, Je Ne Regrette Rien" was French singer Edith Piaf's final hit. If your French is rusty, that song title translates to "No, I regret nothing at all," which Piaf insisted reflected her philosophy. But less than three years after singing that she had no regrets, she was dead at 47—drug addiction and hard living had taken their toll. Her final words were, "Every damn thing you do in this life, you have to pay for."

The woman famous for having no regrets obviously had them. She was far from alone—a public opinion survey of 4,489 Americans conducted with Qualtrics suggests that 99 percent of us at least occasionally look back on our lives and wish we had done things differently, and 43 percent of us do so frequently or continually.

Regrets are viewed as negative forces in our positivity-promoting society. But the secret to life isn't getting through it without accumulating any regrets. It's keeping regrets in perspective…and learning to shape these powerful negative feelings into positive thoughts and actions.

Benefits of Regret

Research suggests that it's possible to derive powerful benefits from regret…

• **Improved decision making.** A 2021 study of senior business leaders by researchers at Bentley University found that reflecting on their regrets improves business leaders' future decisions. The deeply unpleasant feeling of regret likely reminds them not to rush into decisions and/or to remain wary of past mistakes.

• **Improved performance.** A 2019 study by researchers at Northwestern University's Kellogg School of Management found that scientists who narrowly miss receiving prestigious grants go on to produce more hit research papers than those who are narrowly approved for grants. Missing out on grants triggers regret…but that appears to lead to self-improvement.

• **A more meaningful life.** A 2017 study by another professor at Kellogg School of Management found that when people spend time thinking about what might have been if they'd made different choices, they tend to come away feeling a deeper sense of purpose in the life that they're living, as well as elevated levels of spiritual feelings. Similarly, when researchers involved in a 2010 study at University of California's Haas School of Business asked college students to imagine that they had selected a different school—and consequently were on a different campus with different friends—those students ended up sensing greater meaning in their friendships and college choices. When we regret a path not taken, it reminds us that our lives could have gone in a million different ways—that makes the path we did take seem very special, even miraculous.

Regrets Can Work for You

If you push regrets from your mind, they'll probably keep flooding back.

Better strategy: Reshape the pain of regret from a suffocating force that holds you down into a jab with a stick that prods you forward—that's still not pleasant, but it's tolerable and potentially useful. *To do this, complete as many of the following five steps as possible…*

1. Undo the regret. If you regret becoming estranged from a family member, for example, reach out to see if the relationship can be revived. Undoing a regret doesn't mean no trace of it will linger in your mind—even if an estranged relationship is revived, you'll still regret the lost time and hurt feelings—but it does put a positive final chapter on what had been a purely negative story.

If there's no way to fix what's been broken, offer a sincere apology to someone who has suffered due to your mistake. If this person grants you forgiveness, it should help blunt the pain of the regret. If forgiveness isn't offered, your apology could remind you not to define yourself by that mistake.

Regrets that involve long-ago inaction are tricky to undo. If you regret not spending more time with your children, there's no way to undo that once those kids are grown. If you regret not marrying a long-ago love, it's almost certainly too late to do so if he/she married someone else. If you regret not saving for retirement, there's no realistic way to fix that once you're retired.

Regrets of inaction grow more common as we grow older—surveys show that 20-year-olds generally have roughly as many regrets about things they've done as opportunities they've missed. But regrets about missed opportunities dramatically outnumber regrets about actions for people age 50 and up. Perhaps that's because the older we get, the clearer it becomes that a missed opportunity was the best one that will ever come our way.

When it's too late to undo an inaction: At least share the story of this regret with younger people, such as your grandchildren. Encourage them to grab opportunities when they arise. The possibility that someone else could learn from your mistake could add a positive note to your painful memory. Don't be disheartened if these young people don't immediately take the lesson to heart—it still might be useful to them down the road.

2. Search for the silver lining. When a regret comes to mind, complete the sentence, "That went terribly, but at least…" Ask yourself, *In what way could the situation have gone worse?* Maybe an investment you made fell sharply in value…but at least you didn't put all of your savings into it. Maybe your marriage was a disaster…but at least you got some wonderful children out of it.

Finding the "at least"—and calling it to mind whenever the regret resurfaces—helps transform the regret from a wave of negative emotion into a more nuanced situation with plusses and minuses. Even if the minuses vastly outweigh the plusses, this forces you to start to think about the regret rationally.

3. Talk or write about the regret. Many people relive their regrets endlessly but never attempt to dissect them and understand what really happened and why—perhaps because digging deeper into these awful memories seems too painful. It turns out the opposite is true—closely examining negative events tends to reduce the pain they cause.

A 2006 study by a psychology professor at University of California, Riverside found that talking or writing about a negative experience for 15 minutes a day for three consecutive days boosted the writer's psychological well-being in ways that simply thinking about the experience did not. When we think about a regret, we might tell ourselves that we're sorting through what happened, but there's a good chance that we're letting the regret remain a mental abstraction—a big, ill-defined cloud of negativity that we're afraid to examine closely. When we write or speak out loud about the regret, we force ourselves to analyze our thoughts on the subject, and that can help us see our regrets for what they truly are—ordinary missteps, not evidence that we're fools or monsters.

Interestingly, researchers also found that it's best not to talk or write much about life's happy memories. Analyzing these too closely tends to sap the sense of joy they provide, just as analyzing regrets saps their sorrow.

4. Practice self-compassion. Do you dress yourself down about your regrets with endless thoughts such as, *How could I have been so stupid?* Or perhaps build yourself up, filling your inner monolog with mental pep talks such as, *You can overcome this.* It turns out that the best self-talk strategy for rebounding from regret is…neither of those.

Instead, treat yourself with the same understanding you would offer a friend if he/she made the mistake—this is known as self-compassion. When a regret nags at you, remind yourself that you're not the first person to make this mistake and you won't be the last. Self-compassion doesn't let you off

Naming Specific Emotions Helps Control Them

It is common to feel a cascade of emotions at stressful times—such as sadness, anger and anxiety all mixed together. Separating the emotions and giving them names lets you become mindful of what stress-caused feelings you are experiencing. In a study of students, those who differentiated between and named their emotions did not have as high a spike in overall negative feelings as those who did not differentiate.

Elise Kalokerinos, PhD, lecturer, school of psychology, University of Newcastle, Callaghan, Australia, and leader of a study published in *Psychological Science*.

the hook, but it does normalize and neutralize your regrets.

Studies conducted by University of Texas psychologist Kristin Neff, PhD, over the past 15 years found that self-compassion is linked with optimism, happiness, wisdom, initiative, and mental toughness...and it's negatively correlated with depression, anxiety, and shame.

5. Study your regrets from a distance. The powerful negative emotions attached to regret can make it hard to learn from the mistake—the pain and shame overwhelm objective analysis.

Try this: Imagine that your misstep was committed by someone else and that you're a "doctor of regret sciences." Your job is to examine your patient's missteps and prescribe the best response to them and lessons that can be drawn. E-mail your findings to yourself as if sending them to the patient— refer to the person who made the misstep as "you," not "I." Studies conducted by researchers at University of Illinois and University of Pennsylvania and researchers at University of Michigan found that using the pronoun "you" normalizes negative experiences, helps people find meaning in them, and deepens their commitment to improving behavior.

If a regret is a fresh wound, imagine that 10 years have passed and that you're looking back on the event. What really happened? What can you learn from this? A 2015 study by University of California researchers found that this time-shift trick reduces stress and improves problem-solving ability.

7 Strategies to Handle Tough Problems

David Posen, MD, former family physician who specializes in stress and lifestyle counseling and author of five best-selling books including *Always Change a Losing Game* and *Authenticity: A Guide to Living in Harmony with Your True Self.* DavidPosen.com

Do you often feel stymied by obstacles in your career or personal life? It's easy to get mired in the same negative patterns of thinking or action (or inaction) that leave you feeling bad or like you are just spinning your wheels. It's like wearing blinders that keep you focused in one direction even when that's not the best direction to take.

We can shift gears by changing the way we look at, assess and act on a situation. Imagine that you're about to host an outdoor party when suddenly it starts pouring. You would not continue to set up tables and chairs in the rain. You would brainstorm workable alternatives. That's the mindset to bring to any type of problem.

There are three ways to deal with any stressful situation—change the situation... change your attitude toward the situation or the way you think about it...or remove yourself from the situation. The technique for changing your attitude is called *reframing*.

7 Ways to Reframe

Here are seven reframing techniques to try, depending on the type of dilemma you're facing...

•**Choose a positive interpretation of a negative situation.**

Example: You feel disappointed at having to cancel your trip of a lifetime due to a family illness. Remind yourself that disappointments happen and, hopefully, you'll be able to fly again soon. In the meantime, view the booked vacation time as an opportunity to relax, read, pursue a hobby, connect with friends and find other activities to fuel your curiosity and your soul.

• **Choose a more positive interpretation of an ambiguous situation.**

Example: Someone yawns while you're giving a presentation, and you take it as a sign that things are not going well. But that person is just as likely to be tired from a poor night's sleep as he/she is bored by your talk. You can choose to believe it's a tired yawn.

Another example: You try to talk to your spouse about something, but he acts distant and rushes to end the conversation. The knee-jerk reaction is to feel dismissed or to wonder, *What did I do wrong?* It's also possible that he had something else on his mind and the timing wasn't ideal for him to listen.

• **Look for benefits that aren't obvious.**

Example: Company layoffs result in your being given added responsibilities in areas where your skills are limited, and now you're in panic mode. Reframe it as a great opportunity to add to your skill-set and expand your résumé. Talk to your boss about seminars or other training that will help you excel.

• **Wait a beat.** This involves becoming an observer rather than a participant. Take a step back—sometimes literally—and just watch.

Examples: Is your grandchild having a temper tantrum? Remind yourself that kids misbehave when they're frustrated. Is a friend ranting at you over something inconsequential? Let her air her grievances and tell yourself, *This is probably more about her than about me* or *Sometimes people have a bad day.*

• **Reinterpret motives or intent behind someone's behavior.** Sometimes it's better to give the other person the benefit of the doubt than to think the worst.

Example: You sent an important e-mail, but a day later you still haven't received a response and you fear you're being ignored. It could be that your e-mail went to the recipient's spam folder or that she is busy or unwell. A simple follow-up phone call may resolve it.

• **Put events into a wider context.** Is the problem bothering you today going to matter a week from now or impact your happiness or well-being?

Example: If your stock portfolio took a hit, remind yourself that you're still ahead of where you were a year ago.

• **Shift your focus to what's there instead of what's missing.**

Example: You've met several milestones in a yearlong plan for achieving better health…but instead of congratulating yourself, you're doing a lot of hand-wringing over losing less weight than you wanted. Reframe by celebrating the successes. Then create a plan to reach the last goal.

Habits That Hold You Back

To successfully change your thinking, you may have to undo these common "Mind Traps."

• **Holding on to old beliefs.** Any time you make decisions based on what you think you need to, should or must do, you're basing your actions on beliefs that may not be serving you well.

Example: Thinking you must bake a cake for your spouse's birthday despite being so busy with work. You can celebrate just as well with a special selection from the bakery.

• **Negative self-talk.** Many people stay stuck because they berate themselves—*I'll never succeed with improving my diet* or *What will my family think if I go to the gym instead of making dinner for everyone?* Start to believe in yourself and give yourself permission to do things that make you happy. Try a new approach, get over barriers, or let go of the baggage or guilt that's been keeping you and your loved ones blocked. It will take time to change a lifelong habit of negative self-talk to create a new habit of positive self-talk and give yourself permission to change. Stay aware, and when you catch yourself, change the inner conversation.

• **Having unrealistic expectations.** When something's reasonable, that means it makes sense to you. "Realistic" refers to how likely it is to happen. Maybe you constantly badger your introverted spouse about being lively at parties and family occasions, but is it realistic to expect him to do that? Reframe your thinking to accept his personality as it is, and the bickering over this issue will stop.

• **Looking for the "perfect" solution.** Many people ignore possible solutions because they don't want to make trade-offs, but every decision involves some level of trade-off. Waiting for the perfect solution usually means you stay stuck. The least-bad option still could be a great choice.

• **Solutions are rarely all or nothing.** There are many increments between any two extremes. I suggest writing on a white board or a piece of paper five or six steps that can take you from one extreme to the other. Then choose a middle ground you can live with.

Example: Between working 60-hour weeks, which leads to self-neglect, and working the typical 40 hours, which a workaholic might see as laziness, there are options that leave you time for needed self-care. These could include taking formal lunch breaks each day, working late just two nights a week and not working on weekends. If your goal is to get into a more rigorous exercise regimen but you think that means either going to the gym for hours every day, which you don't have time for, or not doing it at all, map out more modest options that will improve your fitness level, such as taking a gym class every few days or weight-training twice a week and doing other activities with your spouse on the other days.

Getting Started

If you're unsure of how to begin to resolve a troubling issue, an effective exercise is to write down why it is stressful, what your current behavior or approach to it is and how

---

The Exercise Cure for Stress and Anxiety

Regular Aerobic Exercise Fights Stress Best

Walking, running, biking and/or swimming at least a few times a week much more effectively strengthens the brain's resilience when stressful events occur than non-aerobic exercise such as weightlifting. And regular workouts are much better than any form of exercise done only when a stressful event occurs—such as doing a 10-mile run the day before something stressful is anticipated. An ongoing exercise regimen leads to an increase in the protein *galanin*, which promotes behavioral resilience after stress occurs. Higher galanin levels do not reduce immediate feelings of stress, but they help the body cope with its impact more effectively.

Study by researchers at Emory University School of Medicine, Atlanta, published in *Journal of Neuroscience*.

Exercise Away Your Anxiety

Participants in a 12-week exercise program that included a 60-minute training session three times a week, including strength-training and aerobic exercises, had improved anxiety levels. Most participants reported going from a moderate or high level of anxiety to a low level. Those who did moderate exercise were three times as likely to report fewer and less severe symptoms of anxiety...and those who exercised strenuously, nearly five times as likely.

Study by researchers at University of Gothenburg, Sweden, published in *Journal of Affective Disorders*.

---

else you can think about it. Stop focusing on the action you need to take—which might seem unpleasant or overwhelming—and shift your thinking to focus on the payoffs.

Losing weight is an example. Rather than write down that you'll have to cut calories and give up high-fat foods (the action), write

111

how this will result in better heart and over-all health, feeling comfortable in clothes and being less out of breath when you exercise (the benefits).

If you think only about the problem, you'll think only of the obvious answer or the one that you already know.

Also: The psychological benefits of writing with pen and paper are more powerful than typing on a keyboard. When you write, other thoughts will come to you.

Anxiety's Hidden Lessons

Carla Marie Manly, PhD, a clinical psychologist and wellness expert in Sonoma County, California. Dr. Manly specializes in the treatment of anxiety, depression, trauma, and relationship issues. She is author of *Joy From Fear* and *Date Smart.* DrCarlaManly.com

On March 4, 1933, Franklin D. Roosevelt inspired a generation with his statement, "The only thing we have to fear is fear itself." While Roosevelt was referring to the immense challenges of the Great Depression, his words still ring true. Most people are indeed afraid of fear and do their best to escape it. But running from the feeling is not the same as eliminating the cause of it. Left unaddressed, fear festers below the surface, where it can transform into anxiety, an ever-present, amorphous sense of dread that is no longer anchored to a specific event or object.

If instead of avoiding fears you learn to confront them, you can do more than banish anxiety: You can use them to better understand yourself and learn to live a richer, fuller life. The following strategies can help you start your journey.

Consider Therapy

If you tell your doctor that you're experiencing anxiety, you're likely to walk away with a prescription. For some people, medication offers an effective quick fix, but it's a partial solution that addresses only the symptoms of anxiety. If pharmaceuticals were the whole answer, we would see a decline in the incidence rates of anxiety that coincides with the dramatic increase in prescriptions, but the opposite is true.

Addressing symptoms alone is clearly not working. To conquer fear and anxiety, you also need to address the underlying causes of anxiety. A therapist can be a valuable partner in this process, while books like *Joy From Fear* offer exercises that you can work on at home.

Avoid Unhealthy Coping Mechanisms

Many people don't know how to feel and process their feelings—or often even recognize them. Instead, they turn to external solutions. Shopping, overeating, drinking alcohol, or using drugs may give people a quicker fix than practicing yoga, walking, meditating, or using psychotherapy, but the benefits are transitory.

Think of fear as a two-sided coin. On one side, destructive fear draws you to unhealthy coping mechanisms, avoidance, and self-doubt. But the other side, constructive fear, helps you see that something isn't right, but prompts you to look for positive solutions. For example, if you are afraid that a relationship is failing, destructive fear could lure you to drinking alcohol or overeating to numb and avoid your feelings. Constructive fear, on the other hand, could lead you to explore options that transform and improve what you're worried about. Instead of overeating, perhaps you could plan date nights to rekindle the romance.

Watch Your Media Diet

There is an old saying, "You are what you eat" that can apply to media, too. Think of it as, "What you consume becomes part of you." If you're constantly reading or watching news that focuses on frightening and upsetting things, you're supplying your brain with endless fuel for anxiety. Studies show that high media consumers have more anxiety and a higher level of body loathing than people who consume less.

It's fine to check the news once a day to be informed about what's going on in the world, but you don't need to know what's going on 24 hours a day in every part of the world.

Also, limit your exposure to social media sites, such as Facebook and Twitter, which often serve as triggers for outrage and frustration.

Exercise

Exercise can boost mental clarity and improve brain function. It stimulates the release of endorphins, dopamine, norepinephrine, and serotonin, all of which can improve mood. A brisk, 10-minute walk has the power to reduce symptoms of depression and anxiety, decrease your stress level, and fight fatigue. Use your walking time to consciously let go of life's stressors—to leave them behind you as you move forward.

Gentle exercises such as yoga, tai chi, and qigong combine gentle movement, stretching, breathing, and elements of meditation that can also help reduce stress.

Positive Messages and Imagery

Find a positive message or mantra that feels strong and calming for you. Repeat it when you are calm so your brain associates the words with a positive, relaxed state. Keep a copy of your statement in your wallet, on your mirror, and on your desk. It can be helpful to repeat the words as you press a specific finger or place on your hand to anchor the calming feeling. At the slightest hint of anxiety or stress, repeat the mantra.

Next, envision yourself in a real or imaginary place that feels serene. Etch the details into your mind. When a stressful situation begins to arise, take a break to imagine yourself in that beautiful, stress-free environment.

Get to Sleep

A report from The National Institutes of Health indicated that "after several nights of losing sleep—even a loss of just one to two hours

per night—your ability to function suffers as if you haven't slept at all for a day or two." Not only does sleep loss affect your mood overall, but exhaustion also makes it harder to resist the destructive side of fear and seek out opportunities for transformation.

Write

If you struggle to fall asleep because your mind is filled with worries or plans, keep a notepad beside your bed where you can write down to-do list items and things you don't want to forget. Once pesky thoughts are on the notepad, the psyche can unwind and rest.

Keeping a journal works in a similar way. Writing down your stresses, anxieties, and fears can help release unwanted energy. Let your emotions and thoughts flow freely; don't self-edit or worry about grammar. When you are finished, close the journal and resist the temptation to reread it, as that can bring up self-criticism and judgment.

Time to Worry

If you are a chronic worrier, make a daily time to worry—ideally a few hours before bedtime. At the set time, sit down with a pen and paper and allow yourself to worry for five or 10 minutes. As counterintuitive as this may sound, it works. Instead of trying to force yourself not to worry, which can actually increase worrying, the busy mind often calms down once it knows it will be allowed to worry at a set time.

Enjoy Yourself

Laughter can relieve stress and elevate your mood. Whether you call a friend to share comical memories or watch a rerun of your favorite funny television show, remember that laughter is a very powerful medicine.

For an added bonus, cuddle up with a loved one or pet. Touch can relieve stress, decrease anxiety, and elevate your mood.

Routines

The routines that we live with day in and day out create hard-wired patterns and felt memories.

Think *nonjudgmentally* about how you begin most of your days. Do you wake to the alarm clock screaming at you? Do your first thoughts take you to work and to-do lists? When it's time to head to work, do you hug your partner or pet goodbye and move out into the world with a smile?

Whatever your routine may be, ask yourself, "Is this how I want to start my day?" Give your evening routine the same objective review. Develop routines that make your home life feel safe and free from the external world's stressors.

As you use these steps, you will find that you enjoy life just a bit more each day. Listen to yourself. Listen to your needs. Move forward consciously and compassionately, taking one small step at a time.

Seeking Mental Health Services

Charles B. Inlander is a consumer advocate and health-care consultant based in Fogelsville, Pennsylvania. He was the founding president of the nonprofit People's Medical Society, a consumer-advocacy organization credited with key improvements in the quality of U.S. health care, and is author or coauthor of more than 20 consumer-health books.

No matter where you may live, mental health services are available to help you get through any difficult period. These services may be as close as your computer or telephone, located at a nearby hospital or associated with a church or other religious-based organization. Some are free services, others may have fees, and many are covered by Medicare or Medicaid or your private health insurance. *Here's how to find mental health services...*

•**Start with your primary care physician.** Your primary care doctor is a good

---

Diet Improves Mood in People with Bipolar Disorder

A 12-week study showed that eating fewer omega-6 fatty acids (red meat and vegetable oils) and more omega-3 fatty acids (tuna, salmon, and flaxseed) reduced mood variability in people taking medication for bipolar disorder.

Penn State Health Milton S. Hershey Medical Center, Hershey, Pennsylvania.

---

starting point. Frankly discuss what you are feeling. Ask for suggestions or referrals to the best mental health professionals in your area that might be appropriate for your needs. Don't be surprised if the doctor suggests a non-physician such as a licensed social worker, psychologist, guidance counselor, or stress management classes run by county or municipal health departments.

•**Widen your search.** There are many possible sources of counseling and stress management you should check out. Many people turn to their pastor, rabbi, or other religious leaders for counseling. You may also find services at locally run senior centers. Check with your local Department of Welfare or Area Agency on Aging (most counties have one) for a list of available services. Go online or have someone search for mental health services in your area.

•**Seeking specialized help.** There are numerous mental health support programs when you may be suffering from severe stress or anxiety. Call 911 if you are feeling suicidal and you'll be connected to a trained professional to help you. There are special services for veterans that can be accessed through the Veterans Administration and/or county government. These services can be found online. Search for "mental health services in your community".

Obsessive Compulsive Disorder Breakthrough

James Greenblatt, MD, chief medical officer at Walden Behavioral Care in Waltham, Massachusetts, and assistant clinical professor of psychiatry at Tufts University School of Medicine and Dartmouth College Geisel School of Medicine. He is the founder of Psychiatry Redefined, an educational platform dedicated to the transformation of psychiatry.

It's human nature to have occasional worried thoughts or to overanalyze important decisions. Normally, these thought patterns dissipate quickly, but in people suffering from obsessive compulsive disorder (OCD), letting go of repetitive thoughts isn't so effortless. Instead, relentless ideas, impulses, or images inundate the brain, mentally imprisoning the individual in recurrent, irrational thought patterns.

These senseless obsessions often drive the individual to ritualistic behaviors or compulsions—like handwashing, hoarding, counting or hairpulling—in an attempt to temporarily relieve their anxiety. A person with OCD staggers through life with a sense of powerlessness—fully aware the behavior is abnormal, but unable to stop.

Treatments Miss the Root Cause

There are two standard treatment options: selective serotonin reuptake inhibitors (SSRIs) and cognitive behavioral therapy (CBT). But even with these two treatments, only one out of five patients experiences complete recovery from OCD, and relapse is common. The reason for this failure: Conventional treatments don't address the root cause of OCD.

An Undertreated Ailment

OCD is the fourth most common psychiatric illness in the United States. In fact, it's estimated that OCD is more common than diabetes. But in spite of its prevalence, it is underdiagnosed and undertreated—with more than half of people receiving no treatment at all.

Inflammation and OCD

Inflammation is a natural feature of the immune system. When there is a virus, bacteria, or other foreign invader, the immune system activates to neutralize the threat, producing the telltale redness, swelling, heat, and pain that are the signs of acute inflammation. But an immune system that is out of balance can generate low-grade, chronic inflammation—including inflammation in the brain (neuroinflammation). In the brain, cytokines produce an enzyme called IDO (indoleamine 2,3–dioxygenase). IDO decreases the level of serotonin, the neurotransmitter that regulates mood and anxiety. (Every medication approved for OCD works by increasing serotonin levels.)

Along with this biochemical understanding, there is a growing body of clinical and scientific evidence that immune dysregulation underlies OCD. Psychiatrists know that autoimmune disease—when the immune system attacks the body as if it were a foreign invader—is rampant among those with OCD. For example, a 2021 study in the *International Journal of Environmental Research and Public Health* showed that people with OCD had triple the risk of developing the autoimmune illness Sjogren's Syndrome than the non-OCD population.

Researchers have identified two other neuroinflammatory disorders that play a role in OCD: pediatric autoimmune neuropsychiatric disorder associated with streptococcus (PANDAS) and pediatric acute-onset neuropsychiatric syndrome (PANS). In PANDAS, children who have had a streptococcal infection go on to rapidly develop OCD, practically overnight, because the immune system attacks the part of the brain (basal ganglia) where OCD is thought to originate. In PANS, other types of infections, such as Lyme disease, mononucleosis, and the flu, are also thought to quickly trigger OCD.

Nutritional Support

Along with neuroinflammation, a number of other factors affect serotonin levels, including genes, diet, stress, and neurotoxins. Those factors can be directly affected by nutritional therapy—a key treatment for OCD that is overlooked by conventional psychiatry.

Integrative psychiatrists, on the other hand, are open to both conventional and natural treatments for OCD. (You can find a list of integrative psychiatrists at PsychologyToday.com/us/psychiatrists/integrative).

Anti-OCD Supplements

An integrative psychiatrist may recommend one or more of the following commonly used supplements. *Always talk to your physician before taking any new supplements...*

• **5HTP.** 5-hydroxtryptophan is a precursor of serotonin that has provided relief for many patients with OCD. The typical dose is 100 to 300 milligrams (mg). In some cases, doses as high as 600 mg may be needed.

• **Vitamin B12.** A deficiency of this serotonin-boosting B vitamin is common in OCD. Although most conventional doctors consider blood levels between 200 to 1,100 picograms per millilitre (pg/mL) normal, any level under 500 pg/mL should be considered low, especially with OCD patients. If a patient is low, a weekly intramuscular B12 injection until the blood level reaches 900 pg/mL can be effective. Some patients experience a dramatic decrease in symptoms with just this treatment.

• **Folate.** This B vitamin is crucial in the manufacture of serotonin, and it can boost the effectiveness of antidepressants. However, some people with OCD can't metabolize

The Little-Known Neurotoxin That Can Trigger OCD

The toxic gut bacteria *Clostridia* can generate 3-(3-hydroxyphenyl)-3-hydroxypropionic acid (HPHPA), a compound that disrupts normal brain function. High levels of HPHPA are a feature of many psychiatric diseases, including OCD. Your doctor can order a urine test for HPHPA from a laboratory that specializes in digestive disorders, such as the Great Plains Laboratory. If HPHPA is detected, consider high-dose probiotics that supply 50 to 300 billion colony-forming units daily. You might also need to take an antibiotic, such as *vancomycin* (Vancocin).

—Dr. James Greenblatt

folate because of a genetic abnormality. If you have OCD, consider having a methylenetetrahydrofolate reductase mutations (MTHFR) test to see if you lack the enzymes to process folate. If the test is positive, you may need to take one to 15 grams of folate daily.

• **Zinc.** This mineral is a crucial cofactor in the production of serotonin. A zinc deficiency also can have a number of other negative consequences for health, such as depression, poor metabolism of essential fatty acids, lower melatonin, more vulnerability to stress, and digestive difficulties. Consider a dose of 30 mg daily.

• **Inositol.** In some patients, supplementing with inositol—a vitamin-like compound that affects the serotonin receptors on cells—is the only treatment needed for OCD. Consider taking 5 to 10 grams (g) daily, starting off with 1 g and increasing by 1 g weekly. Taking too much inositol too quickly can cause gastrointestinal discomfort.

• **Omega-3 fatty acids.** The brain is 60 percent fat, and optimal brain function requires healthy fats such as the omega-3 fatty acids eicosapentaenoic acid (EPA) and docosahexaenoic acid (DHA) found in fish oil. Consider a daily supplement containing 3 grams of omega-3 fatty acids with a slightly higher ratio of EPA to DHA.

• **N-acetylcysteine (NAC).** This compound is a derivative of the amino acid cysteine and helps produce glutathione, a powerful anti-inflammatory antioxidant. In a study published in the *Journal of Clinical Psychopharmacology*, 36 women with OCD who didn't respond to serotonin-boosting medication were divided into two groups: One group took NAC daily and one group took a placebo. A total of 53 percent of the NAC group had significant improvement in OCD symptoms, compared with 15 percent of the placebo group. Consider taking 2 to 3 g of NAC daily.

- **Glycine.** This compound is a precursor to glutamine and gamma aminobutyric acid (GABA), two calming neurotransmitters that can inhibit obsessive thinking. Consider taking 3 to 6 g of glycine daily.
- **Vitamin D.** This vitamin can lower neuroinflammation. Your doctor can test you for vitamin D deficiency (blood level below 30 nanograms per milliliter [ng/ml]). If you're deficient, take 2,000 to 4,000 international units (IU) of vitamin D daily to bring levels to at least 50 ng/ml.
- **Magnesium.** To cool inflammation, take 400 to 800 mg of magnesium citrate or glycinate daily, divided into two or three doses.

Lifestyle Support

Several lifestyle factors can also affect OCD…

- **Poor sleep.** Treat insomnia with improved sleep hygiene. Go to bed at the same time every night and get up at the same time every morning, giving yourself at least seven hours in bed.
- **Stress.** Stress not only causes inflammation but also worsens the symptoms of OCD. Reduce stress by learning and practicing mindfulness-based stress reduction techniques.
- **Eliminate gluten and casein.** People who are missing the digestive enzyme DPP-4 can't adequately break down certain proteins from dairy (casein) and wheat (gluten), producing morphine-like compounds (casomorphin, gliadorphin) that can play a role in OCD. Taking the DPP-4 digestive enzyme, which breaks down gluten, and eliminating dairy and gluten-containing foods (wheat, rye, barley, oats) sometimes significantly or even completely resolves symptoms, particularly in children and adolescents with OCD. The Great Plains Laboratory tests for casomorphin and gliadorphin in the urine (GreatPlainsLaboratory.com).

Dealing with Adult Attention-Deficit Disorder

Richard Gallagher, PhD, director of executive function and organizational skills treatment programs, Institute for Attention Deficit Hyperactivity and Behavior Disorders of the Child Study Center at NYU Langone Health, New York.

Researchers estimate that 4 percent of American adults meet the diagnostic criteria for attention-deficit hyperactivity disorder (ADHD).

This chronic condition can make it difficult to focus, to sit still, to be organized, and much more, affecting sufferers' personal and professional lives. It can lead to depression, anxiety, and a higher risk of substance use.

If You Suspect You Have ADHD

The table below lists some common attributes of the two main subtypes of ADHD. (You can have both in what's called combination ADHD.) If these statements ring true for you, particularly if you've had symptoms since childhood, talk to your physician, a mental health professional, or a neurologist with ADHD expertise for a full evaluation. In some cases, ADHD symptoms become apparent only as life and work demands increase in adulthood.

Hyperactive/Impulsive	Inattentive
I feel compelled to move around..	I don't pay close attention to details.
I get bored easily and crave excitement.	I have difficulty sustaining attention.
I generally feel restless.	I often don't listen when people speak.
I have a difficult time waiting in lines.	I don't follow through on instructions.
I finish sentences for other people.	I have difficulty organizing tasks.
I talk excessively.	I am easily distracted.
I fidget whenever I need to sit still.	I lose things that are necessary for tasks.
I have trouble keeping quiet when working or engaging in leisure activities.	I dislike and avoid tasks that require sustained mental effort.

Treatment Options

While ADHD is a lifelong condition, with the proper recognition and diagnosis, treatments can reduce the impact of the symptoms.

• **Medication.** Daily medication can help ADHD sufferers improve their focus and behavior control. The most effective medications stimulate the brain areas responsible for directing and sustaining attention as well as those responsible for selecting and moderating behaviors and choices. These include drugs like *amphetamine* and *dextroamphetamine* (Adderall) and *methylphenidate* (Concerta). These medications come with potential side effects, however, including sleep problems, decreased appetite, weight loss, increased blood pressure, dizziness, headaches, stomachaches, moodiness, and irritability.

• **Psychotherapy.** Whether it's used instead of, or alongside, medication, cognitive-behavioral therapy can help people with ADHD identify and correct thinking errors. For example, many people with ADHD believe that they work best under time pressure, which can lead to procrastination. A therapist can help those patients understand that they are embracing this mistaken belief to avoid completing tasks that are difficult because of a lack of attention control.

Once patients recognize and accept this common pattern, they can start to learn how to use tools and routines to make tasks more manageable. A psychotherapist can help adults with ADHD learn how to slow down to write things down, develop plans for complicated tasks, manage emotional reactions, and build social skills.

Inviting family members into therapy sessions can help adults with ADHD improve relationships, too.

Next Steps

Researchers are developing and testing tools such as mindfulness meditation training and brain stimulation through the use of low-power magnetic fields and low-power infrared light to ease ADHD symptoms. Initial results are promising, but these treatments are not yet widely available.

How to Say "No" to a Drink at Social Gatherings

Ruby Warrington, creator of the term "sober curious" and author of multiple sober-curious books including *Sober Curious: The Blissful Sleep, Greater Focus, Limitless Presence, and Deep Connection Awaiting Us All on the Other Side of Alcohol* and *The Sober Curious Reset: Change the Way You Drink in 100 Days or Less.* Warrington is host of the "Sober Curious" podcast. RubyWarrington.com

Are you "sober curious"? You're in good company! According to Google Trends, searches for "benefits of quitting drinking" spiked 100 percent in 2021 in the U.S....and sales of nonalcoholic beer have increased 86 percent over the past three years, per Instacart marketplace data. Being sober curious doesn't mean swearing off wine, booze, or beer forever. It simply means that you're questioning your personal relationship with drinking and the way society views alcohol.

But a significant portion of the population continues to drink, and that means you may face pressure to imbibe at social gatherings. *Here are some strategies to take a temporary break from alcohol or quit altogether...*

• **Carry a beverage.** Club soda or sparkling water with a citrus wedge looks enough like a cocktail to dissuade most people from asking, "Why aren't you having a drink?" You don't need to hold one all night long, but if it helps prevent unwanted conversations, go for it.

And thanks to a boom in nonalcoholic beverages, many restaurants and bars are stocked with innovative no- or low-alcohol options, from alcohol-free spirits and beer to creative mocktails. These fun drinks replicate the festive feel of social gatherings, taste delicious and won't cause a hangover.

Verbal Habits for Better Interactions

Count to five before replying to someone to give yourself time to think of the best thing to say. *Avoid immediately reacting* when something upsetting occurs—wait a day or half a day to get your emotions under control. *Ask questions* when speaking to people to get them talking more—do not spend your time talking to or at them. *Repeat back* what another person has told you even if you don't agree—this shows that you are paying attention and trying to understand. *Increase the effectiveness of compliments* by first saying, "You might not know this, but…"—the phrase gets people tuned into what you say next. *Start conversations with specific questions,* not throwaway lines—instead of "How are you?" try saying, "How was your weekend trip?"

Inc.com

• **Craft your "no" script.** If you're empty-handed at a social gathering, chances are someone is going to offer you a drink. Be prepared with a few possible responses. At a business event, a simple, "No, thanks" or "I can't…I'm driving" should suffice. At a family gathering, respond with what feels comfortable. That might be a quick "I'm not drinking this month—like Dry January, only it is Dry [insert current month]."

If anyone pressures you, it likely has more to do with their own relationship with alcohol—perhaps they are concerned that they're boring without a few drinks or they're drinking to escape a personal problem.

• **Enlist your friends.** If alcohol usually makes an appearance at your monthly get-togethers with friends, you may want to mention ahead of time that you won't be drinking.

Examples: "I know we normally drink wine, but would you mind if I bring my own soft drinks? I'd love to feel fresh the next morning"…or "I'm trying something new. Instead of meeting for dinner and drinks, why don't we grab coffee and take a long walk?"

• **Remember your why.** Make a list of the reasons why you're reexamining your relationship with alcohol. Shine a light on what you'll be gaining rather than focus on what you'll be missing. Are you seeking better health? Better sleep? To be more productive or more present for your kids? Have you been disappointed with how you act when under the influence? Write your reasons on a piece of paper or in your phone's notes app, and reread it before entering alcohol-related settings.

• **Celebrate your first successes.** You'll have many "sober firsts"—your first sober wedding, dinner party, vacation. Most people get a wonderful confidence boost after each sober first, as you prove to yourself that you don't "need" alcohol. Let yourself feel proud… and congratulate yourself on prioritizing you.

Sleep Loss Can Cause Mental and Physical Deterioration

Soomi Lee, PhD, assistant professor in the School of Aging Studies, University of South Florida, Tampa.

Getting fewer than six hours of sleep can cause mental and physical symptoms after just one night, with the effects adding up and peaking on day three. Many of us think that we can pay our sleep debt on weekends and be more productive on weekdays. However, results from a recent study from the School of Aging Studies at the University of South Florida, Tampa, show that having just one night of sleep loss can significantly impair your daily functioning.

Hearth and Home Help Mental Health

Ways Baking Boosts Your Spirits

It is meditative—it requires full attention to do simple, repetitive tasks, such as measuring ingredients and mixing them. *It stimulates the senses*—the feel of ingredients, sounds of mixing them and the smell of the final product all can increase the body's production of feel-good endorphins. *It is nourishing, and that feels good*—baking means nourishing ourselves and others. *It is creative*—you can deviate from a recipe or follow it but apply creativity afterward—for instance, by making frosting look as pretty as possible. *It makes other people happy*—sharing baked goods or giving them to other people boosts social connections and makes everyone involved feel good.

Roundup of bakers reported on GoodNet.org.

Cleaning Is Good Therapy

Clutter can lead to decreased focus and to confusion and tension. People who described their living spaces as cluttered were more likely to be fatigued and depressed than those who described their homes as restful.

Reason: Cleaning gives a sense of mastery and control over your environment.

Cleaning also may boost physical health: People with clean homes tend to be healthier than those with cluttered or messy homes.

Roundup of research studies on cleaning and health, reported at VeryWellMind.com.

Seven Types of Rest We All Need

Saundra Dalton-Smith, MD, author of *Sacred Rest: Recover Your Life, Renew Your Energy, Restore Your Sanity*, writing at Ideas.TED.com.

Physical—passive (sleeping, napping) or active (yoga, massage). *Mental*—your mind can't keep exercising all the time, so schedule short breaks in your workday every two hours or so. *Sensory*—noises and lights can take their toll. Close your eyes occasionally and unplug from electronics toward the day's end. *Creative*—if you spend your days solving problems, reinvigorate by appreciating beauty, such as art, music and nature. *Emotional*—each of us, especially the people-pleaser types, need a safe space to express ourselves without worrying about who's judging. *Social*—some relationships are exhausting, so keep in touch with the people who bring you joy. *Spiritual*—include activities that serve a higher purpose and give you a feeling of belonging and love.

DIY Vagal Nerve Stimulation Improves Mood, Cognition in Sleepy People

Communications Biology

Sleep-deprived U.S. Air Force pilots reported feeling more energized and less fatigued after using a noninvasive cervical transcutaneous vagal nerve stimulation device. The gammaCore (electroCore) is approved for personal treatment of cluster headaches and migraines. The pilots demonstrated faster reaction times and improved multitasking after using the product.

Chapter 6

FOOD AND FITNESS

Sneaky Ways to Eat More Vegetables

You need to eat your vegetables for good health, but that can be easier said than done. Even if you really like the taste of veggies—which many people don't—it can be hard to get the recommended amounts into your day. That's where the concept of hiding them in other foods comes in. You can sneak veggies into just about anything you're making, boosting the health value of meals for you and your family—and the pickiest of eaters won't even taste them.

Breakfasts

Add zucchini or carrots to breakfast baked goods such as muffins. Try scrambling your eggs with minced broccoli or grated cauliflower. These additions don't change the texture of your eggs, and they give you your daily dose of anti-cancer cruciferous veggies. Try adding canned pumpkin puree to pancakes.

Smoothies

Add extra greens to a fruit smoothie. A large bunch of raw spinach will wilt down to nothing and the taste is easily hidden if you add other naturally sweet ingredients, especially pineapple and banana.

Sandwiches

Bulk up ground meat with carrot puree or chopped mushrooms. Or replace burgers with grilled portobello mushrooms. Choose Mexican-style tacos or quesadillas: Cut the cheese in half, and add lots of corn, onions, peppers, spinach, beans, and salsa.

Soups, Stews, and Casseroles

Thicken soup and add vegetables with pureed tomatoes, carrots, sweet potato, butternut squash, beans, and greens. Add corn, extra tomatoes, onions, garlic, and peppers to chili. Cauliflower, pumpkin, butternut squash, and carrots are all excellent additions to macaroni and cheese. The colors blend with the traditional dish and provide a nice nutrition boost.

Janet Bond Brill, PhD, RDN, FAND, registered dietitian nutritionist, a fellow of the Academy of Nutrition and Dietetics, and a nationally recognized nutrition, health and fitness expert who specializes in cardiovascular disease prevention. Based in Hellertown, Pennsylvania, Dr. Brill is the author of *Intermittent Fasting for Dummies, Blood Pressure DOWN, Cholesterol DOWN,* and *Prevent a Second Heart Attack.* DrJanet.com

Creamy Pumpkin Pasta Sauce

Ingredients...

    1 tsp. of extra virgin olive oil
    2 shallots, minced
    3 cloves of garlic, minced
    15 oz. can pumpkin purée
    8 oz. cannellini beans
    1 Tbsp. oregano
    1 tsp. cracked black pepper
    15 oz. low-sodium vegetable broth

Directions...

In a small saucepan, heat the olive oil over medium-low heat. Cook the shallots until soft and translucent (about 10 minutes). In a blender, add the cooked shallots and the rest of the ingredients in the recipe. Blend sauce until it is a smooth purée.

Yield: 8 servings (½ cup per serving).

Nutrition information per serving (pasta sauce only): *Calories:* 63 kcal, *Fat:* 1 g, *Cholesterol:* 0 mg, *Carbohydrate:* 12 g, *Dietary Fiber:* 3 g, *Protein:* 3 g, *Sodium:* 158 mg

Baked Goods and Desserts

Greens can be pureed and added into cake and brownie batter. Beets make a great addition to chocolate cake—the cocoa flavor disguises the beet's earthy flavor; plus the beets add sweetness. Sweet breads can be made using zucchini. Cookie batter does well with pureed pumpkin. Dark chocolate brownies taste great with added pureed beans.

Snacks

Instead of potato chips, try making kale chips. You get all the crunch and a huge nutrition boost. Zucchini is an incredibly versatile, mild-tasting vegetable that can be transformed into a variety of snacks. Zucchini chips are super simple to make. Slice and season with salt, pepper, and parmesan cheese; then bake in a hot oven until deeply golden and crisp.

Pasta Sauce

Add canned pumpkin to pasta sauce for large amounts of vitamin A to sustain sharp eyesight, the antioxidant beta-carotene to fight cancer, and vitamin C to maintain a healthy immune system

There's More to Five a Day

Study by researchers at Harvard Medical School and Brigham and Women's Hospital, both in Boston, published in *Circulation*.

Five produce servings a day are not enough to promote good health. The balance of fruits and vegetables also matters—and so do the specific items eaten. Two servings a day should include fruits with high levels of beta-carotene and vitamin C, such as berries and citrus fruits. The other three or more servings of produce should be vegetables—such as spinach, other leafy greens, and carrots. Starchy vegetables—including peas, corn, and potatoes—are not associated with reduced risk for death or chronic diseases.

Skin Nutrition: What to Eat to Keep the Glow

Janet Bond Brill, PhD, RDN, FAND, registered dietitian nutritionist who specializes in cardiovascular disease prevention. Based in Hellertown, Pennsylvania, Dr. Brill is the author of *Intermittent Fasting for Dummies, Blood Pressure DOWN, Cholesterol DOWN,* and *Prevent a Second Heart Attack*. DrJanet.com

Scientists are increasingly learning more about the relationship between diet, skin health and aging. *Let's look at the top foods known to contribute to better skin from the inside out...*

•**Avocado.** Avocados are chock full of healthy monounsaturated fat, which the skin needs to stay supple and moisturized. Avocados also are a good source of vitamins E and C, two of the most important antioxidants for your body. Both vitamins are involved in creating new, healthy skin. Some research links antioxidant compounds in avocado with preventing UV sun damage, thereby warding off wrinkles and premature aging.

• **Fatty fish.** Salmon, tuna, halibut, and herring are full of omega-3. A deficiency of this "good" fat has been shown to cause extremely dry skin, illustrating the necessity of getting this type of fat to keep skin flexible and moisturized. The high-quality protein content in fish contributes to the strength and creation of new, healthy cells. The exceptional amount of omega-3 fat, zinc, and vitamin E in fatty fish tame inflammation—a key cause of skin disorders and wrinkles.

• **Walnuts.** Walnuts are packed with the plant version of omega-3 fat called ALA. Walnuts contain a nice cache of vitamins and minerals such as vitamin E, selenium, and zinc. These nutrients help the skin heal, and they fight off bacteria and inflammation, creating a natural defense system that contributes to clearer, smoother skin. Try the walnut encrusted salmon recipe below to get a double dose of skin-healthy nutrients.

• **Soy.** Soy contains a plant chemical called isoflavones, which can either block or mimic estrogen in the body. Research has shown that consuming soy daily improves wrinkles and skin elasticity. In postmenopausal women, regular soy consumption has been shown to improve skin dryness and increase the collagen content, leading to smoother, stronger skin.

Take care of the largest organ in the body from the inside with a nutritious diet and from the outside by routinely using a good sunblock to prevent UV damage.

Walnut Encrusted Salmon

Ingredients…
    3 cloves of garlic
    ¾ cup walnuts
    ½ cup fresh cilantro
    2 tablespoons extra virgin olive oil

4 wild salmon fillets (about 6 oz. each)
1 teaspoon kosher salt
¼ teaspoon freshly ground pepper
Fresh lemon slices for garnish
Directions…

Preheat oven to 450°F. Mince the garlic in a food processor. Add in the walnuts and process to a fine consistency. Add cilantro until mixture is thick and pasty. Add olive oil and process until blended. Place salmon on a foil-lined baking tray and season both sides with salt and pepper. Spread the walnut mixture evenly over the fish. Bake for 20 minutes or until fish flakes easily with a fork. Garnish with lemon slices.

Yield: 4 servings (serving size: 1 salmon filet)

Nutritional Information Per Serving (1 salmon filet): Calories: 456, *Fat:* 32 g, *Cholesterol:* 94 mg, *Sodium:* 658 mg, *Carbohydrate:* 4 g, *Dietary Fiber:* 2 g, *Sugars:* 0 g, *Protein:* 37 g

Switch to a Vegetarian Diet the Easy Way

Roundup of dieticians reported on Shape.com.

If you're interested in trying a vegetarian diet, start slow—swap one meat serving for vegetables this week, two next week, etc. *Beans are your friends*—they're filling, packed with fiber and protein, and great substitutes for ground beef or chicken. *Eat whole, unrefined grains*—don't overload on empty carbs just because they're meatless… instead choose farro, buckwheat and oats, which have high amounts of vitamins, protein, and fiber. *Don't worry about protein*—a varied vegetarian diet will deliver all the proteins and amino acids you need because nuts, grains, beans, and everyday vegetables all have protein. *Use supplements as needed*—most vegetarians are low on iron and vitamin B-12, which are easily supplied by supplements.

Plant-Based Meat vs. Real Meat

Stephan van Vliet, PhD, is a postdoctoral researcher at Duke University, Durham, North Carolina, and leader of a study published in *Scientific Reports*. DMPI.Duke.edu

Plant-based meat substitutes are not nutritionally the same as real meat. Key differences go unmentioned on the Nutrition Facts panel on labels.

Example: Creatine and anserine, linked to improved cognitive function, are found in beef but not in plant-based substitutes. Occasionally eating substitutes likely is not harmful, but for a full nutritional palette it's best to eat plant and animal foods.

When the Only Food Is Fast Food...

Joel Fuhrman, MD, board-certified family physician and expert on nutrition and natural healing. A seven-time *New York Times* best-selling author, his books include *Fast Food Genocide: How Processed Food Is Killing Us and What We Can Do About It...Eat for Life...*and *Super Immunity*. He also runs the Eat To Live Retreat in San Diego, where guests can lose weight, overcome food addictions, and reshape their lives. DrFuhrman.com

Fast food is never good for you, but sometimes you just don't have a choice. When that happens, knowing the best options at the better restaurant chains means having a meal with the least negative impact on your health...and the least remorse about having to refuel this way.

Many fast-food restaurants still specialize in the equivalent of a heart attack on a bun (think double cheeseburger with bacon), but more progressive chains such as Panera and Starbucks have made improvements to their menus for both their customers' health and the environment. All fast-food chains post nutrition information on every menu choice on their websites, and many, such as Chipotle, allow you to customize their offerings—eliminating cheese, for instance, and doubling up on veggies. It's easy when you order on the restaurant's website or app, and making your selections in advance rules out any last-minute temptation—but also keep these guidelines in mind when you visit in person.

Make-It-Healthier Guidelines

When you can, the best choice is to head for a salad bar, freestanding or perhaps within a supermarket, where you can create your own meal. Search the Internet for salad bar locations when you're close to home or traveling. *But if you must go to a chain restaurant...*

•**Look up nutritional information before making your selections.**

Example: At Chick-fil-A, a packet of Light Italian Dressing has 25 calories while Zesty Apple Cider Vinaigrette has 230 and Avocado Lime Ranch has 310.

•**Choose healthful beans and bean-based menu items instead of meat options whenever possible.**

Example: A bean burrito with avocado and salsa (skip the sour cream) is tasty and filling.

•**Avoid special sauces and salad dressings,** particularly those made with mayonnaise or soybean/canola vegetable oils. Look for olive oil and vinegar or dressings with a base of tahini, avocado, nuts or tomato. Or opt for a plant-based salsa—a nutritional powerhouse naturally low in fat and cholesterol-free...it makes a great topping for almost anything.

•**Avoid foods prepared with toxic cooking methods**—char-broiling, flame-broiling, barbecuing and deep-frying all use high heat, which contributes to the formation of harmful compounds called *advanced glycation end products* (AGEs). The best choice is baked, and lightly grilled is better than flame-broiled. Soups, stews and vegan or beef chilis are good choices because they're made with water-based cooking methods, which limits AGEs. Avoid deep-fried fillets. Instead, opt for sashimi or sushi (order rolls with crab stick and cooked fish or veggie rolls with lots of avocado if you're concerned about the freshness of raw fish).

• **Order platters instead of white-bread/roll sandwiches.** Unless specifically whole-wheat flour, eating foods made with white flour is like eating sugar because they're absorbed so rapidly.

• **Have fresh fruit for dessert,** instead of pies and tarts laden with artificial ingredients and unhealthy fats and sugars.

Caution: Frozen yogurt can have a surprising amount of sugar.

On the Menu

Go with these healthier options at the following popular fast-food restaurants…

• **Panera.**

Breakfast: Fresh fruit, steel-cut oatmeal and Greek yogurt parfaits…or an egg-based baked Spinach and Artichoke Soufflé with red peppers and artichoke hearts.

Lunch and dinner: A wide array of salads with healthy ingredients, including the Mediterranean Bowl with Chicken…and the Baja Bowl with brown rice, quinoa, black bean and corn salsa, and assorted vegetables.

Another option: Slow-cooked All-Natural Turkey Chili with chickpeas and kidney beans, tomatillos and tomatoes (available seasonally). Panera also is known for its soups, such as the hearty Ten Vegetable Soup and the Autumn Squash Soup.

• **Starbucks.**

Breakfast: Variations on oatmeal such as Hearty Blueberry Oatmeal and Strawberry Overnight Grains with oatmeal, quinoa and chia seeds…or a Spinach, Feta and Egg White Wrap made with cage-free egg whites in a whole-wheat wrap. Avoid the baked goods.

Lunch: Chicken & Quinoa Protein Bowl with Black Beans and Greens or Hummus Protein Box…the plant-based Chickpea Bites & Avocado Protein Box with snap peas, mini carrots, dried cranberry and nut mix.

For the ease of a sandwich: Antibiotic-free Turkey & Pesto Panini on a ciabatta roll.

• **Chipotle.**

Chipotle's menu is built on bean-based offerings that can be customized.

Examples: With the Burrito Bowls, you can request extra beans (black and pinto), fajita vegetables (peppers and onions) and guacamole. The Lifestyle Bowls build on greens and guacamole and offer a Keto option, too. Add steak, chicken or pork if you're a meat eater and want the protein, or check out the vegan or vegetarian options. There's both white and brown rice.

• **Chick-fil-A.**

Breakfast: Healthier morning fare is limited to the fruit cup or Greek yogurt parfait.

Lunch or dinner: Grilled chicken comes as no-utensils-needed nuggets, a fillet and slices in salads such as the Spicy Southwest Salad with roasted corn, black beans, poblano chiles and red bell peppers…and the Market Salad with blue cheese, red and green apples, and berries. (Avoid the breaded versions of chicken.)

Also: Traditional Cobb salad…and the Cool Wrap—a flaxseed-flour flatbread filled with grilled chicken breast, green leaf lettuce and Jack and Cheddar cheeses.

• **Subway.**

Stories of no tuna in Subway's tuna sandwiches sparked a lot of news, but the company maintains that its tuna is real and even wild-caught. And it is a better choice than Subway's processed deli meat sandwiches.

Even better: Recently added items such as slow-roasted turkey and rotisserie-style chicken. You can order them in a protein bowl loaded with vegetables or on the multigrain bread made with whole grains, rye, cracked wheat, oats and seeds.

For vegetarians: Veggie Delite wrap. A great add-in is "smashed avocado"—just avocado and sea salt.

• **Taco Bell.**

Not necessarily known for healthy fare, Taco Bell has bean-based offerings that can

Gluten-Free Options Abound

Has your doctor told you to avoid gluten? Don't despair! There are many alternatives to this protein found in barley, rye, and wheat. Start by emphasizing fresh, unprocessed foods. Try homemade soups and stews made with chicken, beef, rice, or vegetables, which don't have gluten at all. If you use canned broth in a soup recipe, just be sure it is labeled gluten-free. For dessert, you can enjoy custard, sorbet, baked fruit, crustless pie, or meringue cookies. You can even bake cakes and cookies with a variety of gluten-free flours, which are now readily available online or in special sections at your local supermarket.

Cheryl Harris, MPH, RD, a registered dietitian with a private practice in northern Virginia.

be customized—order the bean burrito loaded with tomatoes, lettuce, black beans and jalapeño peppers, for instance…or put together your own combo of guacamole and a side serving of black beans with rice and onions.

• **Wendy's.**

The chain offers mostly burgers, but two of its fresh-made salads—the Southwest Avocado Salad and the Apple Pecan Salad—are built around grilled chicken.

• **McDonald's.**

Breakfast: Fruit and Maple Oatmeal with whole-grain oats, diced apples and a cranberry-raisin blend (there's no actual maple in it, but light cream and brown sugar).

Lunch or dinner: A plain hamburger (skip the bun)—far better than the various crispy chicken sandwiches. *Note:* That chicken patty is not pure chicken—it contains flour, oil and more than a dozen other ingredients.

Fast-food places to avoid: KFC…Burger King for anything other than a plain hamburger…Popeyes…and In-N-Out Burger.

Fad Foods

Janet Bond Brill, PhD, RDN, FAND, registered dietitian nutritionist, a fellow of the Academy of Nutrition and Dietetics, and a nationally recognized nutrition, health and fitness expert who specializes in cardiovascular disease prevention. Based in Hellertown, Pennsylvania, Dr. Brill is author of *Intermittent Fasting for Dummies, Blood Pressure DOWN, Cholesterol DOWN,* and *Prevent a Second Heart Attack.* DrJanet.com

From açaí to oat milk, certain foods rise to fame as devotees claim that they have dramatic health-improving qualities. Some of these foods have some promising research behind them, while others just have great marketing. *Here's the lowdown on four of the more recent fad foods…*

• **Sriracha** is a chili sauce made from a paste of chili peppers, vinegar, garlic, sugar, and salt. It is believed to have originated in Si Racha, Thailand, hence the moniker. This iconic hot sauce has a cult-like following. Search the internet and you will find sriracha-themed shirts and other wearable items that broadcast people's love of this addictive condiment. There was even an award-winning 33-minute documentary based entirely on this hot sauce, called "Sriracha!"

There is some evidence of potential health benefits from the capsaicin in chili peppers, which has been shown to raise metabolic rate and help with weight loss. On the flip side, the high sugar and sodium content make this condiment far from a health food. Eat it sparingly if you love it.

• **Oat milk.** Oat milk is a bona fide fad food due to the genius marketing strategy from the Swedish company Oatly. The oat-milk craze started in coffee shops because of its thick, creamy consistency and ability to froth up like full-fat milk in a latte or cappuccino. In fact, oat milk outperforms all other plant-based milks in the all-important froth factor.

So how does oat milk stack up nutritionally against other plant-based milks? Unfortunately, commercial oat milks have less protein than soy milk and can have unhealthy additives such as added sugar and low-grade oils. Always read the label and opt for organic oat milk with minimal ingredients, and if possible, no added sugar or unhealthy additives.

•**Bone broth.** Bone broth is a brewed liquid containing the connective tissues and bones of animals such as cows, chickens, and even fish. Bone broth is low in calories and contains satiating protein, both of which can aid weight loss.

There is some scientific evidence that drinking bone broth can help treat joint and digestive system disorders as well as promote weight loss. Bone marrow contains several minerals that leach into the brew, most notably iron, zinc, and selenium. Brewing connective tissue into bone broth provides the body with collagen from the cartilage.

•**Açaí berries.** Açaí berries are the grape-like fruit harvested from the acai palm tree, native to Central and South America. The deep purple color is a visual cue that these berries are rich in antioxidants. In fact, açaí berries are one of the best sources of antioxidant polyphenols and may contain as much as 10 times more antioxidants than blueberries.

The hype is real: They are an extremely healthy fruit.

Whether they do a better job than other berries in fighting disease and helping with weight control, however, has not been shown, and açaí products are very pricey.

Wild Mushrooms Alert

Warning! Products labeled with wild mushrooms contain few, if any, wild species. A new study used DNA barcoding to test what mushroom species made up 16 food products. Almost all of the products consisted of cultivated species, and one packet of dried wild mushrooms contained a species from a group of fungi that includes the "Death Cap," a poisonous mushroom known to cause renal failure in humans.

University of Utah.

Can Certain Foods Shield You from Pollution?

David Carpenter, MD, the codirector of the Institute for Health and the Environment at University at Albany (State University of New York), a Collaborating Centre of the World Health Organization in Environmental Health.

No matter where you live, you're likely exposed to pollutants such as heavy metals, pesticides, phthalates, and flame retardants. Scientists have found that exposure to these substances can cause oxidation, a kind of internal rust, and put your immune system into overdrive, causing chronic, low-grade inflammation. The end result is cellular damage and a higher risk of disease.

Illnesses linked to pollution include all the big killers, such as high blood pressure, heart disease, and stroke. Exposure to some air pollutants for even one day can quadruple the risk of dying from a heart attack. That's just the start. Pollution is linked to cancer, diabetes, obesity, Alzheimer's disease, respiratory illness, attention deficit and hyperactivity disorder, age-related macular degeneration, infertility, acne, psoriasis, and Parkinson's disease.

Let Food Be Thy Protection

While you can't entirely avoid pollution, you can take steps to protect yourself. Scientists at major universities around the world are rapidly accumulating evidence that some foods can help prevent, slow, or reverse the cellular damage caused by pollutants.

•**Fruits and vegetables.** Polychlorinated biphenyls (PCBs) have been used in hundreds of industrial applications and products, and they permeate the soil, water, and air. Once they're ingested, they're stored in fat. Research links high blood levels of PCBs with a higher risk of type 2 diabetes, but the risk is much lower in people with a high intake of fruits and vegetables, which deliver a wide range of antioxidant and anti-inflammatory compounds, including vitamins, minerals, and phytochemicals (plant compounds). PCBs are also linked to heart disease and cancer, and researchers from the College of Medicine at the University of Kentucky say that eating more fruits and vegetables may lower the risk of pollutants triggering those diseases.

Aim for at least five servings of fruit and vegetables each day. If you're not a fan, try hiding them in other foods. A handful of spinach disappears in chili, while minced cauliflower blends seamlessly into just about any recipe. Also, since PCBs are stored in fat, minimize your consumption of fatty meats, such as strip steak and ribeye.

• **Vitamin C.** One reason fruits and vegetables are protective is that they are rich in vitamin C, which is particularly protective for some of the people most vulnerable to air pollution—those with chronic obstructive pulmonary disease (COPD) and asthma. In one study, researchers from the United Kingdom noted that exposure to air pollution increased hospital admissions in people with COPD and asthma, but people with the highest blood levels of vitamin C had a 35 percent lower risk of being hospitalized. Boost your vitamin C by eating citrus, strawberries, broccoli, and tomatoes.

• **High-fiber foods.** Foods that are high in fiber, such as fruits, vegetables, whole grains, beans, bran cereal, popcorn, and nuts, reduce the absorption of pollutants and help you excrete those that have been absorbed. Aim for 21 to 25 grams a day for women and 30 to 38 grams a day for men.

• **Green tea.** In a scientific paper published in the *Journal of Nutritional Biochemistry*, researchers from the University of Tennessee and several other institutions cited more than 70 studies that detailed how green tea—rich in the phytochemical epigallocatechin gallate (EGCG)—may help protect against environmental toxins of all kinds, including pesticides, smoke, mold, PCBs, and

> Foods that are high in fiber—such as fruits, vegetables, whole grains, beans, bran cereal, popcorn, and nuts—reduce the absorption of pollutants and help you excrete those that have been absorbed.

arsenic. (More than 2 million Americans have well water with a high level of arsenic, a carcinogen.) Try to drink two cups per day.

• **Beer contains hops,** which are rich in *xanthohumol*, an antioxidant and anti-inflammatory phytochemical that can protect cells from pollution-induced damage to DNA, which can trigger cancer. Xanthohumol is also found in yogurt, chocolate, and muesli.

• **Sesame-based foods.** According to a scientific paper recently published in *Reviews on Environmental Health*, sesame is uniquely protective against disease processes triggered by pollutants. The "bioactive" components in sesame seed and oil include lignans, sasamin, sasamol, and sesamolin. These components reduce oxidation, boost the antioxidant power of vitamin E, kill cancer cells and stop them from multiplying, lower high cholesterol and blood pressure, strengthen the liver, a detoxifying organ, protect brain cells against damage, and downregulate inflammatory immune factors.

You can use sesame oil like any vegetable oil. Sesame-based foods include tahini (a nut butter), hummus, baba ghanoush (a dip with mashed cooked eggplant, olive oil, lemon juice, and seasonings), and halva (a dessert).

• **Cranberry.** Several types of air pollutants—including sulfur dioxide, nitrogen dioxide, ozone, carbon dioxide, and particulates—have been linked to a wide range of respiratory problems, including lung and esophageal cancers. According to Bernard Hennig, PhD, at the University of Kentucky, cellular studies have shown that cranberry can protect against those and other cancers, including cancers of the colon, prostate, and brain (glioblastoma). You can ingest cranberry as a food, in juice (choose a low-sugar variety), or in supplemental form.

• **Selenium.** Research shows that this trace mineral binds to toxic metals such as lead, cadmium, and methylmercury, forming a so-called "insoluble precipitant" that is easily ex-

The Power of Fish and Fish Oil

A study published in *Neurology* showed the protective power of fish and fish oil against the cell-damaging, disease-causing particulates in air pollution. A team of researchers from eight leading medical schools tracked 1,315 women, ages 65 to 80, for 10 years and assessed their exposure to particulate pollution, the amount of omega-3 fatty acids in their red blood cells (both docosahexaenoic acid [DHA] and eicosapentaenoic acid [DHA]), and the size of the hippocampus and the white matter of the brain. Brain shrinkage in those areas is a sign of aging and increases the risk of cognitive decline.

They found that the women with the most exposure to air pollution had the greatest degree of brain shrinkage—unless they had high blood levels of omega-3s. The researchers also found that the women with the greatest dietary intake of omega-3s—from non-fried fish and fish oil supplements—had greater brain volume.

In a new study published in the *American Journal of Cardiology,* Chinese scientists found that people who took a fish oil supplement maintained normal biomarkers after exposure to air pollution—but people who didn't take the supplement had several signs of circulatory dysfunction, including blood inflammation, thicker blood, and tighter arteries.

The best food sources of omega-3s are fatty fish such as wild-caught salmon, sardines, and anchovies. The American Heart Association—which has issued a formal scientific statement linking air pollution to cardiovascular illness and death, recommends that all adults eat fatty fish at least twice a week. Omega-3 supplements containing DHA and EPA are also widely available, and research shows they are effective. Look for a supplement that delivers a daily minimum of 250 to 500 milligrams of combined EPA and DHA.

—Dr. David Carpenter

creted. Seniors are more likely to be deficient in the mineral.

Brazil nuts and seafood are the richest sources of selenium. Other good sources include red meat, grains, and dairy products. Seniors may want to include a selenium supplement. Look for a product with at least 55 micrograms (mcg) and take it once a week. (Too much selenium can be toxic.)

•**Quercetin.** Cellular studies show that quercetin can protect the arteries from PCBs. This phytochemical is found in apples, onions, cherries, citrus fruits, red grapes, and green leafy vegetables.

•**Curcumin.** This anti-inflammatory compound is the active ingredient in turmeric. Several cellular and animal studies show that curcumin—also available in supplement form—can help prevent lung and heart damage from air pollution, including diesel exhaust. Curcumin can also prevent inflammation from cadmium, a heavy metal.

Curcumin is very difficult for your body to absorb, so when using it in cooking, combine it with a fat and/or black pepper to boost its bioavailability. If taking a supplement, look for one that is formulated for enhanced bioavailability, such as products with added oil, piperine (a pepper extract), or a smaller particle size.

Potential Risks from Popular Cookware

Andrew Rubman, ND, FABNE, medical director of Southbury Clinic for Traditional Medicines in Southbury, Connecticut. He is a founding member of the American Association of Naturopathic Physicians. SouthburyClinic.com

"Cooking healthy" isn't only about nutritious ingredients—the cookware you choose can have medical consequences as well...

•**Stainless steel cookware can create trans fats**—the least healthy fats, raising bad cholesterol and lowering good cholesterol.

The FDA has largely banned food manufacturers from adding trans fats to foods sold in the US—but some people accidentally add trans fats when they cook in stainless steel. Stainless steel cookware contains nickel, a catalyst in a "hydrogenation" process that can create trans fats from cooking oils.

Self-defense: When cooking in stainless steel, keep oils below their smoke point. Oils with high smoke points—and thus lower trans-fat risk—include avocado, peanut and grapeseed oils. Or switch to enamel-coated cast-iron pots and pans, such as Le Creuset cookware.

• **Uncoated cast-iron cookware can increase the iron level in your blood.** The more acidic the food you are cooking, the more iron that is shed by the pan. That's not a problem for most people, but when iron levels get too high, it can lead to serious health consequences such as liver damage, heart disease or cancer.

Self-defense: Replace uncoated cast-iron cookware with enamel-coated, as above, if a blood test suggests that you have elevated iron levels and/or you have been diagnosed with hereditary hemochromatosis, which leads to high iron levels. Symptoms can include joint pain, abdominal pain, fatigue, weakness and loss of sex drive. An enamel coating prevents the iron from leaching into food.

If you prefer to keep using your non-enamel cast-iron pans, the best way to avoid undue shedding is by "seasoning" the cookware to give it a protective, nonstick-type coat...and using hot water and a "chainmail" stainless steel scrubber to clean it. Soap is not recommended for cleaning cast iron, as it can leave residue and remove the protective seasoning coating.

Also helpful: Ask your doctor to run an "iron panel" blood test for guidance on your personal use of uncoated cast iron.

• **Nonstick cookware can release toxic chemicals.** Cancer-causing chemicals in nonstick Teflon coatings can flake into food if the cooking surface gets scratched...and toxic fumes can be released into kitchen air if this cookware is overheated.

Self-defense: Switch to "nonstick stoneware" or ceramic nonstick cookware, which has a natural nonstick surface but does not come with these cancer risks. It's extremely durable, too. Choose brands described in marketing materials as being completely free of alkylphenol ethoxylates (APEOs) and perfluorooctanoic acid (PFOA). These compounds undercut stoneware's safety advantage.

Are Eggs with Cracked Shells Safe to Eat?

Lynne Ausman, DSc, director of the Master of Nutrition Science and Policy program, Tufts University, Boston.

Not if you bought them that way. Visible cracks are wide enough to let in salmonella, which could make you sick, so check eggs carefully before you buy. But if an egg cracks while in your custody, just remove it from its shell, seal it in a clean container, refrigerate it and use it within the next few days.

Coconut Oil Is Not a Superfood

Roundup of nutrition experts reported in *The New York Times.*

Coconut oil may not be all it's cracked up to be. It's often touted as a superfood, but experts say coconut oil is no better for you than other fats. It has more calories than butter, and more of it is saturated (87 percent) than is butter (63 percent) or beef fat (40 percent), meaning that it can drive up cholesterol levels and clog arteries just like its less glamorous peers.

Best Way to Buy Spices

Lior Lev Sercarz, a spice master who has created custom blends for some of the world's top culinary minds. He is founder of the spice emporium La Boîte in New York City, and author of *Mastering Spice: Recipes and Techniques to Transform Your Everyday Cooking, The Spice Companion* and *The Art of Blending.* LaBoiteNY.com

The right spices make cooking faster and easier yet deliver more taste complexity to your recipes. The best place to shop for quality spices are dedicated spice shops. Don't be afraid of the higher prices—a cheaper product means that you'll need to add more to get the same effect. Buy no more than you'll need for three to six months so that spices remain fresh. If there's no quality spice shop near you, there are wonderful resources online.

Check for Freshness

• **Look for bright, consistent color.** Dried herbs should be green, not brown. Single spices should have a uniform color, not dark and light particles or different shades.

Examples: Ground black pepper shouldn't be gray, and whole black peppercorns should be quite black.

• **Whole spices are fresher than preground generally**—dust at the bottom of a jar is a sign of age.

• **Clumping is good in preground spices**—it signals moisture, which indicates freshness.

When You Bring Home a Spice

• **Inhale the aroma.** Then, to taste it, place a little on your tongue (you could first mix it with a little neutral oil). Not all spices taste great straight, but you'll get a sense of the flavor.

• **Try a sprinkle** on plain yogurt, rice or a cube of cooked meat or fish. Stir some into a cup of hot broth to see how heat changes the taste.

• **Sprinkle a small amount on a familiar dish** so you'll know how it changes the taste. If you like it, the taste will be even better when you cook the whole dish with it.

Turmeric: The Anti-Inflammatory Spice

Janet Bond Brill, PhD, RDN, FAND, is a registered dietitian nutritionist, a fellow of the Academy of Nutrition and Dietetics, and a nationally recognized nutrition, health and fitness expert who specializes in cardiovascular disease prevention. Based in Hellertown, Pennslyvania., Dr. Brill is author of *Intermittent Fasting for Dummies, Blood Pressure DOWN, Cholesterol DOWN,* and *Prevent a Second Heart Attack.* DrJanet.com

Turmeric has been used in India for thousands of years as both a spice and medicinal herb. It lends both flavor and rich color to dishes like curries, and, thanks to a compound called curcumin, provides a solid dose of anti-inflammatory and antioxidant effects, too. *Here are some of its promising health benefits…*

• **Alzheimer's disease and brain cancer.** Curcumin can cross the blood-brain barrier and has been shown to help battle the disease process of both Alzheimer's disease and brain cancer. Curcumin can disrupt the brain plaques that are the hallmark of Alzheimer's disease, and it can inhibit the growth of malignant brain tumor cells.

• **Arthritis.** Because of its anti-inflammatory properties, turmeric has shown promise for easing the joint pain and stiffness associated with both osteoarthritis and rheumatoid arthritis.

• **Irritable bowel syndrome (IBS).** Some research has demonstrated that turmeric can help improve symptoms of IBS, such as abdominal pain. It is also being studied as a treatment for other inflammatory bowel diseases like Crohn's and ulcerative colitis.

•**Type 2 diabetes.** Turmeric has been shown to help fight inflammation and keep blood sugar levels steady.

Studies have shown that just 50 mg of curcumin, consumed over a three-month period, provides significant health benefits. But while curcumin makes up just 3 percent of turmeric, it is best not to consume curcumin by itself, as it is very poorly absorbed. Instead, use the whole spice and add black pepper, which contains a compound called piperine. This natural substance has been shown to increase the absorption of curcumin by 2,000 percent.

One caveat, turmeric contains oxalates, which can increase the risk of kidneys stones. Turmeric may also interfere with the action of drugs that decrease stomach acid. Consult your physician if you have these conditions.

Tofu Scramble with Turmeric

2 Tbsp. extra virgin olive oil
½ cup egg substitute
7 ounces soft tofu
⅛ tsp. black pepper
½ tsp. ground turmeric
½ avocado, cubed
½ tsp. salt-free seasoning blend
½ cup grape tomatoes, quartered

In a large non-stick skillet, heat oil over medium-high heat. Pat the tofu dry with a paper towel, and then crumble into the skillet. Sprinkle with turmeric. Cook, stirring gently, until most of the moisture is cooked out of the tofu, about four minutes.

Meanwhile, in a bowl whisk together the egg substitute, salt-free seasoning blend, and pepper. Set aside.

When the tofu appears dry, reduce the heat to medium. Pour the reserved eggs over the tofu. Cook, stirring occasionally for about two minutes until set. Divide between two plates and serve with avocado and tomatoes.

Makes 2 servings.

Nutrition per Serving: Calories: 208, *Sodium:* 95 mg, *Potassium:* 523 mg, *Magnesium:* 45 mg, *Calcium:* 120 mg, *Fat:* 15 g, *Saturated Fat:* 2 g, *Cholesterol:* 0 mg, *Carbohydrate:* 9 g, *Dietary Fiber:* 4 g, *Sugars:* 1 g, *Protein:* 13 g.

Healthful Garnish

Crispy lentils. Use dried French or beluga lentils—they hold their shape when cooked. Soak the lentils overnight…drain and rinse… shake them dry…then sauté them in olive oil over medium-high heat until crispy. Drain on a towel-covered plate…add salt and seasoning to taste…and use as a garnish on pasta or soup. Store for up to five days.

Epicurious.com

Foods Better Bought Frozen

Roundup of food experts, reported in *USA Today*.

Blueberries—they are picked at their best, when sweet and tasty, while fresh ones can be hard and flavorless out of season. *Butternut squash*—fresh squash is hard to peel and seed, while frozen is easy to use and has the same flavor. *Mangoes*—fresh ones are hard and fibrous until ripe, then quickly become too soft and are hard to peel, while frozen mangoes are easy to use and always tasty. *Raspberries*—they are flavorful only in season, but even then quickly get moldy, while frozen ones defrost nicely and remain firm. *Salmon*—it is frozen when first caught, so frozen is in a sense fresher than at a fresh fish counter…and freezing kills parasites.

Avocados Reduce Dangerous Belly Fat in Women

Study by researchers at University of Illinois at Urbana-Champaign, published in *Journal of Nutrition*.

It is difficult to lose visceral fat, the deep belly fat that surrounds inner organs and raises risk for diabetes.

Recent finding: Overweight and obese women who consumed a daily meal that included one fresh avocado showed a reduction in abdominal fat and improvement in the ratio of visceral fat to subcutaneous fat, indicating that fat was redistributed away from the inner organs. A similar group of women who ate a similar daily meal equal in nutrition and calories that did not include avocado had no change in abdominal or visceral fat…nor did men in the study, regardless of whether they ate avocados.

Avocados and Tomatoes Can Be Frozen

Avocados...

Avocados can be frozen if you plan to unfreeze them for use in smoothies, guacamole or salad dressing. Freezing and thawing makes them unappetizing to eat on their own, but frozen avocados retain most of their nutrients and flavor if kept for no more than four to six months. Cut, mash or purée them before freezing. If freezing halves or pieces, brush the exposed flesh with lemon juice to reduce browning. To mash or purée, prepare the avocado by hand—you can add lemon or lime juice or seasonings but not vegetables such as tomato or onion. To use frozen avocado, thaw it at room temperature for about an hour.

Healthline.com

Whole Tomatoes...

Just put them in plastic bags, and store them in the freezer. The tomatoes will look fresh when taken out months later, although they will shrink and appear less appetizing as they defrost. But their skins will slip right off, and they are fine to use in sauce or anything else that involves cooking.

Mark Bittman, author of the *How to Cook Everything* series, writing at Heated.Medium.com.

Drink Without Derailing Your Diet

Rachel Beller, MS, RDN, founder of Beller Nutrition, based in Culver City, California. She is a spokesperson for the American Cancer Society, and creator of the Beller Method 8-week Transformation Masterclass. BellerNutrition.com

A glass of wine with dinner or a cocktail when out with friends can undermine otherwise healthy eating habits.

If you're watching your calories, it can be confusing to choose the best option: Should you stick to a glass of wine? Have a light beer? Or try a spiked seltzer or seemingly healthy fancy cocktail?

Nutritionist Rachel Beller, MS, RDN, explains how you can enjoy a drink without derailing your diet and packing on the pounds.

Wine

Whether you choose white, red, or rose, a 5-ounce glass of wine contains about 100 to 130 calories. Watch out for port wines or sweet dessert wines, which can contain up to 300 calories in the same serving.

Best choice: Go red. All wine is produced by crushing and fermenting grapes. To produce red wine, crushed red grapes are fermented with the skin, seeds, and stems intact. For white wine, the stems, seeds, and skins are removed before fermentation. Because many of the healthful compounds are found in the grape skin, red wine contains more of the beneficial plant compounds found in those skins, such as resveratrol. Resveratrol contains antioxidant and anti-inflammatory properties, which help reduce heart disease risk, increase HDL "good" cholesterol levels, and slow age-related mental decline.

Beer

Whether it is a pale ale, a lager, a stout, or other type, beer generally contains about 150 calories in a 12-ounce can or bottle. In a bar or restaurant, a pour may be a larger 16-ounce pint.

Best choice: If what really quenches your thirst on a hot day is a nice cold beer, consider choosing a light beer. The calories in a 12-ounce serving typically range from about 50 to 100 calories. Squeeze in a little lime, lemon, or orange for a small shot of vitamin C.

Hard Seltzer

These popular canned drinks, such as Truly and White Claw, are made with brewed cane sugar and/or malted rice, with added soda water and flavorings. A typical 12-ounce can contains about 100 calories. Some hard seltzers contain real fruit juice, but it is not enough for any nutritional benefit.

Best choice: If you want to enjoy this fruity option, feel free to choose your favorite flavored hard seltzer, but don't overdo it. They are easy to overdrink.

Liquor

A 1.5 ounce (shot glass) serving of gin, rum, vodka, tequila, or whiskey is 100 calories. The mixers you choose, however, can quickly add up. For instance, 4 ounces of orange juice will add nearly 60 calories, and many sodas, such as Coke or Sprite, have about 45 to 50 calories in the same amount. A mojito or margarita on the rocks can be as low as 150 calories, but a pina colada, daiquiri, or other frozen drink can pack as many as 500 calories into one drink.

Best choice: If you crave a cocktail, pick no-calorie mixers such as fruit-flavored sparkling water, club soda, or plain sparkling water.

To add some flavor, squeeze in a little lime or lemon. To pack a nutritional punch, try a splash of pomegranate juice, which adds flavor plus the cancer-fighting compound ellagic acid, with few calories. Or consider a teaspoon of 100 percent ginger juice, which contains anti-nausea and anti-inflammatory properties.

Responsible Drinking

The extra calories in alcoholic drinks can really add up. Adding 100 calories a day could potentially result in weight gain of 10 pounds a year. Further, alcohol can increase hunger and lower inhibitions and judgment, resulting in grabbing for more snacks, rich hors d'oeuvres, extra pizza, or other unhealthful choices.

Even when making low-calorie choices, it's important to limit overall alcohol consumption to protect your health. Heavy drinking has been linked to high blood pressure, heart disease, stroke, liver disease, and digestive problems, cancer, a weakened immune system, memory problems, depression, anxiety, and alcohol-use disorders. To avoid overindulgence, think of your drink as a treat to be enjoyed occasionally.

Summer Ginger Zinger

This summer cocktail is low in calories, sneaks in nutritional value, and is delicious.

1½ oz vodka
3 oz soda water
2 Tbsp pomegranate juice
1 tsp 100 percent pure ginger juice
Squeeze of lime
Mix and pour over ice.

Serves one. Per serving: 115 calories, 0 g total fat, 0 g saturated fat, 0 g protein, 4 g carbs, 4 g sugar, 0 g fiber, 0 g cholesterol, 14 mg sodium

Source: Recipe courtesy of Rachel Beller, RDN

Virgin Mojito

Try this mocktail recipe when you want a festive drink, but not the alcohol or extra calories.

6 cups soda water
2 Tbsp lime juice
15 ice cubes
1 cup fresh mint leaves
1 Tbsp pure maple syrup
Mix in a large pitcher.

Serves four. Per serving: 14 calories, 0 g total fat, 0 g sat fat, 0 g protein, 4 g carbs, 3 g sugar, 0 g fiber, 0 g cholesterol, 47 mg sodium

Source: Recipe courtesy of Rachel Beller, RDN

Are "Healthy" Wines Better for You?

Jeff Siegel, the Wine Curmudgeon, is a wine writer and wine critic who specializes in the inexpensive wine, he says, that most of us drink. He is author of *The Wine Curmudgeon's Guide to Cheap Wine* and oversees the award-winning Wine Curmudgeon website (WineCurmudgeon.com). He has taught wine, spirits, and beer at El Centro College and Le Cordon Bleu in Dallas.

The hot new craze in wine isn't about varietal or country or even cost. It's about so-called "healthy" wine—wine that is good for you. Brands such as FitVine, Cupcake Light Hearted, Mind & Body and Kim Crawford Illuminate are part of a new generation of wines that promise fewer calories, less sugar and less alcohol. *These new "healthier" wines have tapped into several market trends…*

- **The backlash against added sugar** that has been gathering momentum in the US for the past 20 years, and the perception that wine has added sugar.

- **The Keto and Paleo diet trends,** which emphasize avoiding carbohydrates—something wine has, thanks to its alcohol.

- **The demand from younger consumers for healthier options,** even for alcohol.

But the question is, are these wines actually "healthier"? *The facts…*

- **These wines have fewer calories and less alcohol than traditional wines.** But that is because most of wine's calories come from the alcohol, so a glass of a lower-alcohol wine may have about 90 calories, as opposed to 125 calories for a glass of traditional wine. To reduce the alcohol content, many of these wines are manipulated using a process called "spinning cone technology." The fermented grape juice is placed in a huge cone that spins at a high speed, separating the alcohol from the grape juice. Then, some alcohol is added back to the grape juice. So wine that starts out with 13½ percent alcohol can be reduced to 9 percent or 10 percent alcohol.

- **The claims about sugar and sulfites are more difficult to pin down.** Most of the "healthy" wines come from California. While sugar occurs naturally in grapes, it's illegal to add sugar during the winemaking process in California.

- **Sulfites are added to wine as a preservative**—white wines usually get more than reds. Some wine drinkers are sensitive to sulfites and may get headaches, but sulfites occur naturally in wine and minimal additional amounts are added.

- **Almost all wine is gluten-free and vegan**—not just the "healthy" ones. Grapes and yeast, after all, are naturally gluten-free…and almost all wine is vegan—made of grapes and yeast.

Your best bet? Find a wine that you like, drink it in moderation…and the rest will take care of itself.

Healthy Drinks for People Who Don't Like Water

Vandana Sheth, RDN, CDCES, FAND, a registered dietitian nutritionist, certified diabetes care & education specialist, and certified intuitive eating counselor based in Los Angeles, California.

Drinking water replenishes lost fluids, lubricates joints, and moisturizes the skin. It's important to your mood, sleep, digestion, cognition, and energy levels. But if you don't like the taste of water, it can be difficult to drink enough to reach your daily needs. This is especially problematic in older adults because, with age, one's sense of thirst diminishes, increasing the likelihood of dehydration.

Fortunately, you can satisfy much of your daily hydration needs by drinking liquids that are just as thirst- and body-quenching as water, but run the gamut of flavor, texture, and temperature.

Jazzed-Up Waters

You may find water more palatable with just some simple twists…

• **Sparkling water** is just as hydrating as tap water, but it comes in dozens of flavors, such as grapefruit, lemon-lime, cherry, blackberry, and watermelon. The tingly bubbles can make drinking water feel more exciting. Experiment with different brands to see which bubbles you like best. Some brands have more powerful carbonation, and others boast more delicate, "softer" bubbles.

Sparkling waters don't contain phosphoric acid, an ingredient in carbonated soft drinks that can reduce bone density. In fact, many brands contain trace amounts of calcium, so they may have a positive effect on bone.

Check the label and avoid sparkling waters that contain sugar, which adds needless calories, or artificial sweeteners, which can cause stomach trouble and have been shown to cause sugar cravings in some people.

• **Fruit-infused water.** Make your own flavorful infused water, sometimes called spa water, by adding your favorite sliced fruits, vegetables, and herbs to a pitcher of water. Let it steep in the refrigerator for four to six hours or, even better, overnight. The flavor of your berries, citrus, or cucumber slices will permeate the water, making it more enjoyable to sip. Strawberry-basil and cucumber-mint are two winning combinations. Crush the herbs before adding to intensify the spa water's flavor.

• **Tea.** With 2 billion cups drunk every day, tea is the second most consumed beverage worldwide. (Water is number one.) Green, black, oolong, and white tea all come from the same *Camellia sinensis* plant. They taste and look different from each other thanks to how the leaves are processed. All four are caffeinated but still contain less caffeine than coffee, so if java gives you the jitters, tea is a smarter bet.

> ## Coconut Water
>
> The clear fluid found inside young coconuts is highly hydrating thanks to three electrolytes: potassium, sodium, and magnesium. This means it can lower blood pressure. In fact, patients scheduled for surgery should avoid coconut water for two weeks beforehand to avoid possible complications.

They also contain antioxidant compounds called polyphenols which, when consumed regularly, lower the risk of several chronic diseases, including heart disease and cancer. Habitual tea drinkers have better cognition, and a new University of California, Irvine, study found that compounds in green and black tea relax blood vessels and reduce blood pressure.

For extra health benefits, try matcha, a type of green tea that is made by crushing green tea leaves until they reach a powdered consistency, then whisking with water. This means you consume the actual green tea leaves when sipping matcha, along with all of their great-for-you compounds. Matcha has high levels of L-theanine, an amino acid known for promoting a calm sense of mental alertness. It has a grassy, non-bitter flavor.

Avoiding caffeine? Herbal teas like chamomile, peppermint, rooibos, and ginger are made from the flowers, leaves, and roots of various plants. They each offer unique health perks, such as improving digestion (peppermint) or soothing a sore throat (slippery elm).

Enjoy tea hot or iced for equal hydration and health benefits. Just be sure not to load it up with excess sugar or you'll negate many of the health advantages.

Black Coffee

Despite the old wives' tale about coffee being dehydrating, it actually counts towards your daily water quota. In fact, when a group of UK researchers asked 50 men, all regular coffee drinkers, to consume four mugs of black coffee a day for three days, followed by three days during which they consumed an equivalent amount of water, they found no difference in hydration status.

Regular coffee intake confers some protection against cancer and cognitive decline thanks to its high antioxidant content. It can also reduce the risk of developing type 2 diabetes. A 2021 study published in *PLOS Medicine* linked coffee consumption with a reduced risk of stroke and dementia. That same study found that drinking two to three cups of coffee and two to three cups of tea a day reduced stroke risk by 32 percent and dementia risk by 28 percent. Again, steer clear of excess added sugar or cream.

Kefir

Kefir (pronounced "KEE-fir") is a tart, tangy, slightly effervescent, fermented dairy drink that offers two to three times more probiotics than yogurt. Probiotics are helpful bacteria that help regulate gastrointestinal health, immunity, mental health, and more. Kefir is also anti-inflammatory, antimicrobial, antidiabetic, antihypertensive, and antioxidant. It's high in protein and calcium for strong muscles and bones.

Some commercially available kefirs are high in added sugars, so check the label. The American Heart Association recommends a maximum of 36 grams of added sugar per day for men and 24 grams for women.

(*Note:* This differs from the total sugar content, which can be high in dairy products thanks to naturally occurring milk sugars. Just pay attention to added sugars.)

Coffee Makes Sweets Taste Sweeter

Alexander Wieck Fjældstad, MD, associate professor of clinical medicine, Aarhus University, Holstebro, Denmark, and leader of a study published in *Foods*.

Researchers tested the taste sensitivity of 156 subjects before and after they drank coffee.

Result: Participants reported increased sensitivity to sweetness and blunted sensitivity to bitterness after consuming either reg-

ular or decaf, thanks to the bitter substances found in coffee.

Wise: If you've been trying to switch to dark chocolate to reap its health benefits but can't handle its bitterness, eating it as you sip coffee might get you over the hump.

Effective Ways to Halt Sugar Cravings

Roundup of nutritionists and dietitians reported at EatThis.com.

Eat well-balanced meals—the desire for sugar often is because some important food component, such as protein or fiber, is deficient in your diet. *Do not skip meals—* that causes the body to need fuel quickly and so it may crave sugar. *Stay well-hydrated—* the body sometimes misinterprets thirst as a sugar craving. *Avoid high-salt foods—*they can trigger a desire for sweetness to balance the salt. *Figure out the reason for the craving—*it often is emotional or habitual. Try to determine if you tend to want sweets when you are unhappy or bored or upset, and then find ways to deal with the underlying feeling. *Give in to the craving, and then move on—*if you really want some chocolate or ice cream, have a modest amount and go on with your day. Trying to deflect the craving or restrict what you eat only makes the desire stronger.

When to Eat Chocolate for Weight Loss

Study of 19 women led by researchers at Brigham and Women's Hospital, Boston, published in the Federation of American Societies for Experimental Biology's *The FASEB Journal.*

Chocolate for breakfast may help you get skinny.

Recent finding: Women ate either 100 grams of milk chocolate in the morning, in the evening or abstained from chocolate for two weeks. There was no weight gain in either of the chocolate-eating groups...and women who ate chocolate at breakfast had improved metabolism, increased fat-burning and lower blood glucose levels.

Keep It Simple to Lose Weight

Giles Yeo, PhD, is principal research associate, Metabolic Research Laboratories & MRC Metabolic Diseases Unit, University of Cambridge, United Kingdom, and the author of *Why Calories Don't Count.*

There is no magical one-size-fits-all solution to weight loss, but there are three biological principles that may make choosing a diet that suits you easier...

To lose weight, you need to eat less.

Food that takes longer to digest will travel further down the gut, which results in a release of hormones that make you feel fuller. If you feel fuller, you will eat less and will lose weight.

Foods have different levels of caloric availability, which is the number of *usable* calories we can get out of a food.

The two components of food that take the longest to digest and have the lowest caloric availability are protein and fiber.

Protein Power

Protein is the most chemically complex macronutrient, so your body uses more time and energy to digest and metabolize it. It has a caloric availability of 70 percent, which means that for every 100 calories of protein that you consume, you use only 70 because you spend 30 on metabolism. By comparison, fat has a caloric availability of 98 percent. Complex carbohydrates (whole grains, vegetables) have 90 percent availability, while refined carbohydrates (white flour, white sugar) have 95 percent. This is why a calorie

of protein makes you feel fuller than a calorie of fat or carbohydrate, and why high-protein diets work well for some people.

Fiber

Fiber is a type of plant-based carbohydrate that is structured in a way that humans cannot digest. From the perspective of caloric availability, it slows down the rate of digestion, which causes the release of nutrients over a longer period of time and reduces the absolute number of calories absorbed.

An illustration of the impact of fiber can be seen when you compare drinking a glass of orange juice to eating an orange. When you drink OJ, the sugar, which, incidentally, is at the same concentration as that of soda, is absorbed almost immediately. When you eat an orange, however, the sugar is interlocked in the fiber, so it takes energy and time for our digestive system to extract it, thus we feel fuller. This is why dietary approaches that are high in fiber, including plant-based, low-glycemic index, and Mediterranean plans, work for weight loss.

Losing Is the Easy Part

People often say that 95 percent of diets don't work, which is not technically true. A more accurate statement is that 95 percent of diets are ones we can't stick to. Losing weight (which is the easier part of the process) and keeping it off (this is undoubtedly the more difficult part) requires a long-term change to one's eating behavior and pattern.

Whatever approach you choose can't be extreme, because then it won't be sustainable.

It also has to suit your life situation: *What can you afford? Do you have kids? Do you work shifts? How do you get to work? What foods do you enjoy?*

Keep it simple: Eat adequate protein—about 16 percent of your total daily intake—from either animal or plant-based sources, and try to include as much fiber as possible. That's the foundation of a healthy, effective, and (hopefully) sustainable weight-loss diet.

Selenium Protects Against Weight Gain

Andrew Rubman, ND, medical director of Southbury Clinic for Traditional Medicines, Southbury, Connecticut, commenting on a study by researchers at Orentreich Foundation for the Advancement of Science.

Mice fed high-fat diets lived longer and were less obese if their diet included selenium. The selenium group also showed physiological benefits similar to consuming a vegan diet. Selenium is known to decrease gut inflammation, which contributes to weight gain.

Food sources of selenium: Nuts, fish, beef, and poultry. Selenium supplements also are available. The safe upper daily limit for selenium is 400 micrograms.

Keto Quick Start

Amy Lee, MD, chief medical officer of Lindora Weight Loss Clinics and head of nutrition at Nucific. She is board certified in internal medicine, medical nutrition, and obesity medicine.

The ketogenic diet is soaring in popularity with its promises of dramatic and rapid weight loss.

The diet works by restricting carbohydrates so your body will burn fat instead. Burning fat creates ketones, which the body uses for energy in a process called ketosis, hence the name ketogenic diet.

While the plan can be very effective, some of the popular advice can make it challenging to maintain a healthy, well-balanced diet—and to stick with the program long-term. *Here's how to turn the ketogenic diet into a healthy lifestyle that will yield lasting results...*

•**Don't be overly strict.** The ketogenic diet was developed in the 1920s to treat children with epilepsy. In that version, which some people still follow, carbohydrates were limited to just 10 grams (g) per day. That's about one small orange. It can be difficult to adhere to such a strict regimen and to get adequate fruit and vegetable intake. Most people can stay in ketosis and lose weight with up to 50 to 80 g of digestible (also called net) carbohydrates per day.

•**Think net carbs.** To calculate net carbs, take the total carbohydrate content of a food and subtract both the fiber and sugar alcohols, neither of which are digestible. For example, one cup of broccoli contains about 6 g of carbohydrates, but 2.5 g are from fiber, leaving a net carb value of 3.5 g.

•**Bacon is still not healthy.** A common mistake people make is to load up their plates with fatty or processed meats, oils, and butter. But just because you are in ketosis, it doesn't mean a diet is healthy.

Instead, base your meals on lean protein sources (lean meats, poultry, eggs, whey),

Eating on the Run

While home-cooked meals are the healthiest choice, the reality is that we get busy, we go out, and we sometimes get hungry far from our own kitchens. The key to getting through these moments is planning. You can keep nonperishable snacks like almonds and protein bars in your car, but that doesn't mean you'll always reach for them. If you have to stop at a quick-serve restaurant, look for a low-carb option and don't be afraid to ask for modifications. *Here are a few examples...*

Panera	Greek salad
Chick-fil-A	Grilled chicken club without the bun
Subway	Protein bowls
McDonald's	Burger without ketchup or bun
Jersey Mike's Subs	Sub in a tub (everything from a sandwich but the bread)
Starbucks	Egg bites

non-starchy vegetables (broccoli, greens, squash), and low to moderate levels of healthy fat (avocados, nuts, coconut).

• **Fruit is part of a healthy diet.** In the beginning, or induction period, of a ketogenic diet, you may have to skip the fruit to help your body get into ketosis. But once you're there, you can gradually increase fruit without affecting your body's ability to burn fat. Some fruits, like berries, are lower in carbohydrates, making it easier to stay within your daily net carbohydrate budget.

• **Avoid an all-or-nothing mentality.** Following a ketogenic diet can be difficult, and you might make mistakes—especially in the beginning. It takes time to give up beloved foods. If you slip up, don't give up. At your next meal, return to low-carb eating.

Can't Lose Weight? Don't Blame Your Metabolism

Herman Pontzer, PhD, associate professor of evolutionary anthropology at Duke University, Durham, North Carolina, lead author of a study titled "Daily energy expenditure through the human life course" published in *Science* and author of *Burn: New Research Blows the Lid Off How We Really Burn Calories, Stay Healthy, and Lose Weight*.

People have been blaming a faulty metabolism for their extra pounds for as long as there's been an obesity epidemic. But a "slow" or "faulty" metabolism is an unlikely culprit. *Here's the truth about metabolism and how to get on the right track with losing weight…*

Just What Is Metabolism?

It's a broad term that covers all the work your cells do, primarily pumping molecules, such as enzymes, hormones, neurotransmitters, and DNA, in or out of cell walls and converting one kind of molecule into another. We measure metabolism as energy expenditure—the amount of energy needed for all the cells in your body to do that work.

The total energy your body burns in a day is the sum of two things—your basal metabolic rate (BMR) plus everything else that you consciously do. Your BMR is the energy used to keep you alive. *There's a general formula to figure out how many daily calories this amounts to…*

BMR for women = 5 × weight + 607
BMR for men = 7 × weight + 551

Now here's the tricky part: Your BMR number could easily fall above or below that total by 200 calories per day, mostly because of your body composition. Tall people burn more than short people…lean people burn more than people who have more fat. But some people just burn more energy than others.

All these variables point to the limitations of online BMR and daily-expenditure calculators—if the calculation you get is off even by the equivalent of a bag of M&Ms, you could overeat enough to put on a pound every two weeks.

Your metabolism does change over the course of your life span but not at the times people think (or even are taught in medical school)…

• **Infancy.** A baby's metabolic rate is the highest of any other time in his/her life. A one-year-old burns calories 50 percent faster for his/her body size than an adult.

• **Childhood through adolescence.** Metabolism slows by about 3 percent each year, even during the teen growth spurt.

• **20s through 50s.** Energy expenditure is stable—a "slowing metabolism" can't be blamed for extra weight, whether you're a woman entering menopause or a man hitting the big 4-0.

• **Age 60 and beyond.** Metabolism does start to decline, but at a very gradual 0.7 percent a year. By age 70, your calorie requirement is down by 7 percent. In your 90s, you need about 26 percent fewer calories than you did in midlife.

Blame Your Brain

When we curse our metabolism for struggles with obesity or fall for the latest metabolism-boosting scam, we are making a fundamental mistake about the way metabolism works. It's your brain—and specifically your hypothalamus—that's pulling the strings. Unlike our primate relatives who store excess calories as lean muscle, our bodies are wired to store these calories as fat—it's our evolutionary burden, designed as a safeguard for a rainy day (e.g., famine). And once you've put on that fat, your hypothalamus doesn't want you to lose it. The brain is very good at getting you to make up for any increase in energy expenditure by increasing hunger.

Research has found that people the world over burn roughly the same number of calories each day, yet the Hadza, the hunter-gatherer people I've studied extensively in Tanzania, for instance, are lean while Americans aren't. To understand why, you need only look at the foods we eat. Take the typical packaged foods at our supermarkets—fiber, protein, and anything else that will make you feel full are removed. Sugar, fat, salt, and other things to tempt you are added.

Food triggers our brain's reward system. The variety at our fingertips sabotages our ability to judge our intake because we jump from one set of reward neurons in the brain to another.

Example: Ordering dessert even though you're full from the main course. That savory main course lit up the reward neurons for fat and salt. By the time you've finished it, your hypothalamus has successfully extinguished the reward of savory food—you think you couldn't eat another bite. But dessert is sweet, and those reward neurons are open for business.

What to Do to Lose Weight

You can't "reset" your metabolism, but you can make diet changes to help thwart your hypothalamus…

•**Pick any diet.** If you look at the research on various diets—low-fat or even one based on eating Twinkies (done just to prove a point)—the bottom line is you have to reduce the overall number of calories you eat. The diet that will work best for you is one that will satisfy you most on the fewest calories. That said, it's healthier to eat foods that fill you up—vegetables, fruits, meat and fish—and avoid foods that prod you to overconsume, such as sugar, salt and unhealthy fats.

Be suspicious of diets that target one specific nutrient as a weight-loss hero or villain. Any calories that aren't burned—no matter if they come from starches, sugars, fats or proteins—will wind up as extra tissue (fat) in your body.

•**Pare down the options at home.** If you don't have potato chips in the house, you can't eat them.

•**Set boundaries.** Some people do well with hard and fast rules.

Example: Decide that you won't look at the dessert menu when it's offered…you will shop only the perimeter of the supermarket where healthier options are displayed.

•**Change your habits.** People often eat because of rituals they've created. Yours might be to unwind in front of the TV at 9 pm…with a sugary snack. Change the snack, or change the habit.

•**Weigh yourself every day.** This simple act helps you be more conscious about what you're eating.

Also: Studies have shown that people underreport and underestimate how much they eat, so keeping a log can help.

•**Have a plan to keep the weight off.** Weight loss lowers our daily energy needs, but the hypothalamus-based hunger and satiety systems continue to push you to eat more calories than you burn and put those pounds back on until your weight and daily energy expenditure are back where they were before you lost weight.

•**Harness the power of exercise.** There's a reason that exercise is called free medicine—it helps to fend off heart disease, diabetes and other consequences of a sedentary lifestyle. A complete absence of physical activity seems to mess up our body's ability to regulate its metabolic jobs, including the regulation of eating. Basic tasks of cellular hygiene, such as breaking down lipids in the blood or trafficking glucose into cells, start to fall apart.

The only thing that exercise can't do is move the needle on metabolism in any meaningful way. Getting in those 10,000 steps per day, for instance, burns only about 250 calories—roughly the equivalent of a 20-ounce bottle of soda or half of a Big Mac.

Exercise becomes even more important after weight loss, helping to prevent weight regain.

•**Keep your guard up indefinitely.** As you've likely heard before, it takes lifelong change to avoid regaining those lost pounds.

5:2 Diet Plan Is an Easier "Sell"

Study of 300 adults with obesity by researchers at Queen Mary University, London, England, published in *PLOS ONE*.

*R**ecent finding:* Participants with obesity who participated in a weight-loss program were given instructions for either a traditional weight-management diet and exercise...or the 5:2 diet, which involves two nonconsecutive days a week of calorie restriction and five days of sensible eating. Both groups lost about the same amount of weight—15 percent of participants in the standard group and 18 percent in the 5:2 group lost at least 5 percent of body weight in a year. But those on the 5:2 diet said they were more likely to recommend that approach to others and were more willing to continue the diet after the study ended. Researchers suggest that at least some of the appeal of the 5:2 plan is that it can be explained briefly, which makes it seem less complicated.

Intermittent Fasting: Eat Less, Get Healthier, Live Longer

Janet Bond Brill, PhD, RDN, FAND, is a registered dietitian nutritionist, a fellow of the Academy of Nutrition and Dietetics, and a nationally recognized nutrition, health and fitness expert who specializes in cardiovascular disease prevention. Based in Hellertown, Pennsylvania, Dr. Brill is author of *Intermittent Fasting for Dummies, Blood Pressure DOWN, Cholesterol DOWN,* and *Prevent a Second Heart Attack.* DrJanet.com

W hat's all the buzz about intermittent fasting providing health and longevity benefits? Is there scientific proof that a program of intermittent fasting can help prevent disease and even help us live longer? The answer is a resounding *yes.* A review article recently published in the prestigious *New England Journal of Medicine* revealed that intermittent fasting has many health benefits.

What Exactly Is Intermittent Fasting?

Years ago, scientists discovered that mice put on a low-calorie diet or caloric restriction (CR) lived longer and were healthier than mice on a regular diet. Intermittent fasting is a remake and much more palatable form of fasting that consists of repetitive, short-term fasts. Methods of intermittent fasting dictate *when* you eat rather than *what* you eat. There are a variety of recommended strategies, but one of the most popular is the 16:8 method, which stands for 16 hours of fasting and eight hours of eating each day. You may eat breakfast at 8 a.m. and finish your final meal of the day by 4 p.m. and abstain from any foods or drinks with calories until 8 a.m. the next morning. Or you may eat your first meal at noon and finish by 8 p.m., not eating again until noon.

Effects on the Body

Once you're done eating for the day, the body transitions into a fasted state and the liver converts fat into ketones for use as fuel. The phenomenon is called the metabolic switch, which affects two important hormones: insulin and norepinephrine. Insulin levels increase when you eat and decrease dramatically when you fast. Lower levels of insulin increase fat burning. (Long-lived people tend to have unusually low insulin levels.) When you're fasting, your nervous system also sends norepinephrine to your fat cells. Norepinephrine increases your metabolism and helps cells break down body fat to be burned for energy.

Numerous additional health benefits that have been associated with intermittent fasting include improved cellular stress response to free-radical damage; reduced inflammation and oxidative stress; improved markers of cardiovascular disease such as blood pressure, resting heart rate, and levels of high-density and low-density lipoprotein (HDL and LDL) cholesterol, triglycerides, glucose, and insulin; and prevention and treatment of autoimmune diseases such as arthritis, asthma, and multiple sclerosis. Intermittent fasting can also promote brain health by enhancing production of a protein called brain-derived neurotrophic factor, a substance that prevents stressed neurons from dying. This boosts cognition in multiple domains, including spatial, associative, and working memory.

Get Started

If you'd like to try intermittent fasting, first get your doctor's go-ahead and stock up on plenty of fruits and vegetables, lean meats, nuts, and seeds to follow a healthful plant-based Mediterranean dietary plan during your eating hours. Set your eating window for the time that works best for you. If you wake up hungry, set an early window. If nighttime hunger is a problem, move your eating window later so you can eat when you are most hungry. To stave off hunger in your fasting periods, drink plenty of calorie-free liquids and keep busy with hobbies and exercise. Also, remember that it takes about a month for your body to adjust to fasting.

Why You Still Feel Hungry After Eating

HealthLine.com

If you frequently have the munchies soon after a meal, here are likely reasons. *Not enough protein*—a high-protein meal helps you feel fuller than a high-carb or high-fat meal. *Not enough fiber*—fiber takes longer to digest than other carbs and slows your stomach's emptying rate. *Not enough volume*—"stretch receptors" in your stomach sense how much you've eaten. Vegetables, chicken breast and turkey are good high-volume/low-calorie choices. *Eating too quickly or while distracted*—not chewing thoroughly and not focusing on your eating make you feel less full. *Leptin resistance*—your brain may have trouble recognizing the hormone that signals fullness. Plentiful sleep and exercise helps, but see a doctor if you suspect this is the problem.

Exercise Could Make Up for Bad Sleep

Insufficient sleep, insomnia, snoring, and daytime sleepiness increase risk for stroke, coronary heart disease and death.

Recent study: Getting the recommended amount of weekly physical activity (75 minutes vigorous/150 minutes moderate) offsets the serious health consequences of poor sleep.

Emmanuel Stamatakis, PhD, professor of physical activity and population health at University of Sydney, Australia, and leader of an 11-year study of 400,000 adults, published in *British Journal of Sports Medicine*.

Sleeping More Could Help You Lose Weight

Study titled "Effect of Sleep Extension on Objectively Assessed Energy Intake Among Adults with Overweight in Real-Life Settings," by researchers at the University of Chicago Sleep Center, published in *JAMA Internal Medicine*.

When it comes to fighting the battle of the bulge, research has shown that dieting (eating less calories) is more effective than burning calories through exercise. But dieting is difficult in the land of plenty, so researchers continue to search out unique ways to help people lose weight. These researchers include those who study sleep. One of the interesting discoveries from sleep research is that people who slumber less than the recommended seven to eight hours a night tend to eat more and gain more weight. Lack of sleep leads to increased appetite.

A team of researchers led by the University of Chicago Sleep Center wanted to see if the opposite was true. Would people who sleep more—called sleep extension—take in less calories? To find out, 80 overweight adults who averaged less than 6.5 hours of sleep per night were recruited for a four-week study.

More Sleep Resulted in Less Calorie Intake

Half of these volunteers received personalized instruction in sleep hygiene to help them sleep longer. The other half made no changes in their hours of sleep. Neither group increased their activity level or made any changes in their diet. At the end of the study, the sleep extension group had increased sleep by 1.2 hours and decreased calories by 270 per day. Over three years that decrease in calories would amount to about 25 pounds of weight loss.

During the first two weeks of the study, body measurements, calorie intake, and hours of sleep were recorded for all the participants. Their ages were 21 to 40 and they were about equally divided between men and women. Their BMIs ranged from 25 to 29.9. BMI (Body Mass Index) is a measure of weight health based on height and weight. A BMI between 25 and 29.9 is considered overweight. After establishing baselines for sleep and calorie intake, half of the group were given sleep hygiene instructions to extend their sleep to up to 8.5 hours per night. Sleep hygiene includes steps such as going to bed at the same time every night, keeping your bedroom quiet and dark, avoiding caffeine late in the day and using your bed only for sleep and sex. The intervention that seemed to work best was avoiding electronic devices before going to sleep. The study is published in the journal *JAMA Internal Medicine*.

Hours of sleep were measured by a motion sensing device worn at night. Calorie intake was measured with a urine-based test that has been shown to reliably measure daily energy use, along with daily weights and a type of body-composition imaging called dual-energy x-ray absorptiometry.

Sleep Extension = Safe, Easy Weight Loss

The results of the study show that sleeping more results in less calories taken in, probably due to a decrease in appetite, since nothing else was modified. Those in the sleep extension group who added more than 1.2 hours of sleep took in even less calories, up to 393 calories for the longest sleepers. The control group, who did not change their sleep habits, had no change in calorie intake.

The research team concludes that sleep extension for people who are overweight and sleep less than the recommended seven to eight hours per night is a safe and effective way to help people lose weight and could be part of obesity prevention or weight loss programs. So if you'd like to lose weight and you enjoy late-night scrolling and media binge-watching, try to cut back, hit the hay earlier, and see how your appetite responds.

Copious Protein Doesn't Build Extra Muscle

Nicholas Burd, PhD, is associate professor of kinesiology at University of Illinois at Urbana-Champaign and leader of a study published in *American Journal of Physiology: Endocrinology and Metabolism.*

The Recommended Dietary Allowance for protein is about 0.36 grams of protein per pound of body weight per day (about 56 grams for the average man, 46 grams for the average woman). In a study of 50 weight-lifting novices ages 40 to 64, those on a high-protein diet saw no benefit in strength or body composition after 10 weeks of training versus those on a moderate-protein diet.

Lift Weights to Burn Fat

Researchers discovered that strength training for 45 to 60 minutes three times per week cuts the same amount of body fat as an equivalent amount of cardiovascular exercise. After analyzing 58 studies, they found that five months of exercise leads to an average fat loss of 1.4 percent of body weight.

University of New South Wales, Kensington, Australia.

Limitations of BMI

William Yancy, MD, professor of medicine, Duke University School of Medicine, and medical director of the Duke Lifestyle & Weight Management Center.

Body mass index (BMI) has become the most commonly used measurement to assess the relative healthiness of one's weight.

It delineates where normal weight crosses into overweight, and where obesity—and its associated health risks—begins. But taken as a single measure, its accuracy and validity can vary widely.

BMI Basics

BMI is calculated as (weight in kilograms [kg]) / (height in meters [m] squared). Ideal BMI is between 18.5 kg/m2 and 25 kg/m2 (BMI is usually written without the unit of measure.) A person with a BMI between 25 and 30 is considered overweight, and a person with a BMI 30 or over is considered obese. Generally, people with higher BMIs have a higher risk of diabetes, arthritis, fatty liver disease, hypertension, some cancers, high cholesterol, and sleep apnea.

Studies show that BMI can accurately reflect the health risks of obesity at high levels (over 30), but is less reliable in the overweight (25 to 30) category. That's because BMI only represents weight by height. It doesn't differentiate between lean and fat mass. A weightlifter or athlete, for example, could be very lean and muscular but show a high BMI because of overall weight.

Further, BMI doesn't take into account the location of fat. Visceral (or belly) fat is associated with more health risks than higher fat in other parts of the body. The value of BMI has also been questioned in older adults because height and body composition change as we age.

Even one's ethnicity can affect the validity of BMI. Asians have higher health risks at substantially lower BMI levels, so different risk cutoffs are used. In addition, studies have shown that at the same BMI, people who are African American have lower levels of body fat than those who are Caucasian.

Other Measures to Consider

•**Waist size.** The National Institutes of Health concluded that a waist larger than 40 inches for men and 35 inches for women increases the chances of developing heart disease, cancer, or other chronic diseases. Waist measurement is fairly easy to use, but there is less information available about race/ethnic variations.

Body-Fat Scales

Scales that use bioelectric impedance are widely available and inexpensive. They send a small electric current through the body and measure the resistance. (The current faces more resistance passing through body fat than it does passing through lean body mass and water.) These measurements can be affected by hydration, so be careful hanging your hat on one measurement. Following a trend may be more useful.

•**Waist-to-hip ratio.** You can also take your waist measurement and divide it by your hip measurement to get a waist-to-hip ratio. According to the World Health Organization, a healthy result is 0.9 or less in men and 0.85 or less for women. Waist-to-hip ratio is not substantially more accurate at determining risk than waist size alone but is more difficult to interpret.

•**Relative fat mass index (RFM).** Researchers at Cedars Mount Sinai developed a formula to compare height and waist circumference…

Men: 64 - (20 x height/waist circumference) = RFM

Women: 76 - (20 x height/waist circumference) = RFM

Men who score over 30 and women who score over 40 would be considered obese and at elevated risk for health problems and even death.

There are more technical ways to measure body fat, but many are fairly expensive and therefore reserved for research purposes. BMI remains one of the easiest ways to determine risk and is accurate in a large percentage of people. Having said that, it is probably more useful for health providers and researchers than it is for patients.

Core Curriculum: 5 Pilates Exercises to Maintain Strength and Vitality

Erica Christ, founder/owner of FMR Wellness in Port Chester, New York. Erica is a fully certified, advanced Pilates instructor, exercise physiologist, health and fitness instructor certified through the American College of Sports Medicine, certified diabetes educator (CDE) and registered dietitian (RD). EricaChrist.com

If you want to be able to turn around in your car and grab something in the back seat without throwing out your back…if you want to be able to pick up a heavy, oversized box without getting hurt…if you want to keep doing all the things you were able to do when you were 20 years old when you reach 90, consider taking up a Pilates routine at home.

The Pilates method is an excellent form of low-impact exercise to strengthen the multitude of muscles that surround the spine, from the top of your neck to the tip of your tailbone. In addition, Pilates can improve posture and balance to help protect your body from falling and other injuries.

Core Principles of Pilates

Pilates, developed by Joseph Pilates, a German physical trainer, in the 1920s, often is associated with the use of large pieces of studio equipment with bars, straps and springs that create resistance. But you can also do Pilates exercises at home using just a thick padded mat.

The Pilates philosophy has evolved substantially beyond Joseph Pilates' original concept of using movement to help people heal their bodies from injury. Today, there is a distinct intellectual component to the practice of Pilates, in which participants are encouraged to continuously think about their body alignment as they do each exercise to ensure proper movement and avoid further injury. *The core Pilates principles…*

•**Centering.** All Pilates movements start from and are sustained through the Center, known as the core or Powerhouse. This is true even if you are working other muscle groups such as the arms or legs. Your Powerhouse includes all of your musculature from shoulder to shoulder and hip to hip, from the front to the back of the body.

•**Concentration.** With Pilates, the mind guides the body. Razorlike focus on what you are doing is essential to executing the exercises to their fullest benefit.

•**Precision.** To gain the most benefit from each exercise, you have to do them precisely. Pay attention to the form, structure and quality of your movements. If you are doing an exercise in the optimal manner, you don't need a lot of repetitions to tire the muscle.

•**Control.** Gravity must never be allowed to control the exercises. You can control gravity by moving slowly through the motion.

•**Breath.** Pilates breathing is about increasing your lung capacity, inhaling to increase oxygenation of muscles and exhaling to rid the body of stale air. By supplying fresh oxygen during an exercise, the muscles of the Powerhouse become stronger and more flexible.

•**Flow.** As you progress with your Pilates practice, your goal is to move continuously and gracefully from one exercise to the next.

Essential Exercises

This powerful five-exercise workout takes a mere 15 minutes. It stretches and strengthens nearly every muscle in your body—all the muscles of the Powerhouse in your core as well as neck, legs and arms, glutes (buttocks) and inner thighs, hamstrings (back of the thighs) and hip flexors. It even massages the spine. Do the exercises at least once a week formally, but try to bring the principles of the practice into your everyday movement as often as possible. As explained above, do them slowly and thoughtfully with an emphasis on maintaining good form—keep your abdominal muscles pulled in and your spine lengthening rather than compressing.

You don't want to increase repetitions...you want to enhance the effort by engaging the muscles with more depth and control. You may not feel like you're moving very much at first, and that's OK. Your goal with each exercise is to fatigue your muscles without feeling pain—which could mean as few as five repetitions. If your muscles shake, that's also OK—it is a sign of painless fatiguing.

Helpful: Look online for a beginner Pilates mat class, or book a virtual session with an instructor to learn proper form so you do the exercises safely.

My favorite online resource: Pilates Anytime.com, $22 per month after a 15-day free trial.

If a move hurts, stop doing it—never try to work through pain. Part of the progression with Pilates is learning how to self-correct if something hurts. Meeting with an instructor also can help you learn how.

Warning: Yoga mats are too thin to cushion pressure points and protect the back.

Preferred mat: EcoWise ⅝-inch thick ($65, Aeromats.com).

I. Hundred

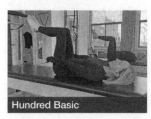
Hundred Basic

Lie on your mat, and center your body. Bring your knees into tabletop position (knees over your hips, shins parallel to the floor), and raise your head and neck up toward your knees. Be sure to raise your head and neck from your core and not by simply tucking your chin, which can put undo strain on your neck. Vigorously pump your arms up and down to above the level of your hips and then down to the floor while you inhale deeply for five counts and then exhale deeply for five counts up. Start with one to five repetitions, and work up to a max of 10 repetitions, which is 100 pumps.

Important: Inhale through your nose, exhale through your mouth as if you're breathing through a straw to support your upper

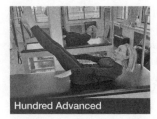
Hundred Advanced

body. If you feel neck strain, lower your head and neck a bit and continue the exercise. Count breaths, not hand pumps.

To advance the movement: Perform the exercise with your legs straight, toes relaxed. The higher your legs, the more you support your back.

2. Single Leg Circles

Lie on your back on your mat, arms at your sides, palms down. Extend one leg up to the ceiling as high as you can. The bottom leg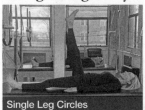
Single Leg Circles
can be straight, or bend it to support the back and help straighten the lifted leg. Keep the knee soft, and push the heel of the lower leg gently into the mat to stabilize the hips. Start making a circle with your extended leg, staying within the frame of the body. Your goal is to keep the hips stable on the mat. Repeat five times, and then reverse the circle for five repetitions. Switch legs, and repeat on the other side.

To advance the movement: Straightening the bottom leg and/or increasing the diameter of the circle can both increase the challenge of this exercise, but you never want to go wider than your shoulders, and your hips always should stay on the mat.

3. Rolling Like a Ball

Sit on your mat, knees bent, feet on the mat. Place your hands behind your knees, and lift your feet off the mat a few inches. With a small rhythmic rocking motion, gently roll back as far as feels comfortable and then come back up in a continuous flow. The motion drives from the abdominals. Keep your

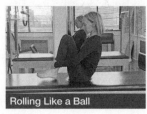
Rolling Like a Ball

abdominal muscles pulled in and up. Inhale as you rock back, and exhale as you rock forward. Progress to rolling farther back toward the floor and back up again, keeping arms behind your knees.

To advance the movement: Hug your shins so your body is in a tighter ball. Repeat five to 10 times.

4. Single Leg Stretch

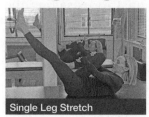
Single Leg Stretch

Lie on your mat, and bring your knees into your chest. Lift your head and shoulders off of the mat using your abdominal muscles rather than your neck muscles to avoid straining your neck. Place both hands on one knee with your elbows out wide. Extend the other leg out at no more than a 45-degree angle while you continue to hug the knee toward your chest. Exhale and pull the extended leg toward your shoulder. Inhale and shift your hands, and extend the other leg. Exhale and pull the extended leg toward your shoulder. If your neck is compromised with lifting, keep your head on the mat. Repeat eight to 10 times for each leg.

To advance the movement: You can hold your position during your breath work and increase the movement flow.

5. Spine Stretch Forward

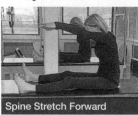
Spine Stretch Forward

Sit up tall on your mat. Open your legs a bit wider than your mat, keeping your knees slightly bent and your feet flexed, so that the heels are digging into the mat. Reach both of your arms forward at shoulder height and shoulder-width apart with your fingers stretching toward the end of the mat. The arms should be at shoulder height and parallel to the mat at all times during this exercise. Shoulders should remain neutral. Inhale and lift your spine. Exhale and curl your nose toward your naval and the top of your head toward the mat. Let the shoulders move naturally, and keep your lower back straight as you stretch forward—curl from your upper back and shoulder blades. Inhale as you roll back up to sitting tall. Exhale and repeat three to five times.

To advance the movement: Deepen your exhalation so it reaches further into the abdominals to deepen the stretch of the spine.

Exercise photos courtesy of Erica Christ.

Tired of the Gym? Try Golf

Carrie Ali, editor, *Bottom Line Health*. BottomLine Inc.com

The gym isn't for everyone. It's good news, then, that enjoying a day on the golf course provides a complete workout with aerobic, strength, and balance activities. A study presented at the International Stroke Conference last year found that it's associated with longevity, too. Regular golfers have a significantly lower rate of death over

10 years than non-golfers: 15.1 percent compared with 24.6 percent.

In the International Consensus Statement on Golf and Health, 25 experts outlined multiple health benefits of the game…

•**Golf can provide moderate-intensity physical activity.** Over an 18-hole game, golfers walk from four to eight miles, racking up 11,245 to 16,667 steps. Even golfers who use carts still take about 6,280 steps. As a result, golfers expend 531 to 2,467 calories during the game.

•**Golf boosts physical health.** Regularly playing golf lowers total and low-density lipoprotein cholesterol and improves body composition, cardiorespiratory performance, and trunk muscle endurance.

•**Golf reduces risk factors for cardiovascular disease** by improving blood lipid, insulin, and glucose levels while increasing physical activity and aerobic fitness.

•**Golf is associated with mental well-being,** including lower stress, more energy, and increased socialization.

•**Golfers have better strength and balance.** Shifting weight while swinging a golf club and walking on uneven terrain may be responsible for this fall-preventing benefit.

From fresh air to friends, steps to stress reduction, there are many reasons to hit the links. The pace is perfect for people to continue as they age, even after major health events, such as stroke or heart attack. But if you start soon enough, you just may hold major health problems at bay.

Save on a Gym Membership

Use a guest pass—use a free pass to check out a gym before signing up. The site FreeFlys.com can help you find guest passes in your area. *Join a minimalist gym*—if you need only the bare minimum and can skip the juice bars, child care and other perks, check out gyms with low-cost options, often locally owned…or Planet Fitness, which has plans that start as low as $10/month. *Check with your insurance*—it may offer a discount on a gym membership. *Consider community recreation centers*—these often offer low yearly membership deals or daily rates and generally have a lot of the same exercise equipment and classes that are available at local gyms.

LivingOnTheCheap.com

Afternoon Workouts Are Better for You

Study by researchers at Maastricht University Medical Center, the Netherlands, published in *Physiological Reports.*

If you struggle to drag yourself out of bed for an early-morning workout, you can stop beating yourself up.

Recent finding: Of 32 men at risk for or who had type 2 diabetes, those who worked out between 3:00 pm and 6:00 pm did better on tests of insulin sensitivity, body composition, weight loss and exercise performance than those who worked out between 8:00 am and 10:00 am.

Try Tai Chi

Rudolph Tanzi, MD, Joseph P. and Rose F. Kennedy Professor of Neurology, Harvard Medical School, and Tara Stiles, founder of Strala Yoga, and author of *Clean Mind, Clean Body: A 28-Day Plan for Physical, Mental and Spiritual Self-Care.*

Tai chi is a gentle, low-impact exercise that involves a series of graceful movements accompanied by deep breathing. It is gentle enough for anyone, and research suggests that it offers substantial benefits.

- **Cognitive functioning.** A study led by Peter Wayne, PhD, a professor of medicine at Harvard Medical School, reported that tai chi shows potential to enhance cognitive function in older adults by improving attention and processing speed.

- **Osteoarthritis.** Tai chi can reduce pain and stiffness while increasing physical function. The American College of Rheumatology recommends it for osteoarthritis of the hip and knee.

- **Lung disease.** Several review articles reported that tai chi can improve asthma and chronic obstructive pulmonary disease, according to a report in *Canadian Family Physician.*

- **Stress relief.** The exercise can also promote the relaxation response, which can help lower blood pressure, heart rate, breathing rate, oxygen consumption, adrenaline levels, and levels of the stress hormone cortisol.

Give It a Try

All of these benefits are pretty impressive for an exercise that won't cause you to break a sweat. *Here are a few simple exercises you can try at home...*

Avoid These Workout Mistakes

Stretching same-hand to same-foot. When doing a seated one-leg stretch, always reach for your toes with the opposite-side hand. ***Leaning forward when you squat.*** If you tend to bend forward at the waist while doing squats, try crossing your arms in front of your chest to correct your form. ***Working your neck during ab exercises.*** You should never feel strain in your neck while you're doing crunches. If you do, you're probably pulling upward on the back of your head with your hands. Instead, make an X in front of you by crossing your forearms at the wrists, palms inward, and move this X behind you to the base of your neck to use as a cradle during the exercise. It'll keep you from tugging up on your head.

Celebrity trainer Joel Harper. JoelHarperFitness. com

- **Breathing exercise for relaxation.** Sit or stand comfortably. Close your eyes and relax your knees, elbows, and shoulders. Remain soft and moveable. Imagine that if someone nudged you gently, you would sway like a tree in the wind. Stay in this state for a moment before taking a single, deep breath through your nose. Notice your body lifting up and expanding with your inhalation. Exhale through your mouth and notice your body relaxing downward. Repeat this breathing twice more. Notice how your body moves after your breath. The movement follows the breath. Keep your eyes closed. How does your body feel? Softer? Do you feel tension anywhere? Take note. When you're ready, gently open your eyes.

- **Movement exercise.** Stand comfortably, with your knees, elbows, and shoulders soft. Let your arms hang by your sides. Move your hips from side to side, letting your arms

Small Bouts of Exercise Work for Good Health

Four Seconds Is Good...

Bouts of intense exercise lasting as little as four seconds can have surprising benefits—especially for people who spend hours at a time sitting at a desk, which can make it harder to burn fat even during exercise. A small study found that such micro-sessions conducted five times per hour over an eight-hour period improved fat metabolism and lowered triglycerides. Study participants used a specialized exercise bike that allowed them to hit maximal energy exertion quickly.

Study by researchers at University of Texas at Austin published in *Medicine & Science in Sports & Exercise*.

12 Minutes a Day Is Better...

Twelve minutes a day of strenuous exercise can be enough to boost life expectancy and lower the risk for heart disease and diabetes. After a 12-minute burst of intense physical activity, levels of the biomarker DMGV—which is linked to risk for diabetes and fatty liver disease—dropped 18 percent. And levels of glutamate—associated with heart disease, diabetes, and shorter life expectancy—decreased 29 percent. The exercise needs to be intense and done on a regular basis—but does not need to continue for a long time.

Study of 411 men and women by researchers at Massachusetts General Hospital, Boston, published in *Circulation*.

soft. As you exhale slowly and deeply, lower your arms to your sides.

Tai Chi Sequences

Tai chi instructors create routines that combine a variety of gentle movements with fanciful names, such as Grasp the Bird's Tail, White Crane Flashes Its Wings, and Step Back to Repulse the Monkey. These more advanced programs, which you've likely seen in movies or television shows, offer additional benefits as you shift your weight from side to side, stretch, and gently strengthen muscles. There are different styles and sequences, and a class is an excellent place to learn them. Look for programs at the local hospital, fitness center, or community center, or find instructional videos online.

A Single Exercise Session Boosts Metabolism

Oregon State University

Sedentary people who rode a stationary bicycle at a moderate pace for one hour showed enhanced mitochondrial activity in a laboratory study. They burned 12 to 13 percent more fat-based-fuel and 14 to 17 percent more sugar-based fuel.

For Better Health, Walk with a Purpose

Study of the walking habits of more than 125,885 people, ages 18 to 64, by researchers at The Ohio State University, Columbus, published in *Journal of Transport & Health*.

People who walk from home to work or for other specific purposes, such as to the grocery store, report better health than those who walk for leisure. Those who walk for targeted purposes walk faster—an average of

sway gently like windshield wipers. Let your breath guide your motions.

• **Touch the sky.** Sit up straight in a comfortable chair. Place your hands in your lap, palms up. Take a slow, deep breath and raise your hands in front of you to chest level. Then turn your palms outward and lift your hands above your head. Keep your elbows

2.7 miles per hour, versus 2.55 miles per hour for people who walk for recreational reasons. Trips from home also are longer—64 percent last at least 10 minutes, compared with 50 percent of walks that begin elsewhere.

Pogo Sticks Keep Grown-Ups Fit

OutdoorSportsLab.com and PogoSticks.club.

If you bounced on one of these as a child, consider taking it up again—not just for fun, but for great health benefits. Pogo sticking is especially good for improving back muscles, which help maintain balance, as well as strengthening muscles of the stomach, legs, hips and butt.

Bonus: One hour of pogo sticking burns 600 calories.

Cost: Pogo sticks suitable for adults are available on Amazon and start at about $130.

Fun fact: Pogo sticking is now a professional sport. Called Extreme Pogo or "Xpogo," the highest recorded bounce by a professional player is more than 11 feet. Learn more at PogoSticks.club.

Foot Muscles Need Exercise, Too

Lifehacker.com

Strengthening moves: Stand barefoot with feet flat on the floor, and pull your arch upward to shorten your footprint and raise your instep.

Toe scrunch: Place a dish towel on the floor, and stand barefoot on it, then scrunch your toes to bunch up the towel.

Run on uneven terrain: Running on trails, sand or grass gives your feet a workout because they need to support your body at a variety of angles on varied terrain.

Once You Build Muscle, Your Body Never Forgets

Kevin Murach, PhD, assistant professor, University of Arkansas, Fayetteville, Arkansas.

Good news for anyone who took a break from strength training during the pandemic: Previously trained muscles respond to exercise with more sensitivity and grow more rapidly than previously untrained muscles, thanks to DNA memory.

Chapter 7

GET THE BEST MEDICAL CARE

Telehealth Transformation

Before the pandemic, seeing a doctor meant being limited to health-care providers in a drivable distance, trudging to the office, and sitting for up to an hour in a germy waiting room—even after you were told to arrive 15 minutes early. But the widespread acceptance of telehealth—the use of telecommunication technologies and electronic information to deliver care—has changed everything.

With telehealth, you receive care from home, appointments are usually on time, and you can see a provider from anywhere in the country if you live in a state that has waived in-state doctor requirements. That's because the federal government responded to the overwhelming need for care and a shortage of health-care providers in any given place by easing restrictions on telehealth and providing more money for the visits.

From Acute to Chronic Care

In the simplest form of the technology, you can use a phone or computer to have a doctor's visit using a platform such as Zoom. These programs are easy to use, and most doctors' offices will walk you through getting set up. You and the doctor can see each other during the visit.

A growing number of health-care providers are going a step further and using technology to better monitor chronic health conditions to keep you well and out of the hospital. At home, you can use tools such as wireless blood pressure cuffs, pulse oximeters, scales, a glucometer, and wearables such as Fitbits or Apple Watches to gather data and upload it into software and services that run on the Internet (the Cloud). Your doctor's office can then monitor that data manually or with the use of artificial intelligence. When a nurse navigator (a nurse who serves as a liaison between you and your doctor) sees a trend that could suggest worsening symptoms, he or she can intervene before those symptoms become a full-blown problem.

Consider a patient with congestive heart failure (CHF). When CHF worsens, patients may have a sudden weight gain in a short time and have shortness of breath that leads

---

David Wilcox DNP, MHA, BSN, RN-BC, LSSBB, author of *How to Avoid Being a Victim of the American Healthcare System: A Patient's Handbook for Survival.* Dr. Wilcox has a doctorate in nurse executive leadership with a focus on using technology to improve patient care.

to walking less due to increased retention of fluid. If a wireless scale detects a 5-pound weight gain in a few days, a pulse oximeter shows low oxygen levels, and a Fitbit shows that a person's steps have dropped dramatically, a nurse navigator can set up a telehealth appointment for the patient with the doctor to address those concerns before they worsen.

I would strongly encourage you to manage any chronic disease using these tools. They will increase your quality of life and allow you to avoid nasty germy hospitals and doctors' offices. It should decrease the amount of time you spend going to doctor's appointments and should cost you only minutes a day of your time.

Hospital at Home

Telehealth isn't limited to routine doctor visits: It's affecting hospitalization too. Hospital-at-home can make any room in your house into a hospital room complete with oxygen tanks, medical supplies, and almost anything else you may need. Many of these programs are linked to a 24/7 monitoring system to monitor your vital signs and other pertinent health-care data in real time. Your health-care team can go over your data and communicate with you remotely, and send a nurse when you need one. Plus, you'll have a button you can press at any time for emergency help.

For people with lower-level health issues, this is the perfect combination of technology and clinical care in which patients can derive the benefit of staying at home while

Technology and Medication

For Americans ages 65 and older, 33 to 69 percent of hospital admissions are due to patients not taking their medications. Another 40 percent of nursing home admissions occur because Americans are unable to reliably self-medicate at home. With one in four people over 65 living alone, telehealth solutions could allow them to live independently longer. If a home health nurse visits a patient once a week and loads their medication-monitoring device with a week's worth of their medications, the system can notify the patient when to take their medication by several means. It could be an alarm, text message or if the device is interfaced into Google Mini or Alexa, it could be delivered verbally. These systems are also capable of alerting the home health agency, a relative, or the doctor's office when the patient doesn't take their medications.

Excerpted from *How to Avoid Being a Victim of the American Healthcare System: A Patient's Handbook for Survival.*

their chronic care is being managed or they are recovering from an illness. Patients sleep better in a quiet home, fall less often, are more mobile, and can eat whatever they want. And studies are showing that patients recover just as well at home as in the hospital.

In the future hospitals will consist only of emergency departments, intensive care units, stepdown beds which is where a patient is cared for before they become a low-acuity (less sick) patient, and home care.

Telehealth Considerations

The technology that doctors are using is streamlined and quick to learn and use—even for people who don't consider themselves to be tech-savvy. But access isn't equally available to everyone. People in rural areas may not have the broadband internet access that is necessary for video. A telephone call may be adequate in some cases, but not all. As such, in October 2020, the Federal Communications Commission introduced a $20 billion fund to improve broadband access in rural America. The Coronavirus Aid, Relief, and Economic Security (CARES) Act of March 2020 included another $200 million to help provide devices to patients who don't have phones or computers to access telehealth.

A New Model of Care

Telehealth will play a key role in the transformation from fee-for-service health care (where doctors are paid according to how many tests and procedures they perform) to value-based care (where doctors earn more by keeping patients healthy and out of the hospital). Value-based care is provided by groups of health-care providers called accountable care organizations (ACO). In the model, a health-care team is paid a set amount of money for each person they treat—no matter what care that person needs.

If the group spends less than they've been given for a patient, they get to keep the difference. The best way for these groups to save money on a patient's care is to keep them healthy and out of the hospital. Technology makes it easier for patients and providers alike to stay in touch and on top of chronic health conditions, reducing the likelihood of hospitalization.

The Power of Prevention: A Guide to Health Screenings

Multiple members of the United States Preventive Services Task Force, including Michael Silverstein, MD, MPH, Boston University School of Medicine; John B. Wong, MD, Tufts Medical Center; Aaron B. Caughey, MD, MPP, MPH, PhD, Oregon Health & Science University, et al.

Health screenings help healthy people stay well. Physicians use them to look for signs of potential problems before they become symptomatic and when they're easier to treat. A multitude of health-care organizations develop screening guidelines, but they don't always agree. That's where the United States Preventive Services Task Force steps in. This independent, non-governmental body digs deep into the research to compare the benefits and harms of a wide variety of preventive screenings. *Here's a look at the Task Force's recommended screenings...*

•**Abdominal aortic aneurysm.** The USPSTF recommends one-time screening for abdominal aortic aneurysm (AAA) with ultrasonography in men ages 65 to 75 years with

a history of smoking. Men in this age group who have never smoked may be screened selectively taking into consideration a patient's medical history, family history, other risk factors and personal values. There is insufficient evidence to assess the balance of benefits and harms of screening for AAA with ultrasonography in women ages 65 to 75 years who have ever smoked or have a family history of AAA. Women who have never smoked should not be screened.

•**Breast cancer.** Women should have a mammogram every other year starting by age 50. Some women in their 40s may benefit from screening and should discuss what's best for them with their doctor. The current evidence is insufficient to assess the balance of benefits and harms of mammography in women ages 75 years or older. (But see page 22 and discuss with your doctor.)

•**Cervical cancer.** Screening is recommended every three years with the Pap test (cervical cytology) for women ages 21 to 29. Women ages 30 to 65 have three options: screening with the Pap test alone every three years, screening with high-risk human papillomavirus (hrHPV) testing alone every five years, or with both tests every five years.

Cervical cancer screening is not recommended in women who are older than age 65 who have had adequate prior screening and are not otherwise at high risk, or for women of any age who have had a hysterectomy with removal of the cervix and no history of cervical cancer or no history of high-grade precancerous lesions.

•**Colorectal cancer.** Screening should begin at age 45 and continue until age 75. The frequency of screening depends on the test used. Stool-based tests should be repeated every one to three years (depending on the specific stool test used), whereas CT colonography (the use of CT scanning to produce images of the colon) and flexible sigmoidoscopy (an endoscopic examination of the rectum and lower colon) are recommended every five years. Flexible sigmoidoscopy can occur every 10 years if stool testing with a fecal immunochemical test (FIT) occurs every year. Colonoscopy, which lets your doctor see the entire colon, should be repeated every 10 years.

The USPSTF recommends that clinicians selectively offer screening for colorectal cancer in adults ages 76 to 85.

●**Hepatitis B.** Screening is recommended for people at increased risk, including those born in countries with a high prevalence of hepatitis B, unvaccinated people born in the United States to parents from a high-risk country, current or previous users of injected drugs, men who have sex with men, people with HIV, and those with household contacts or sexual partners of hepatitis-B-positive people.

●**Hepatitis C.** Screening should be done at least one time for adults ages 18 to 79. People who continue to have risk factors, such as injected drug use, should be routinely tested.

●**Human Immunodeficiency Virus.** Screening should occur in everyone ages 15 to 65. Adults older than 65 should be screened if they have risk factors for HIV. Risk factors include sexually active men who have sex with men, people with an HIV-positive sex partner, injectable drug use, commercial sex work, and having other sexually transmitted infections.

●**Hypertension.** The USPSTF recommends screening blood pressure in a clinician's office for people ages 18 or older who do not have known hypertension.

●**Lung cancer.** Screening with low-dose computed tomography (a procedure that uses a computer linked to an x-ray machine that gives off a very low dose of radiation to make a series of detailed images) is recommended for adults ages 50 to 80 years who have smoked the equivalent of a pack of cigarettes a day for 20 years and currently smoke or have quit within the past 15 years. Screening should be discontinued once a person has not smoked for 15 years.

●**Osteoporosis.** Bone measurement testing is recommended in all women ages 65 and older, and in postmenopausal women who are younger than 65 but are at risk based on a formal risk assessment. Risk factors include a parental history of hip fracture,

smoking, excessive alcohol consumption and low body weight. It's unclear how often this testing should occur, but limited evidence suggests that re-testing women with normal bone mass in four to eight years offers no additional benefit.

●**Prostate cancer.** Men ages 55 to 69 should talk with their physicians about undergoing periodic PSA-based screening for prostate cancer. Patients should consider family history, race and ethnicity, and other medical conditions to determine if screening is appropriate. Men 70 and older should not be screened for prostate cancer.

●**Type 2 diabetes.** People ages 35 to 70 who have a BMI of 25 and over should be screened for prediabetes and type 2 diabetes.

Keeping Your Own Medical Record

Charles B. Inlander is a consumer advocate and health-care consultant based in Fogelsville, Pennsylvania. He was the founding president of the nonprofit People's Medical Society, a consumer-advocacy organization credited with key improvements in the quality of U.S. health care, and author or coauthor of more than 20 consumer-health books.

The longer you live, the more encounters you have with the health care system. After a while, you may forget or get confused about procedures or illnesses you had when you were younger. Was it measles or chickenpox, mumps, or whooping cough? Have you had your tonsils removed? Did you have cataracts removed from one or both eyes? And what about medication allergies?

Remembering these issues and other important occurrences related to your health is important. The more information about your health history you can pass along to a health-care provider, the better that professional can treat your current or future problems. You're likely thinking that your doctor has all that information because he or she has been treating you for years. And that may be true for your primary care doctor. But what about specialists you see? While most of those doctors now use electronic medical record systems, those systems are often unable to communicate with doctors or hospitals outside their own system, so it's up to you to provide them with all the information.

That is why I recommend keeping your own medical record. It's easy to assemble and maintain, and you'll find it to be one of the most useful efforts you can make to ensure the best health treatment. *Here's how to do it…*

•**Create your record format.** You can keep your record on a computer or on paper. I prefer both. If you use a computer, create a health record file in a program like Word. If you are doing it exclusively on paper, use a loose-leaf binder. Make a single page for each important topic, such as childhood diseases, surgical procedures, major diagnoses, medications, inoculations, family history of conditions, and provider office visits. Focus on one topic at a time to make this task easier and quicker. By assembling your record in this manner, you will be able to quickly find out the information you or your provider is seeking.

•**Gather your data.** For each topic area, start by listing the information you remember. For example, I had mumps when I was less than 10 and my tonsils removed when I was five or six. Going way back, you may need the help of a sibling or other relative who might remember your ailments. Try to put things down chronologically from the earliest to the latest. The exact dates are not that important, but a general timeframe might help. If you have copies of medical records created by your doctor or from a hospitalization, review them for any pertinent information. Under federal and state laws, you have a right to access and review medical records maintained by your doctor or a hospital. Don't be afraid to ask for it.

•**How to use it.** Keep your record as up-to-date as possible. For example, under medications, keep an active list of current medications you take, noting the dose and frequency. Under that same topic, keep a list of adverse reactions to any medications you

Smartwatch Can Monitor Symptoms of Parkinson's Disease

A system called the motor fluctuations monitor for Parkinson's disease (MM4PD) uses the Apple Watch's accelerometer and gyroscope data to continuously track changes in resting tremors and involuntary muscle movements. A study found that the MM4PD measurements correlate well with in-clinic evaluations and capture symptom changes in response to treatment in 94 percent of participants.

Jamie Adams, MD, assistant professor, department of neurology, movement disorders, University of Rochester, New York.

have taken in the past. I bring my loose-leaf binder with me any time I am seeing a new doctor or medical professional. This saves my time and theirs as they assemble my medical history. If you have the information on a computer, transfer it to your smartphone or a tablet when you see someone new so that you can quickly access it.

Health care is a partnership between you and your providers. The most accurate and complete information available to each of you will only make your care better.

Find the Doctor Who's Right for You

R. Ruth Linden, PhD, founder and president of Tree of Life Health Advocates, where she helps clients with serious illnesses navigate the health-care system. She is a former professor at the University of California, San Francisco; Stanford University; and Tufts University; and has advised the FDA on developing policy to facilitate expanded access to experimental therapies. TreeOfLifeHealthAdvocates.com

here are many reasons why you might need to find a new doctor: You moved. Your doctor retired. Your insurance changed. You're dissatisfied with your care.

You have trouble scheduling an appointment with the physician and always end up seeing a nurse practitioner or a physician's assistant.

Knowing that it's time to move on is the easy part, but simply finding a new doctor isn't enough: For your health and well-being, you need to find the doctor who is right for you.

The Challenge

Finding the right primary care physician or specialist may not be easy. In fact, it's likely to be extremely difficult. The best primary care doctors often have full practices, and they may not be taking new patients. A growing number of physicians accept only direct payment, not insurance. Among those who do take insurance, you have to find one who is in your network. And then you need to find one that you both like and trust.

Smart Tips for Finding the Right Doctor

Taking a step-by-step approach can help you work through these challenges to find the best partner in your care.

•**Identify candidates.** Start by asking your family and friends for recommendations. Try the app Nextdoor, which offers local recommendations for a range of services. If several people on the app say they love a doctor in town, there's a higher probability that he or she is a gem. Yelp also may give you useful info, but negative reviews based on experiences such as an encounter with a surly receptionist or parking challenges may have nothing to do with the quality of the doctor's care.

•**Set up consultations.** Once you've identified doctors you want to consider, call and request a new patient consultation. The front desk staff can verify if your insurance is accepted. If so, it should cover the cost of the visit, minus the copay for which you are responsible. But don't go to the consultation

thinking you'll sit in the doctor's office and interview the doctor. Rather, go to the visit with a specific problem or process, such as a concerning symptom or a refill of a prescription. Most new patient consultations last about 45 minutes, so you'll have plenty of time to see how the doctor interacts with you.

•**Ask questions.** During the visit, ask the doctor at least one specific question. Any question will likely elicit more than the response to the question itself. Because the doctor doesn't know the question in advance, you'll get a sense of how well he or she responds to the unexpected—whether they're reassuring and humorous (good) or defensive and snarky (bad).

What to Look For

The two most important elements in the doctor-patient relationship are good communication and trust. If good communication is missing, you may withhold information that is critical in formulating an effective treatment plan. If trust is missing, you may not adhere to your doctor's recommendations, or you might habitually cancel appointments.

But trust isn't always obvious. It's a feeling created by actions, not words, based on how your doctor engages with you. Signs of trustworthiness include being authentic and demonstrating integrity, compassion, kindness, and humility. Another factor that contributes to trust may be "cultural concordance." For example, you may feel more trust in a doctor who shares your gender or cultural identity, or—for non-English speakers—is fluent in your native language.

Your Concerns Matter

Another important factor is the doctor's ability to convey that he or she takes your concerns seriously. That is, if you bring a problem to the doctor and he or she says something like, "I wouldn't worry about it," without further explanation, find another doctor. Any doctor who is unwilling to order a test to rule out a serious problem that concerns you is not the right doctor for you. Rather, the doctor might say something reassuring and respectful like, "I don't think this is anything to worry about, but I can see how concerned you are. Let's explore this further."

Competence

You want to feel confident in your doctor's level of competency, which means you want an expert diagnostician who is well-informed about the latest evidence-based treatments. But the right doctor is also willing to say, "I don't know but I will find the answer to your question and message you by the end of the week." You can't expect your doctor to know everything, but it's important that he or she honestly tells you when more digging is needed.

Know Your Criteria

You should also know your specific criteria. For example, maybe you tend to be anxious during a doctor visit and think of questions only once you get home. Is the physician available for post-visit calls? Does the practice offer an online portal where you can send questions or request refills?

Post-Visit Evaluation

After the visit, evaluate whether or not the doctor is someone you'd like to work with. *The best way to do that is to ask yourself the following questions…*

- **Did I feel listened to?**

- **Did I feel like I could trust the doctor with my body and my life?**

- **Did I get all of my questions answered?**

- **Did the doctor's recommendations make sense to me?**

- **Did I feel like the doctor gave me enough time?**

- **Did the doctor say anything that rubbed me the wrong way or put me off?**

If you answered yes to those questions (except for the last one, where the right answer is no), you have likely found a doctor who is right for you. If you feel relieved of anxiety and confident about the future—trust your instincts. On the other hand, if you don't feel right about the doctor, keep looking.

First Visit with a New Doctor?

Tziporah E. Rosenberg, PhD, LMFT, associate professor in the departments of psychiatry and family medicine at University of Rochester Medical Center, Rochester, New York, director of the Institute for the Family's Strong Family Therapy Services, and physicians' coach in the Medical Center's Patient- and Family-Centered Care Coaching Program.

It's an uncomfortable reality—at some point, or even many points, in your lifetime, you will have to start a relationship with a new health-care provider. Perhaps your primary care doctor retires, or a health condition makes it necessary for you to see a specialist. *The prospect may fill you with anxiety, but there are key steps to help you make the most of that first visit…*

The Match Game

For many people, the right doctor has expertise and a comfortable bedside manner—being a good communicator may be as high on your list as being a good practitioner. Even if you've been referred to a new doctor by your current doctor and/or have consulted the in-network practitioner list from your medical insurance, also do some research to find more potential health-care providers in your area.

Ask friends and family members you trust which doctors they think might be good choices for you. List for them the three things that are most important to you—perhaps the amount of time the doctor devotes to each office visit…his/her philosophies regarding lifestyle changes as well as medication…and his ability to communicate in a way that will resonate with you.

Many health systems and practices have profiles of their clinicians online that include their philosophies along with details of their training. Read through these descriptions to help you narrow down your choices.

Example: If you need a specialist or a general practitioner with a certain expertise, see if the health-care providers you are considering went beyond the requirements needed to practice medicine to focus on these. Becoming board-certified, taking additional fellowships, doing research and/or being actively involved in clinical trials demonstrate investment and proficiency in their fields.

Caution: It can be impressive when a doctor is affiliated with a large academic institution and runs a fellowship training or a lab or is the chair of a department. But find out how available that doctor is for his patients. How might the practice accommodate you if you need to be seen for an acute problem or regularly for a chronic condition but the doctor is in the office only twice a week? He might be backed up by someone else or otherwise work alongside a team of other providers, but you will want to know this up-front rather than learn it when you call the office for an urgent matter.

Another consideration: You may want to choose a doctor within the same health system as your other practitioners. This makes coordination of care easier because your health record will be accessible—there's less onus on you to bring lab results and medication lists to the new doctor, and an opportunity for all of your providers to have a fuller picture of your health.

Warning: Be cautious about relying on any crowd-source websites with "patient satisfaction" ratings. Ratings can be based on a group of one and can be skewed to a negative or positive extreme.

On the other hand—once you're a patient, receiving a patient satisfaction survey after a visit indicates that the practice is interested in finding out what can be done to make future visits better.

Call My Office

Gone are the days when you could talk to a new doctor in advance by phone to get a sense of his or her style. But you still can call a doctor's office and ask the receptionist or office manager questions that can help set your expectations. Some offices have specific staff devoted to helping new patients become established. *Questions to ask…*

What is the protocol for urgent needs, and how does it differ during and after business hours?

Also: How long might you typically wait for a call back? And how will you know whether you need to go to urgent care or the ER?

What is the doctor's preferred style for communication between visits—e-mails or phone calls?

Can a loved one accompany you to office visits?

Does the doctor tend to run on time or late for patient appointments? Many people develop preconceived notions about a doctor based on the amount of time spent in the waiting room and then are agitated when they get into the exam room or office. What matters most is the experience you have when you're in the room with your provider and his/her presence and focus on you.

Note: If the office staff is too rushed to take the time to address your questions, that could reflect on the doctor and/or the pace of the practice.

Define Your Agenda

You won't know until you're in the exam room if a new provider relationship is going to work, and even then, you might not know right away. But keep in mind two things about every practitioner—a doctor isn't a mind reader, and he probably has an agenda for how he conducts office visits. *What to do to get the most out of your first office visit…*

• **Bring a list of three things that you need to get done.** Your agenda and your doctor's agenda might be different, but you can agree on what will be accomplished during the appointment. You can start off by saying something as simple as, "These are the things I am hoping we can accomplish today." The best scenario is that the practitioner will respond with what he feels is most important and say that he will also address what's on your mind.

• **Tell the doctor about yourself as a person.** Say, "Here are things I'd like you to know about me that will help you to better partner with me." You might communicate that your biggest health fear is about cancer...or that you have an analytical mind and will research everything he says...or that you really want to be given recommendations for what to do and how to make decisions.

• **Be as honest as you can be about everything.** Be straightforward when you describe your health condition or answer questions—from symptoms and how bad they are...to sex, drinking, depression and drug use.

One approach: Start small by saying, "There's something I want to talk about, but I'm scared [or embarrassed] to tell you." This provides structure to the conversation. It's even helpful for the doctor to know if you don't want to take action about what you're sharing, such as "I know I drink too much, but I don't want to stop now."

• **Review communication options with the doctor.** Rather than waiting for a follow-up visit, using a portal is a way to ask questions to optimize a care plan and share important feedback, such as drug side effects or clarifying the need for new referrals or labs. Ask if that's the doctor's preferred method or if you should call the office. Also ask about the average time frame for getting a reply.

If Things Aren't Working

As with any relationship, it can be difficult in the moment to recognize that it's not going well. You might feel stressed, agitated and scared but find it hard to give voice to that. Tune into yourself...do a gut check...and try to put words to what's not going well. If you can articulate what's going off the rails,

you may be able to remedy the situation. *Examples...*

• **If you feel that you're not being heard** or that the practitioner is just going through the motions without making a connection with you, you might say, "Can we slow down? I'm not sure you've had a chance to review my full history, and I'd like to share things that are important."

• **If you are overwhelmed by the doctor's jargon** or rapid-fire recommendations, ask for clarification by saying, "Can you give me an example that I can better relate to?"

• **If something doesn't feel right** while you're in the exam room, you are under no obligation to proceed. Call a time-out and say, "I don't feel comfortable going forward." The doctor might be willing to alleviate your concerns, but if not, you can leave or not schedule a follow-up.

After the Appointment

What if after leaving the office, you feel the appointment went so badly that the relationship can't be recovered?

• **Ask yourself if you're making too quick a conclusion.** The more anxious we are about a doctor visit, the more we want an instant connection, and we may be disappointed when it doesn't happen as we expected. Like all of us, health-care providers can have bad days.

• **Think about whether you can collect more data**—perhaps by trying again with a second visit or communicating with the doctor via e-mail. You might send a message saying, "You used words I didn't understand, and I left scared. Can you explain it in language I can understand?" or "I don't feel that all my questions were answered—can you tell me what to do about X until our next visit?" Most people who go into the health-care field want to help, and many will acknowledge that a first visit may have gotten off on the wrong foot.

If you don't like the response you get, you may not want to invest more effort trying to make it work, especially if your condition is long-term or serious enough that you don't have time to waste.

How to Avoid a Missed Diagnosis

David E. Newman-Toker, MD, professor at the Johns Hopkins University School of Medicine, Baltimore, Maryland, the director of the Armstrong Institute Center for Diagnostic Excellence at Johns Hopkins, and the president of the Society to Improve Diagnosis in Medicine.

Most people will experience at least one missed diagnosis or diagnostic error at some point, according to David E. Newman-Toker, MD, president of the Society to Improve Diagnosis in Medicine. Women and minorities are misdiagnosed most often.

Misdiagnosis can lead to needless suffering, untreated diseases, serious harm, or death. In addition, many misdiagnosed patients have been told that the problem is all in their heads.

Protect Yourself

To help reduce the risk of misdiagnosis, Dr. Newman-Toker recommends taking the following steps...

•**Make a list.** Before your appointment, put together a one-page, easy-to-read list of your symptoms and the timeline during which they occurred. Instead of the doctor spending time finding out about your symptoms, he or she can spend that time thinking about what caused your problem. It also helps you avoid talking about what previous doctors have said, which may affect your physician's views.

•**Ask:** *"What is the worst problem this could be and why is it not that?"* This simple question guides the doctor to give you a detailed explanation about what he or she thinks is going on and to provide specific information. For instance, if your major symptom is dizziness, you're hoping to hear something like: "I suspect vestibular

The Importance of Second Opinions

Research from the Mayo Clinic shows that 88 percent of patients who seek a second opinion leave with a refined or changed diagnosis.

Investigators examined the records of 286 patients who had been referred from primary care providers (nurse practitioners, physician assistants, and physicians) to Mayo Clinic's general internal medicine division. The Mayo Clinic's final diagnosis confirmed the referring provider's initial diagnosis in just 12 percent of patients. About 21 percent of people received an entirely different diagnosis, and 66 percent had their initial diagnosis refined or redefined.

The Mayo Clinic

neuritis, an inflammation of a nerve in your ear, which causes dizziness. The problem I'm most worried about is stroke, but there is substantial evidence that my findings in this exam confirm your problem is vestibular neuritis."

This shows that the doctor is thinking clearly and systematically about the problem and can articulate the rationale for the diagnosis. It also shows that he or she is thinking about making sure you don't get harmed by a diagnostic error.

If the doctor instead says something like, "You don't need to worry about that," or "I see a lot of this, and it is very common," you should immediately find another doctor or at least get a second opinion.

•**Don't give up.** During your visit, your doctor will give you a treatment plan. When it doesn't work, patients tend to think they have received the wrong treatment. But you might have the wrong diagnosis instead. If you're not getting better, keep the possibility of a diagnostic error on the physician's radar by giving the office a call.

Many Doctor Reviews Are Fake

A growing number of medical practices, doctors, dentists, and other businesses buy and sell fake reviews that appear on sites such as Google, Yelp, and Trustpilot. The reviews come from businesses that offer reviews for pay, employees, and other business owners who trade reviews with doctors.

Medical Justice

How to Remedy Massive Medical Bills: A 6-Step Plan

Caitlin Donovan, senior director of the National Patient Advocate Foundation, a nonprofit organization based in Hampton, Virginia, that provides case management and financial aid to Americans facing chronic, life-threatening and debilitating illnesses. PatientAdvocate.org

Even though Congress passed legislation, which took effect at the start of 2022, to address surprise out-of-network medical expenses at in-network hospitals, there still are many ways that seemingly well-insured patients can be subjected to burdensome health-care costs.

Examples: Out-of-network doctor visits...ambulance rides, which are excluded from the legislation (though air ambulances are included)...and treatments the insurance company or Medicare deems not medically necessary or when patients are uninsured.

Here's a six-step plan for what to do if you receive a massive medical bill—it's often possible to pay much less...

1. Check the "Explanation of Benefits" (EOB) statement before paying. This document details how much your coverage will pay and how much you must pay. It will be mailed to you by your insurer or Medicare and typically is marked "This Is Not a Bill." When you receive it, compare the amount listed under "patient responsibility" or "you owe" with the amount the provider is billing you. These figures should match. If they don't, call both the health-care provider's billing office and the insurer/Medicare until you get an explanation for the discrepancy.

Among the potential explanations: The care provider might have mailed your bill before your insurance/Medicare paid its share...the provider might have submitted its claim incorrectly to your insurance/Medicare...or it might have failed to submit an insurance/Medicare claim at all. If necessary, make sure your health-care provider refiles the paperwork properly.

Also: Medical billing errors are very common. Read the bill and the EOB in search of procedures that do not seem relevant to your treatment—a coronary angioplasty if you were in the hospital for a hip replacement, for example—and contact the provider to question whether you actually received these services.

2. Ask your insurer/Medicare why a procedure was not well covered.

Among the explanations your coverage provider might offer: The health-care provider wasn't in network...the procedure wasn't medically necessary...or the provider failed to submit the information required to process the claim. Don't back down if you believe their explanations might be inaccurate—they often are.

Examples: If you're told the provider isn't in network, you might say, "I confirmed that this provider is in network through your website—why is it being coded as out-of-network?" If you're told the procedure wasn't medically necessary, ask, "How does this need to be coded for you to cover it?" and/or ask your doctor to provide a written "letter of medical necessity" explaining why the procedure actually was necessary in your case. If you're told the claim wasn't submitted properly, contact the health-care provider and ask for it to be resubmitted.

Helpful: If you have Medicare, call 1-800-633-4227 to ask these questions...or visit Medicare.gov, click "Claims & Appeals" at the bottom left of the screen, then click "Talk to Someone."

3. File formal appeals with your coverage provider. You have a legal right to submit at least two formal written appeals per medical bill with your insurer/Medicare if you believe it is not covering a bill properly. For information on how to file an a Medicare appeal and to find the appropriate forms, go to Medicare.gov/claims-appeals. When you complete these appeals documents, keep in mind that you are essentially making a legal argument that the insurer/Medicare is failing to provide the coverage to which you are entitled, not an emotional argument that your bill is crushingly large. Approach this as you would any legal contract, using professional language.

4. Request financial assistance with hospital bills. Ask the hospital's billing department if you qualify for any financial assistance. Most hospitals have programs that can reduce or waive bills for people who can't afford to pay. Eligibility rules vary, but even people with incomes above $100,000 may qualify when bills climb into five figures.

5. Negotiate. You can negotiate medical bills—if you can't pay, the provider will have to sell your debt to a collection agency for pennies on the dollar, a result that the provider wants to avoid.

Strategy: Look up the typical cost paid for the procedures you received. Hospitals now are required to list their negotiated rates on their websites, or check HealthcareBlue Book.com (a membership site benefit provided by some employers) or Medicare.gov/procedure-price-lookup. Compare the prices you find to your bill. Even if you're not going through a hospital system, you still can use your local hospital's list to get an idea of a reasonable charge. Generally, a hospital charge will be more than an in-office service at an independent provider.

Next, call the provider's billing office. Explain that you can't afford to pay the amount billed, then use the lowest price you uncovered for the procedures—that's usually the

Medicare price—as the starting point for negotiations. If you can afford to pay immediately, ask if the provider offers prompt-payment discounts or cash discounts.

If you can't afford to pay in a lump sum, ask the provider for a payment plan that fits your budget after you have negotiated a price. Whatever terms you negotiate, get the agreement in writing before making any payment. This written agreement should confirm that the amount you are paying will be considered payment in full…and, if possible, that your failure to pay the entire amount originally billed will not be listed as a late or unpaid debt on your credit reports.

6. Enlist outside help. There are nonprofit organizations that help people find financial assistance or other means of support, such as negotiating a lowered rate. Locate organizations that might help you on PatientAdvocate.org (select the "National Financial Resource Directory" button under the "Explore Our Resource" tab). Also ask any religious and fraternal organizations you belong to whether they have programs that could help. Your town or county might have programs that provide assistance to residents facing financial challenges as well.

Helpful: If you have a chronic, life-threatening and/or debilitating disease, the Patient Advocate Foundation might be able to provide access to a case manager who can review your bills for errors, help you locate financial assistance and negotiate bills on your behalf. We've helped patients with cancer, HIV/AIDs, lupus and diabetes. (You must be receiving care or have received care within the US, and we don't handle behavioral/mental health, accidents or pregnancy.) If you don't qualify for this assistance, you can engage a for-profit medical billing advocate who can vet and negotiate bills on your behalf for a fee—potentially $50 to $100 or more an hour…or 25 percent to 35 percent of the amount the advocate gets your medical bills reduced.

Also contact area newspaper and TV reporters who cover consumer advocacy and/or health-care issues. If a reporter starts pok-

Save on Your Meds

Prescription drug prices typically aren't negotiable—but there often are ways to save. Your pharmacist isn't going to haggle...but before filling a prescription, it is worth asking for both the cash price of the drug and your out-of-pocket cost if you pay with your insurance/Medicare—the cash price sometimes is lower.

Also use the drug-discount website GoodRx.com to search for coupons that could lower the cash price and to compare the cash prices charged by various pharmacy chains in your area. Prices for a drug can vary dramatically from pharmacy to pharmacy.

If it's a name-brand drug, not a generic, investigate whether the pharmaceutical company that makes it has a "patient-assistance program." These programs sometimes dramatically discount the price of expensive drugs for patients in financial need. Patient-assistance program details can be found on pharmaceutical companies' websites, or you can search for them at NeedyMeds.org.

Also, look into charitable copay relief organizations, such as the Patient Advocate Foundation (PatientAdvocate.org). Programs such as these can be even better than the manufacturer programs because you may be instantly approved and the funds can be used to cover anything to treat your condition, including medications for pain, copays, over-the-counter medications, even your insurance premiums.

Caitlin Donovan, senior director of the National Patient Advocate Foundation, a nonprofit organization that provides case management and financial aid to Americans facing chronic, life- threatening and debilitating illnesses, Washington, DC. PatientAdvocate.org

ing into your case, there's a good chance that the provider or insurer may back down and offer better terms to avoid negative publicity. Reporters can't cover everyone who has huge medical bills, however, so when you reach out to them, stress the ways in which your bills are especially egregious and/or your situation especially heart-wrenching.

Medical Tourism

Lydia Gan, PhD, professor of economics, University of North Carolina at Pembroke.

Patients from developing nations have long traveled to the United States to access care they couldn't get at home, but the high cost of U.S. care is now sending some Americans in the opposite direction.

As the COVID-19 pandemic winds down, people are showing renewed interest in medical tourism, the practice of traveling to places like Mexico, Thailand, Singapore and many more countries for a wide variety of procedures, from cardiac, cosmetic, bariatric, spinal, and orthopedic surgery to cancer treatment, dentistry, and infertility care. We spoke with Lydia Gan, PhD, to learn more about medical tourism.

Cost Savings

For Americans, saving money is the top motivator to travel for health care. Consider heart bypass surgery. In the United States, a patient without health insurance can expect to receive a dizzying array of opaque and confusing bills that add up to between $70,000 and $133,000. But the identical procedure can be performed by Western-trained surgeons in a high-tech hospital in Singapore for about $16,000 or India for less than $9,000—including medical costs, airfare, and hotel. Americans regularly cross the border to Los Algodones, Mexico, also known as Molar City, to save 70 to 80 percent on dental services such as crowns ($180 vs. $1,250), and dentures ($250 vs. $1,850).

The Hospital Experience

Saving money isn't the only benefit of medical tourism. In many cases, hospitals that cater to medical tourists also offer a more luxurious experience, from private rooms and more personalized attention to dedicated centers that offer assistance with scheduling, interpretation, sightseeing, travel arrangements, and accommodations.

Further, instead of recovering at home, you can combine recovery with a vacation (as long as you stay within doctor-approved activities).

The best hospitals provide Western-trained health-care providers, but not every hospital in every country meets American standards. To ensure safety, seek care only from hospitals that are accredited by Joint Commission International (JCI), which is related to the Joint Commission that accredits hospitals in the United States. Any JCI-accredited hospital meets the same standards as those in America. In addition, seek hospitals that are affiliated with reputable American brands such as Johns Hopkins, Harvard Medical Center, and Mayo Clinic.

Consider a Medical Middleman

While you can arrange for international medical care on your own, it can be helpful to work with a domestic medical tourism facilitator (DMTF), which is essentially a medical travel agency. These companies match you with a doctor or hospital, make your travel plans, pick you up at the airport, offer translation services, secure your medical visa, and may arrange excursions. Look for a DMTF that is based in the United States, is certified by the Better Business Bureau, and works only with JCI-accredited hospitals. A trustworthy DMTF should have physicians on staff or be managed by someone who has an extensive career in health care.

Tips for Success

Careful preparation can make medical tourism safer and more successful.

- **Plan ahead.** Before you travel, meet with your health-care provider to discuss your health status, the procedure, and travel restrictions before and after the procedure.

- **Make sure you can get any needed follow-up care in the United States.** Call your insurance company, if applicable, to discuss your coverage.

- **Identify where you will be staying immediately after the procedure,** and make sure you have a long enough recovery period. If you have chest or abdominal surgery, cosmetic procedures of the face, eyelids, or nose, or laser treatments, do not fly for at least 10 days to avoid risks associated with changes in atmospheric pressure.

- **Find out what activities are not permitted after the procedure.** Sunbathing, drinking alcohol, swimming, or engaging in strenuous activities may be prohibited.

- **Make sure you're up to date on all vaccinations for your home and destination countries.** Consider adding a hepatitis B vaccine.

- **Buy travel health insurance that covers medical evacuation home.**

- **Take copies of your medical records to your destination,** and bring any new records home with you.

- **Pack enough medications to last your whole trip,** plus a little extra in case of delays. Keep your medication in your carry-on bag.

- **Be aware of antibiotic resistance risks.** The risk of antibiotic resistance varies by location. For example, India has the highest rates of antibiotic resistance in the world.

- **If you are traveling to have a procedure that is not available in the United States,** understand that you may have difficulty getting insurance to cover any post-procedure complications.

Sample Price Differences		
PROCEDURE	**COST IN U.S.**	**COST ABROAD**
Hip Replacement	$40,000 - $65,000	$7,000 - $13,000
Knee Replacement	$45,000 - $60,000	$7,500 - $12,000
Face & Neck Lift	$8,000 - $15,000	$2,500 - $4,000
Tummy Tuck	$6,000 - $12,000	$3,800 - $5,200
Source: MedRetreat.com		

Asking Dr. Google: Find Reliable Health Info Online

Kapil Parakh, MD, MPH, PhD, author of *Searching for Health: The Smart Way to Find Information Online and Put It to Use.* He is a cardiologist based in the Washington, DC, area, adjunct associate professor at Georgetown University, and medical lead for Google Fit, a health and fitness app. Google.com/fit

It's tempting to ask Doctor Google for advice given how costly and annoying the health-care world is. But a recent survey found that online medical advice was reliable less than 40 percent of the time and actually increased worries for 74 percent of people who accessed it.

The Internet can be a valuable source of health information—but only if you know where to look…how to determine which medical conditions truly match your symptoms…and what online health advice is best used to supplement treatment from medical professionals, not replace it.

We asked Kapil Parakh, MD, MPH, PhD, a practicing doctor, search engine expert and author of the book *Searching for Health*, how to best use the Internet to find reliable and appropriate health information and avoid the potential traps…

•**Write down your symptoms before searching online.** Track your symptoms when you don't feel well, noting what you feel and when and how severely you feel it—"strong burning sensation in throat after dinner," for example. This written log reduces the odds that you'll misremember symptoms when you later go online and try to figure out what health problem you might have. You're probably thinking, *I wouldn't misremember*, but it's surprisingly common for people to convince themselves that they have experienced symptoms when they read about them, in part because many symptoms are subjective—it's easy to think, *I did feel bloated after eating the other day…*or *I have felt fatigued* even if you really didn't feel any more bloated or tired than usual. Also track the symptom over time—how long have you had it? Does it come and go? Is it growing more severe or fading away?

It isn't just untrained Internet searchers who do this—medical students so often convince themselves that they have the diseases they're studying that this tendency has been dubbed "medical student syndrome" and has itself been the subject of medical studies.

•**Collect potential diagnoses before digging deep into any one.** The Internet makes it easy to identify diseases that could fit a set of symptoms. Enter a symptom into a search engine such as Google or Bing… or into a "symptom checker" such as Isabel Symptom Checker (SymptomChecker.Isabel HealthCare.com)…Mayo Clinic Symptom Checker (on MayoClinic.org, click the "Symptom Checker" button)…or WebMD Symptom Checker (on WebMD.com, scroll down to "WebMD Symptom Checker"), and in seconds, you'll have a list of potential diagnoses. Rather than getting sidetracked and delving deep into the details of a particular disease, compile a list of diseases that could potentially fit. Sort this list by approximate likelihood, doing your best to factor in not only how well the symptoms seem to fit yours but also how common the condition is in the US… how likely someone of your age, gender and physical health is to get it…and whether it's a condition that already exists in your medical history and family medical history.

Example: If you search for the symptom "loss of feeling in hands and feet," beriberi, a severe thiamine deficiency, might be among the diseases you come across—but beriberi is extremely rare in the US, except among extreme alcoholics. It should be marked as very unlikely on your list.

•**Start with a terse search.** It's tempting to enter every symptom you've experienced when you use search engines as diagnosis tools. If you have a sharp jabbing pain under your ribs, mild headache and slight stomachache, surely giving Google all of that info increases the odds that the web pages it locates will be about the condition you have, right? *Not so!* Adding details often detracts from the quality of search engine results. When a search includes more than six to eight symptoms, a high percentage of the results often are from obscure and potentially unreliable websites as the search engine struggles to match all of the search terms. And if a health search includes multiple symptoms, the search engine won't know to prioritize the main symptom.

Instead, your first search should include only the main symptom you are experiencing and perhaps a detail or two about that symptom. Rather than search "chest pain," for example, you could search the phrase "jabbing chest pain after eating." This simple search isn't necessarily the only search worth trying, but it should be where you start because it's the least likely to lead you down unhelpful Internet rabbit holes.

Try additional and longer searches only after this simple initial search. Longer searches produce less reliable results, on average, but now and then they do turn up possible diagnoses that shorter searches miss. When you do these longer searches, it's especially important to pay attention to results that come from only trustworthy websites—more about evaluating the quality of health websites to follow. Details worth adding to the main symptom during subsequent searches include your age or gender, such as "jabbing chest pain after eating for man in his 70s"… details about how long the symptoms have persisted, such as "jabbing chest pain for a week"…medication names—the symptom could be a side effect…or a secondary symptom or two. You could also repeat the search described above, replacing your primary symptom with a different symptom that's also troubling you. If both of those searches turn up the same potential diagnosis, that could be your answer.

•**Beware of "symptom checker" scares.** A study published in *The BMJ* tested 23 online symptom checkers and found that the correct diagnosis was listed first only 34 percent of the time. The misdiagnoses were not random—most pointed patients toward health problems more serious than they actually had, inducing needless anxiety. Liability concerns are one possible explanation why these web tools tend to favor worst-case scenarios—if someone died after a symptom checker suggested there was no reason for concern, it could lead to a lawsuit.

Example: If you enter "chest pain" into a symptom checker, there's an excellent chance that the first result will be "heart attack" even though there are many less serious health problems that also can cause chest pain.

•**Use the end of web addresses to gauge the reliability of health information.** As a rough rule of thumb, information about health issues found on official government sites ending .gov… the website of the British National Health Service, ending in *nhs.uk*… or Canadian national health services, ending in *Canada.ca/en/health-canada*—tends to be very reliable. Health info from sites ending .edu or .org usually is trustworthy as well—those generally are the websites of medical schools, hospitals, medical centers and health-related professional organizations, such as the American Heart Association (Heart.org). There are trustworthy sources of health info ending in the more familiar .com, too—WebMD.com and Healthline.com both do a solid job providing largely accurate info, for example. But proceed with caution when reading health information on unfamiliar .com websites…especially sites that seem to be selling the treatments they're recommending or community-based message board sites.

• **Stick with truly trusted sites for info about alternative medicine.** There are plenty of effective traditional and alternative treatments—the challenge is determining which ones. These treatments often are not discussed on mainstream health websites, and some have never been proven to be safe and effective in large-scale studies, though many have been "proven" by the test of time. Fortunately, there are a few websites that are very authoritative on alternative medicine, including the sites of the National Center for Complementary and Integrative Health (NCCIH.NIH.gov)…The University of Arizona's Andrew Weil Center for Integrative Medicine (IntegrativeMedicine.Arizona.edu) …the National Cancer Institute's Complementary and Alternative Medicine (Cancer.gov/about-cancer/treatment/cam)…and the National Institutes of Health's Office of Dietary Supplements (ODS.od.nih.gov).

Find a primary care physician and a pharmacist who are open to alternative treatments, and discuss these treatments before trying them. These professionals can confirm that the treatment is well-regarded and that it won't interfere with your other prescriptions or treatments.

• **Health-related personal blogs and social-media posts can be wonderful sources of moral support.** It's easy to feel alone when you have a worrisome symptom or serious health problem—even your loved ones might not understand what you're going though. On the Internet, you can find blogs and social-media user groups and posts by people who have had symptoms or diagnoses similar to your own. The accuracy of the medical guidance offered on these can be uneven, but the community they offer could be invaluable.

Warning: Don't be frightened if all the blogs or social-media posts that mention your symptom link it to a serious health problem—that's just the nature of the Internet. If someone has a rash and it turns out to be cancer, she blogs about it…if she has a rash and it clears up in a few days, she forgets about it.

Beware DIY Genetic Tests

Gillian Hooker, PhD, ScM, LCGC, past president of the National Society of Genetic Counselors. She is an adjunct associate professor at Vanderbilt University Medical Center and chief scientific officer at Concert Genetics, both in Nashville. ConcertGenetics.com

If you are considering genetic testing because of a family history of a specific medical condition or some other concern, it's wise to stick with tests ordered by your physician or with the support of a genetic counselor. So-called "direct-to-consumer" tests, including those advertised by such companies as 23andMe.com and Ancestry.com, check for only a few common mutations.

Example: 23andMe's test for BRCA1/BRCA2 mutations, which are linked primarily to elevated risk for breast and ovarian cancers, looks for just three of more than 1,000 variants of these genes known to increase cancer risk.

Among the types of doctor-ordered genetic tests you might encounter…

• **Focused tests or panel tests** search only a small number or multiple number of genes, respectively, related to a specific medical problem, such as genes associated with breast and ovarian cancers, genes associated with kidney disease or genes associated with high cholesterol.

• **Whole genome/whole exome tests** are much broader than focused tests. Whole genome tests examine the patient's complete DNA…while whole exome tests examine every gene that provides instructions for making specific proteins. Either is sufficient to identify all currently known genetic health risks. These could be appropriate when a patient has mysterious symptoms and her doctor is searching for its cause.

Somatic tests examine the DNA of a tumor or a specific part of the body, which is different from the patient's hereditary DNA. An oncologist might order this test to learn more about a patient's cancer and potentially to choose a treatment.

Fake Drugs

Jack E. Fincham, PhD, RPh, professor at the Osher Lifelong Learning Institute, University of Arizona, Tucson, and dean emeritus, University of Kansas School of Pharmacy, Tucson, Arizona. He is a *Bottom Line Health* editorial board member.

As the cost of drugs skyrockets in the United States, Americans are increasingly turning to the Internet to look for better prices. Tens of thousands of online pharmacies advertise discounted drugs, on-site prescriptions, and even access to controlled drugs with no prescription at all. But in a large percentage of cases, what they're really offering is counterfeit drugs.

Chalk Dust to Concrete

Counterfeit medications may contain incorrect, insufficient, or inactive ingredients, active ingredients that are different from those described on the package, and a wide range of impurities, such as road paint, floor wax, rat poison, concrete, boric acid, road tar, and antifreeze. They may be real drugs that have expired or contain nothing but chalk dust. These counterfeit components of a medication may cause the drug to have no effect, a negative effect, or even to be lethal.

These drugs span the therapeutic landscape and include lifestyle medications, such as those for weight loss and erectile dysfunction, anesthetics, pain medications, contraceptives and fertility treatments, drugs for diabetes, high cholesterol, high blood pressure, HIV, hepatitis, malaria, and cancer, heart medications, psychotropics, antibiotics, generic drugs, over-the-counter medications, herbal remedies, and medical devices.

Widespread Issues

The problem isn't limited to just a few rogue players. The National Association of Boards

---

Online Pharmacy Resources

If you want to buy online, use the following websites to ensure that the pharmacy you are considering is legitimate...

- **The NABP Verified Internet Pharmacy Practice Sites program** https://NABP.pharmacy/programs/accreditations-inspections/digital-pharmacy/accredited-digital-pharmacies/

- **NABP** https://safe.pharmacy/buy-safely

- **National Association of Pharmacy Regulatory Authorities** https://napra.ca/online-pharmacies

- **LegitScript** http://legitscript.com

Look for online pharmacies with a web address that ends in ".pharmacy". These pharmacies are vetted by the NABP and, where applicable, local authorities.

—Dr. Jack E. Fincham

---

of Pharmacy (NABP) reports that 62 percent of medicines purchased online are fake or substandard and less than 5 percent of the estimated 35,000 pharmacies you can find online comply with U.S. laws and practice standards. Half offer foreign or non-FDA-approved drugs, one-quarter list a physical address outside of the United States, and 42 percent have server locations in foreign countries.

Canadian pharmacies are a popular choice for Americans seeking safe and affordable drugs, but they're often not what they seem: The FDA found that 85 percent of the online pharmacies purporting to be in Canada were based in 27 other countries. India, China, Vietnam, Indonesia, Pakistan, and the Philippines appear to be the main producers of counterfeit pharmaceuticals.

Even physicians have been duped into buying counterfeit drugs. In 2015, the FDA contacted close to 1,000 physicians and medical practices in 48 different states to let them know they may have purchased a counterfeit cancer drug called *bevacizumab* (Avastin). Investigators traced some of the counterfeits to Montana Health Care Solutions, a pharmaceutical distributor owned by a Canadian company and a British citizen, which imported the fake drug from Turkey and sold it to doctors at low prices.

Canadian Pharmacy Drug Differences

Even if you buy medications from a Canadian pharmacy, you're not guaranteed to get what you expect. In fact, the official-sounding Canadian International Pharmacy Association (CIPA) website is itself questionable. The CIPA website claims to list "certified" Internet drug access sites; however, the pharmacies listed on that site have not been verified by independent and valid inspections. Many of the listed locations sell drugs that are sourced from unreliable countries and have never had to pass through Canada's equivalent of the FDA (Health Canada) regulatory process for assurance of safety and efficacy.

The NABP notes that there are no Canadian online pharmacies that consistently dispense Health Canada-approved medicines to American customers: The drugs you buy from a Canadian pharmacy are not the same ones a Canadian is getting at the pharmacy counter.

How to Protect Yourself

If you're looking to save money on medications, before you go online, talk to your physician and pharmacist to see if they can offer alternatives such as generic or therapeutically equivalent medications. Look into pharmaceutical company assistance and other discount pharmacy programs, such as GoodRx.com. Lastly, compare prices at different pharmacies, as costs can vary dramatically.

Avoid Rogue Pharmacies

Don't shop from an online pharmacy site that engages in any of the following practices...

- **Does not require a prescription**
- **Does not provide verifiable contact information**
- **Sells prescriptions after a patient answers only a few health questions**
- **Does not fill orders through licensed pharmacies**
- **Does not have a licensed pharmacist dispensing prescriptions**
- **Offers to sell controlled substances**
- **Does not protect personal and financial information,** as rogue pharmacies are increasingly stealing information for identity theft
- **Do not use CIPA.com to verify Canadian pharmacies.**

DEA Issues Warning

In September 2021, the U.S. Drug Enforcement Agency (DEA) issued a public safety alert warning of an "alarming increase" in lethal counterfeit pills containing *fentanyl* or *methamphetamine*. More than 9.5 million counterfeit pills were seized by September 2021, which was more than the prior two years combined. Further, there's an increasing number of counterfeit pills that contain at least two milligrams of fentanyl, which is considered a lethal dose. These pills, which look identical to drugs like *oxycodone* (OxyContin, Percocet), *hydrocodone* (Vicodin), *alprazolam* (Xanax), and *amphetamines/ dextroamphetamine* (Adderall) are mostly being made in clandestine Mexican laboratories using chemicals from China and India.

"Reports of deaths from counterfeit opioids often portray the victims as street drug addicts looking for a high. While no person deserves to die from counterfeit opioids, we need to better understand all of the issues that may lead to patients seeking these opioid medications through the black market," Mark Coggins, PharmD, CGP, FASCP, wrote in *Today's Geriatric Medicine*. Intense scrutiny of opioid prescribing has led many physicians to stop prescribing the drugs entirely, even to patients who have responsibly used them for months or years. In some cases, patients weren't properly weaned off or given other suitable treatment options to manage their pain. "As scenarios like this occur, more patients are likely to turn to risky online pharmacies and street dealers in an attempt to obtain relief," Dr. Coggins notes.

New Drug for Psoriasis Patients

Kristian Reich, MD, dermatologist, is professor of translational research in inflammatory skin diseases at University Medical Center Hamburg-Eppendorf, Germany, and co-leader of two clinical studies totaling more than 1,200 psoriasis patients, published in *The New England Journal of Medicine*.

The new drug *bimekizumab* was 20 percent more effective in inducing full skin clearance than *secukinumab* (Cosentyx) after 48 weeks...and 35 percent more effective than *adalimumab* (Humira) at 24 weeks. The only significant side effect was yeast infection. At press, bimekizumab is awaiting for FDA approval.

The Risks from Steroids

Joshua Levitt, ND, naturopathic physician and founder and medical director at Whole Health, a natural family medicine practice in Hamden, Connecticut. He has served as a clinical preceptor for medical residents from the Yale School of Medicine. He is a cofounder and medical director at the natural-products company UpWellness.

Steroids are so routinely prescribed that odds are you've used an oral or topical steroid—a corticosteroid such as *prednisone, cortisone,* and *dexamethasone*—at some point...or even several points...in your life. And that could have put you at risk! While most doctors think short-term treatment with steroids is safe, recent research indicates that may not be the case.

These powerful, fast-acting drugs are prescribed for bronchitis, asthma, chronic obstructive lung disease (COPD) and other respiratory conditions...musculoskeletal aches and back pain...flare-ups of rheumatoid arthritis, inflammatory bowel disease and other autoimmune diseases...and topical versions for rashes and other problems.

Most doctors avoid long-term treatment with corticosteroids because these drugs can cause high blood pressure, diabetes and osteoporosis as well as negatively affect digestion, the eyes, skin and the nervous system. But new research indicates that even short-term bouts of steroids could be dangerous. We asked naturopathic physician Joshua Levitt, ND, about the dangers of steroid use and how to avoid taking them in the future.

The Trouble with Steroids

In a three-year study published in *The BMJ*, University of Michigan Medical School researchers analyzed data from more than 1.5 million Americans. They found that 21.5 percent had been prescribed a short-term dose of oral steroids during the study period. The most common reasons for a steroid prescription were upper and lower respiratory tract infections, allergies and back pain. Participants taking steroids—even at low doses for less than 30 days—were 5.3 times more likely to develop life-threatening sepsis...3.3 times more likely to develop a life-threatening blood clot...and 1.9 times more likely to break a bone up to 90 days after they started taking the steroid.

Researchers now urge doctors to be cautious about prescribing steroids. But prescription of short-term steroids still is common. In a study published in *The BMJ Open*, steroid use had increased by 14 percent over a recent eight-year period.

I see patients suffering from the side effects of steroids in my practice every day. *Here are the natural ways I help them avoid steroids altogether...*

•**Practice an anti-inflammatory lifestyle.** Many of us have chronic, low-grade inflammation that makes acute inflammation from an infection or back pain even worse. By using the following lifestyle methods to control chronic inflammation, you're less likely to need an anti-inflammatory steroid.

• **Eat minimally processed foods.** Increase consumption of plant-based, minimally processed foods (which are anti-inflammatory), and decrease consumption of factory-farmed meats, trans fats and polyunsaturated vegetable oils (which promote inflammation).

Also helpful: Good oils rich in monounsaturated fats including olive oil, avocado oil and macadamia nut oil.

• **Move more.** A minimum of 20 to 30 minutes a day of movement—whether it's a brisk walk or a stint of gardening—reduces inflammation.

• **Get enough deep sleep.** Insomnia increases inflammation. Sleeping seven to eight hours a night reduces inflammation.

Best: Go to bed and get up at the same time every day. Over time, your wake-sleep cycle will match this habit, and you'll start to sleep well.

• **Look on the bright side.** A positive mindset is anti-inflammatory. New research shows that awe—a feeling of wonder—reduces an inflammatory biomarker. Other research shows that gratitude reduces inflammation.

Smart idea: Keep a daily gratitude journal.

• **Minimize toxin exposure.** Use all-natural products, including personal-care products such as soap and shampoo…laundry and dish soap…and cleaning products (an alternative is white vinegar).

• **Ingest anti-inflammatory nutrients and herbs regularly**—increasing amounts when you're experiencing a condition caused by inflammation. *They include…*

• Omega-3 fatty acids. Corticosteroids decrease the cascade of biochemical events that leads to inflammation. The omega-3 fatty acids docosahexaenoic acid (DHA) and eicosapentaenoic acid (EPA)—primarily found in fatty fish such as salmon and sardines—do the same without side effects. Eat a serving of fatty fish

Remember Hydrogen Peroxide?

This old home remedy is still good to have on hand. Keep a small bottle in your first-aid kit to clean wounds when soap and water isn't available. Put a few drops of peroxide in your ear to clear clogged earwax—wait a few minutes, then gently swish your ear canal with warm water. Treat swollen gums by rinsing daily for 30 seconds with one part 3% peroxide mixed with two parts water.

Also: Hydrogen peroxide effectively disinfects sinks, counters, cutting boards, toilets, toys and more. Just don't get it on your clothes or furniture, as it can bleach them.

MedicineNet.com and ClevelandClinic.org

such as wild-caught salmon two or three times a week. During an acute inflammatory attack, consider taking a high-potency fish oil supplement at a dose of three to five grams daily.*

• Turmeric and curcumin. The golden-yellow spice turmeric and its active ingredient curcumin are powerful anti-inflammatories. Add turmeric to soups, stews and other recipes —a teaspoon or so per day. *Dose:* For acute inflammation, a curcumin supplement at a dose of 100 milligrams (mg) to 500 mg two or three times per day.

• Boswellia (frankincense). Look for a product that supplies 65 percent boswellic acid. *Dose:* 250 mg to 500 mg two or three times per day for chronic inflammation…and just until symptoms subside for acute attacks.

• SAMe. This anti-inflammatory amino acid is useful for ongoing joint and muscle pain and depression. *Dose:* 400 mg to 1,200 mg per day, divided into two doses.

*Before starting any supplement, check with your doctor about potential interactions with your medications.

Don't Throw Away Good Medicine

Sharon Horesh Bergquist, MD, associate professor of medicine, Emory University School of Medicine, Atlanta, Georgia.

We all have medications we needed for a one-time concern that end up being shoved in the back of the medicine cabinet: the drug for motion sickness bought for a cruise, the anti-diarrheal bought after a meal at a questionable food vendor, the jumbo bottle of ibuprofen that was a great deal at Costco three years ago.

When you need them again, your relief at not having to run to the store may be tempered by disappointment when you realize that they expired while on standby.

Expired Doesn't Mean Spoiled

The good news is that, based on testing of government stockpiles of drugs stored for national security, many of those drugs are still likely safe and effective after the expiration date. When the U.S. Food and Drug Administration tested 122 expired medications for the Department of Defense, researchers found that almost 90 percent of them maintained their quality a full year after their expiration dates. In fact, the FDA found that the average expiration date could be extended by 5½ years.

An expiration date doesn't mean that a drug goes bad, like perishable food. Rather it's the date through which the pharmaceutical company guarantees the medication's full potency. Because it's expensive to repeatedly test a drug's potency for many years, most manufacturers stop testing at one to five years and set the expiration date based on their testing time. The American Medical Association has pushed for extended expiration dates, and the FDA occasionally extends a drug's expiration if there is a shortage of that medication, but no widespread changes have taken effect yet.

These Drugs Are Safe

How long a drug remains safe and effective past an expiration date depends on many factors, including how it was stored. If kept in a cool, dry place, many medications that are in a solid form, like tablets, could be taken for at least one year past the expiration date. That includes medications for cold and allergy symptoms and nonsteroidal anti-inflammatory drugs.

While the FDA found that certain lots of drugs like the cold medicine *guaifenesin* or the antibiotic *ciprofloxacin* lasted more than 10 years, it's important to note that in the study, the medications were stored in ideal circumstances, which can't be replicated at home.

Throw These Away

While solid-form medications generally hold up well, creams, liquids, and ointments do not. After cough syrups, nasal sprays, eye drops, and topical ointments expire, toss them to avoid bacterial contamination from expired preservatives, or changing composition from evaporation. Probiotics should also be replaced before they expire, as they contain living organisms.

Any medication that you use for a serious medical issue should also be replaced upon expiration. If a drug like *nitroglycerin*, *albuterol*, insulin, or an *epinephrine* pen undergoes even a small decrease in potency, it could be dangerous.

Medication Storage

The way you store medications can affect their potency even if they're not expired. Never store medications or diagnostic strips in the bathroom, where heat and humidity can affect their performance. Avoid extreme temperatures. Most medications can safely be stored from 58 to 86 degrees unless they require refrigeration. Those temperatures can easily be exceeded if you leave medications in your car while running errands on the way home from the pharmacy or if you pack them in a checked suitcase when flying.

When storing medications, take care not to mix them up. Eye drops and ear drops look very similar, so keep them separated or clearly marked. When in doubt, look for the word ophthalmic before putting anything into your eyes and otic before putting a medication in your ears. Keep pets' medications clearly marked or stored in a separate location.

Medication Mishaps

Mixing up ear and eye drops isn't the only medical error you need to watch out for. Something as seemingly harmless as taking a prescription sleep aid while also taking an over-the-counter allergy medication can be dangerous since they can both cause sedation. Some herbs and dietary supplements can alter the effectiveness of prescriptions too. *Every time you fill a new prescription or start taking a supplement, spend a few minutes with your pharmacist to ask the following questions...*

• **Will this new medication interfere with my other medication(s)?**

• **What should I do if I miss a dose?**

• **What should I do if I accidentally take more than the recommended dose?**

• **Are there any foods, drinks, other medications, or activities I should avoid while taking this medicine?**

• **How long should I take it?**

• **What are the possible side effects?** What should I do if they occur?

• **Can I cut this pill?** Some medications are specially coated to be long-acting or to protect the stomach.

• **Can I crush this pill to take with food instead of swallowing?**

Make sure any physician you see, including specialists, has a complete list of all of your current medications and supplements along with dosages. Keep a written record of your prescriptions, or use your smartphone to take photos of the labels

---

What to Bring to the ER

When you have a medical emergency, a quick and accurate diagnosis is critical. Having a written list of certain information ready to hand to the ER physician helps ensure that happens.

Information to include: A list of illnesses, surgeries and injuries—including the dates for all...whether you are being treated for a medical problem...names and contact information for your doctors and the dates of your scheduled follow-up visits....recent diagnostic tests or imaging studies...a list of all your medications and doses...your pharmacy's phone number...your next-of-kin contact...and of course, your insurance information.

Kenneth V. Iserson, MD, professor emeritus, department of emergency medicine, The University of Arizona, Tucson, and a *Bottom Line Personal* subscriber.

If Your Doctor Has Prescribed Oxygen Therapy

American College of Chest Physicians, ChestNet. org, and American Association for Homecare, AA Homecare.org.

The Oxygen Toolkit from the American College of Chest Physicians and the American Association for Homecare is designed for both patients and doctors. It includes a guide to oxygen therapy, including how to pay for it...an explanation of what to do before, during and after delivery of oxygen equipment...and travel guidance for oxygen-therapy users. There also is information that clinicians can use to help determine whether oxygen therapy is appropriate. The guide is available online at Foundation.chest net.org/lung-health-a-z/oxygen-therapy.

Checking Out Hospitals

Charles B. Inlander is a consumer advocate and health-care consultant based in Fogelsville, Pennsylvania. He was the founding president of the non-profit People's Medical Society, a consumer-advocacy organization credited with key improvements in the quality of U.S. health care, and is author or coauthor of more than 20 consumer-health books.

There is an old saying that the last place you want to be when you are sick is in a hospital. While there is a lot of truth to that statement, it's likely that, at some time in your life, you will need a hospital, and a little research now can make sure you go to the best facility.

As recently as 30 years ago, there was virtually no publicly available information about the safety and quality of individual hospitals. Patients went to the facilities where their doctors put them, not knowing if it was the right hospital for their needs. As a result, facilities had no impetus to improve.

But because of consumer demand, that has all changed. Today, consumers can access numerous sources that rate and even compare hospitals by patient safety, quality of care, and outcomes.

Patient Safety

Patient safety is a major problem in many hospitals. Up to 20 percent of patients leave a hospital with a condition they did not have when they entered. That includes potentially deadly infections (called nosocomial or hospital-acquired infections), injuries because of falls, or reactions to inappropriate or wrongly administered medications. Hospitals are required by law to keep track of these issues and make them public. An independent, nonprofit organization called the Leapfrog Group uses that information to give hospitals patient safety grades that you can access for free. Just go to HospitalSafetyGrade.org and enter a city or zip code.

Quality Outcomes

The federal government and most states have excellent websites that help you compare the quality of hospitals. Go to Medicare.gov and click the "Find Care Providers" button and you will find ratings of just about every hospital in the country. The site also provides ratings for nursing homes, home care agencies, and medical practices. Most states also provide hospital outcome data. Do an online search asking for hospital outcomes and your state name. You can also call your state or local health department to help you find information.

Ask Questions

Don't be afraid to ask questions at your local hospitals. If you are contemplating surgery, contact the hospital's medical director and find out how many of the same surgeries they perform each year. The more a procedure is done at a hospital, the better they get at it.

The Best Hospitals

Several websites purport to rank the best hospitals in the country by areas of specialty, such as heart disease, cancer, or pediatrics, but no two sites use the same criteria. The magazine *U.S. News & World Report* publishes one of the most popular and extensive surveys at Health.usnews.com/best-hospitals. It's a good source to review as part of an overall assessment strategy.

How to Stay Safe in the Hospital

R. Ruth Linden, PhD, founder and president of Tree of Life Health Advocates, where she helps clients navigate the health-care system and access the best possible care. TreeOfLifeHealthAdvocates.com

Every year, an estimated 20,000 Americans die unnecessarily in hospitals, according to a recent study from doctors at the Yale School of Medicine.

Prior studies suggest the death toll could be even higher. In 1999, the Institute of Medicine estimated that 44,000 to 98,000 people die from medical errors each year. A paper in the *Journal of Patient Safety* suggested that the true figure could be as high as 440,000 people per year. In 2016, Johns Hopkins University researchers released their estimate of 250,000 people. These earlier studies, however, have been subject to controversy over their methods, while the Yale study took a more conservative approach.

Common Risks

When you enter a hospital, you face a variety of risks…

• **You could be misdiagnosed,** especially in the emergency room.

• **You could receive the wrong treatment** or your condition could be poorly monitored and managed.

• **You could be the victim of a surgical error.** A 2015 study from Massachusetts General Hospital found that some sort of mistake or adverse event occurred in half of all operations.

• **You could receive the wrong drug,** the wrong dose of a drug, or the drug you need might not even be ordered.

• **The Centers for Disease Control and Prevention estimates that there are 1.7 million hospital-acquired infections a year.** You could get an infection from difficult-to-treat bacteria, such as *Clostridium difficile* or *methicillin-resistant Staphylococcus aureus* (MRSA).

• **You could develop a pressure ulcer (bedsore) that becomes infected.**

• **You could fall,** usually while going from the bed to the bathroom.

• **You could develop deep-vein thrombosis,** a blood clot that typically forms in the leg, but can travel to the lungs or heart, threatening your life.

All of these possibilities increased during the pandemic, when family members, friends, and professional health advocates were rarely permitted to enter hospitals and hospital staff were often spread dangerously thin. Now, more than ever, you need to look out for yourself or have someone else looking out for you. Here are several straightforward and commonsense strategies to do that:

Choose the Best Hospital

If possible, choose a university-affiliated teaching hospital over a public hospital or for-profit hospital. At teaching hospitals, you'll be asked the same question about your care many times—by medical students, interns, residents, fellows, and your medical team. This type of redundancy, where everybody is checking everybody else's work, is the best way to keep a patient safe. If you don't live near a city, use tools like Hospital SafetyGrade.org to research the best hospitals near you. (See previous article for more information on choosing a hospital.)

Choose an Experienced Surgeon

The best way to prevent errors during elective surgery is to choose an experienced surgeon. Ask, "How many such procedures have you performed in the past 12 months?" If it's a relatively low number, find another surgeon. And always get a second opinion before any surgery. ProPublica, a nonprofit that conducts investigative journalism, publishes Medicare-based data on surgeons' procedures and complication rates at Projects. propublica.org/surgeons/.

Have a Designated Advocate

Arrange to have an advocate who is tasked with knowing the daily details of your condition and your treatment plan, and to maintain regular communication with nurses and physicians who are supervising and delivering your care. Your advocate can be a family member, a friend, or a paid professional.

To find a professional, visit the website Advoconnection.com, which provides a free directory of independent patient advocates. Interview one or more people to find out if you have a rapport with the advocate, if they've worked with patients with a similar problem to yours, and what the process of advocacy will entail. Ask about their credentials, references, and the cost.

Ask for a Consultation

If you have or develop a symptom that you want evaluated by a specialist rather than the hospitalist (the physician who is managing your care in the hospital), ask for a consultation. If the physician says no, insist.

Demand Sanitization

This is always important to help prevent hospital-acquired infections, but it has taken on added importance during the pandemic. If a clinician or caregiver wants to come into your room but you haven't seen them wash their hands or hit the hand sanitizer dispenser, insist they do so. If they say they have done it, insist they do it again, if only to "humor" you. Likewise, ask the nurse or doctor if they have sanitized the stethoscope before putting it on you.

Prevent Falls

If you're unsteady on your feet or have any question about your balance, or if you're taking a medication that has drowsiness as a side effect, always get a nurse's assistant or nurse to help you to the bathroom. About 40 percent of falls in hospitals occur when a patient tries to get to the bathroom unassisted. If you go to the bathroom by yourself, or otherwise move about the room, always bring your hospital call button so if you do fall, you can get help as soon as possible.

Prevent Bedsores

Bedsores can develop when you don't move enough and there is pressure on your skin for long periods of time. People who are frail, bedridden, or diabetic have the highest risk. To prevent a bedsore, you should turn and reposition yourself at least every two hours to relieve the pressure on any one part of

your body. Your heels and tailbone are particularly risky spots.

If you can't move yourself, call for a nurse to help you. Ask if the hospital can provide a pressure-relieving mattress or other protective devices. If you do develop a bedsore, you will need regular wound cleaning, dressing changes, and good nutrition to speed the healing.

Know the Details of Any Drug You Take in the Hospital

If the nurse wants to give you a pill or injection that you're not familiar with, ask about it. Who ordered it? What is it for? What are the side effects? If the answers aren't satisfactory, demand to speak with your physician before you take the drug.

Ask About Your Medications at Discharge

Medications are often added or changed while you're in the hospital. To ensure drug safety when you are being discharged, ask the nurse, hospitalist, or hospital pharmacist the following questions…

Have any medications been added, stopped, or changed while I was in the hospital, and why?

What medications do I need to keep taking, and why?

How do I take my medications, and for how long?

How will I know if my medication is working, and what side effects do I watch for?

Discharge and Beyond

Also ask the following questions at discharge…

What is my diagnosis?

What medical equipment will I need? Can the hospital order it for me?

What follow-up care will I need?

When and how will I receive test results?

Are my records available to me through a patient portal?

Whom should I call if I have a question or problem?

How soon should I make a follow-up appointment?

Help Nurses Help You

Carrie Ali, editor, *Bottom Line Health*. BottomLine Inc.com

The health-care system is under immense strain, and nurses are working at—and beyond—maximum capacity. I asked a group of nurses what we, as patients, can do to get the best care possible. *Here are their thoughts…*

•**Maintain a healthy weight.** Being obese is linked to the leading causes of illness and death, including diabetes, heart disease, stroke, and some types of cancer. It can make illnesses like COVID-19 worse.

But that's not all: It can affect hospital care, too. Lifting a fallen patient or repositioning someone in bed is much more difficult when that person is very heavy.

"I don't think anyone realizes that severely obese people don't get the same quality of care simply because one little nurse can't move them as often as they need or keep them as clean and dry," Anna Carlyle, RN, BSN, told me.

•**Stay mobile and active.** Simple exercises like tai chi, walking, or resistance training reduce your risk of falls, increase your physical independence, and reduce your chances of having to wait for assistance for simple things like going to the toilet. "The number of patients who come in to the hospital for something like an ankle fracture and are then bed-bound is too high," shared Amy Evans, RN.

•**Get vaccinated.** Both studies and anecdotal experiences clearly show that people who have been vaccinated against COVID-19 are much less likely to need hospitalization. If they do wind up in the hospital, they are

Demand Better from Hospitals

The staffing crisis doesn't come only from nurses retiring or from not enough people entering the field, though these are certainly important issues. Hospitals have increasingly moved toward lean staffing models to save money and boost profits. If you notice that the nurses are scrambling to help all of their patients and being called away from your room because there aren't enough people to help in another room, let the hospital know by filling out the survey at the end of your hospital visit.

less likely to need intensive care. COVID-19 isn't the only vaccine you need. Talk to your doctor or pharmacist about recommended vaccinations for flu, shingles, and pneumonia, too.

•**Be patient.** If you do find yourself in the hospital, have realistic expectations about how quickly a nurse can get to you.

"You need to give a nurse about 30 minutes to respond to a call," explained Elizabeth Gamble, RN. "It can take that long to help somebody to the bathroom and back, and you can't really hurry that up. A nurse can't be in two places at once." The more patients each nurse has, the less time she can spend with each one.

Nurses are trained to prioritize the limited time they have. "You may need to go to the bathroom, which is uncomfortable, but a patient down the hall may be having trouble breathing, which could be life-threatening," she added.

•**Do what you can on your own.** Whenever possible, do as much as you can yourself. If you have someone with you in the hospital, ask them to help with simple tasks that don't require a nurse's specific skills, like fluffing your pillows, brushing your teeth and hair, or refilling an ice pack.

For Appendicitis, Surgery Still Is Best

In recent years, treatment with antibiotics has emerged as a viable alternative to surgery for people with acute uncomplicated appendicitis. But in a new study, patients who received IV antibiotics until their symptoms improved, followed by a five-day course of at-home antibiotics, did worse than those who simply had their appendices removed surgically. One-quarter of the antibiotic group had another case of acute appendicitis within one year and reported a significantly lower quality of life during follow-up than the surgery group.

Study of 186 patients by researchers at Royal College of Surgeons in Ireland, Dublin, published in Annals of Surgery.

• **Plan ahead.** When you do need a nurse, try to ask for everything you need at once. It's a good idea to have a pen and notepad so you can write down what you need. Ask your nurse when she or he is planning on coming back so you can gauge whether you can wait while he or she does rounds.

• **Trust the experts.** Because nurses treat patients all day, every day, they have developed a wide range of strategies to perform tasks safely and efficiently. Let them do what they do best. "I promise I've had dozens of patients with this illness, injury, or surgery," said Sienna Reader, RN. "I'm telling you the easiest and safest way to do whatever it is."

• **Don't harm your nurse.** Almost every hospital-based nurse has experienced physical violence or verbal abuse. Nurses caring for COVID-19 patients have been at the highest risk.

"I experience verbal abuse from patients on a daily basis," shared Roseann Garber, RN. "The worst is when they get combative. …On the bright side, I am so good at dodging punches from patients."

This behavior is never appropriate and never justified. Nurses deserve to do their jobs without fear of being harmed or berated.

"Some nurses are working lots of extra shifts, staying late all the time, not getting enough sleep, we are being asked to work while sick, and we are TIRED," Jana Rice, RN, told me. "Your nurse may be feeling worse than you are."

Antibiotics Are Linked to Parkinson's Risk

Filip Scheperjans, MD, PhD, adjunct professor of neurology at University of Helsinki, Finland, and leader of an analysis of Parkinson's cases from 1998 to 2014, published in *Movement Disorders*.

Doctors have long known there is a connection between the bacteria in a person's gut and Parkinson's disease (PD).

Recent finding: Extensive use of oral antibiotics that wipe out gut bacteria is strongly associated with increased risk for PD. The finding was particularly robust for *macrolides* (such as *erythromycin*) and *lincosamides* (such as *lincomycin* and *clindamycin*). People whose medical histories included five or more courses of these classes of antibiotics within a five-year period had about a 40 percent greater risk for PD 10 to 15 years later than the general population.

Researchers aren't sure how gut bacteria affects PD risk.

Theory: Antibiotic use leaves the gut wall susceptible to inflammation, which allows the naturally occuring protein *alpha-synuclein* to accumulate in the gut wall's nerve cells. Over years, the alpha-synuclein travels to the brain, where it kills dopamine-producing cells. The brain chemical dopamine is involved in many basic functions, including motor coordination. Coordination problems are a major symptom of PD.

After any course of antibiotics, rebuild your gut bacteria by consuming a healthy plant-based diet. The microbiome typically will return to its original state within three months, but in some cases, it may take up to a year or may never return.

There is no evidence that probiotic supplements can help gut bacteria return to normal, although there is some evidence that probiotics can shorten/prevent antibiotic-associated diarrhea.

Don't be afraid to take an antibiotic if your doctor says it's the best treatment for your condition, but don't pressure caregivers to prescribe antibiotics without sound medical justification.

Also: Don't panic if you have taken antibiotics extensively in the past. PD is a multifactorial disease with strong genetic and environmental components that contribute to risk.

The Promise of Palliative Care

Joe Rotella, MD, MBA, chief medical officer of the American Academy of Hospice and Palliative Medicine (AAHPM).

Palliative care aims to prevent or treat the symptoms of a condition and the side effects from its treatments. This relief is often sorely needed by those who are seriously ill, even when they are getting treatments that may result in a cure.

People with cancer, heart failure, and chronic obstructive pulmonary disease may spring to mind as a good fit for palliative care, but so are people with many other serious illnesses, such as kidney failure, liver disease, Alzheimer's disease, neurological illnesses, and those with multiple chronic conditions who are not thriving.

For example, palliative care would be perfect for Alice, an 80-year-old woman living alone at home with joint pain and trouble walking due to arthritis, difficulty breathing due to heart failure, and memory loss due to the early stages of Alzheimer's disease.

Palliative Care Coordination

Many patients who've just been discharged from the hospital don't know the basics about their condition and treatment options, ways to stay out of the hospital, or even when they'll see their doctor again. But if you have a palliative care team, one of the first things they will do is hold a meeting with you and whomever you consider family to fill any gaps in knowledge, identify your goals for your care, and develop a care plan that includes coordination with all who are involved in your care. They will also conduct a careful review of medications. It's not uncommon for the palliative care team to find that a patient has a shoe box full of medications, some of which may no longer be needed, may be causing side effects, or may be doing more harm than good. After the palliative care team discontinues medications that are harmful or unnecessary and perhaps adds a few for comfort, patients often feel and function much better.

—Dr. Joe Rotella

Practical Considerations

Distress related to chronic or life-limiting conditions isn't only physical. Serious illness often brings with it emotional, spiritual, social, and practical problems that are just as important to address as pain, weakness, or trouble sleeping. A person may need a ride to treatments, help understanding insurance coverage, assistance with finances or childcare, or counseling to ease depression and anxiety.

Palliative care uses a team of experts—doctors, nurses, pharmacists, social workers, psychologists, chaplains, and others—to place the person with serious illness and their family at the center of the process and explore their unique needs, values, and preferences. Alice, for example, fears that she'll be forced to leave her home, and her family worries about her safety. The palliative care team would meet with Alice and her family to discuss these concerns and develop a care plan to relieve her physical discomfort, coordinate her care with her other doctors, and keep her safe at home and functioning the best she can.

No Need to Wait

You don't have to wait until all treatments and potential cures have been exhausted to benefit from palliative care. This approach makes sense any time, from diagnosis, when symptoms or distress first appear, to later in an illness, when a change of course may be needed, or in the survivor stage, when you're dealing with lingering pain or side effects. It's beneficial to people with serious illness at any age in any stage. Depending on insurance coverage, this coordinated care may be handled like any other treatment.

Hospice at the End of Life

Hospice is essentially an intensive form of palliative care that is specifically designed for people who are likely to be in their last months of life. The focus is on comfort and quality of life, but, in some cases, it may be provided along with treatments that help control the underlying illness.

As with palliative care, a trained team that includes physicians, nurses, social workers, chaplains, and mental health professionals converge to smooth the patient's and family's path on a variety of levels, easing physical pain as well as addressing emotional, spiritual, and other needs. Hospices may also provide trained aides and volunteers who can assist with personal care and housekeeping services.

This support helps a person focus on living the best they can and sharing meaningful moments with friends and family. Hospice supports hope for living life to its fullest. Indeed, research shows that those in hospice care live just as long as others at the same stage of illness, and more comfortably as well.

Medicare and insurance plans often cover all related charges. In some cases, it may be difficult to estimate a person's life expectancy and eligibility for hospice. Whatever the reason, if hospice is not the best choice at the moment, you can still ask for palliative care.

Planning Ahead

When it comes to health care, it pays to plan ahead. Let your family and your medical team know what's important to you, what treatments you would or would not want to try if you were very ill, and who you would want to speak for you if you couldn't speak for yourself. These conversations may feel awkward at first, but they can make a big difference for your loved ones should they find themselves in the unfortunate position of having to guide major medical decisions on your behalf. It's a good idea to put your wishes in writing in the form of a living will and durable power of attorney for health care.

Don't wait for your doctor to tell you it's time for palliative care. If you're in physical, emotional, or spiritual distress, or face practical challenges or caregiver issues, speak up and ask. Being proactive will help you remain in the driver's seat regarding your health.

Chapter 8

HEART HEALTH

Protect Your Heart During Menopause

Menopause is known to cause plenty of unpleasant symptoms, such as hot flashes, vaginal dryness, disrupted sleep, and mood changes. But what many women don't know, and often aren't told by their doctors until they're in their 50s, 60s, and beyond, is that menopause—defined as the absence of a period for 12 consecutive months—is also a powerful driver of heart disease.

Estrogen Protects the Heart

During the reproductive years, naturally high estrogen levels help keep the heart humming smoothly. Estrogen helps boost high-density lipoprotein (HDL, the heart-protective, "good" cholesterol) and decrease low-density lipoprotein (LDL, the "bad kind" of cholesterol). Estrogen keeps blood vessels and arteries supple, elastic, and dilated so blood can flow easily through them. It also absorbs free radicals, molecules in the blood that can damage the heart and other organs. For all these reasons and more, women in their 30s and 40s are less likely than men to be di-agnosed with cardiovascular disease (CVD), also known as heart disease.

But in perimenopause, the eight to 10 years leading up to menopause, as well as during and after menopause itself, fluctuating and then decreasing hormone levels cause troubling changes that double a woman's risk of heart disease.

• **An increase in cholesterol.** As estrogen drops, LDL cholesterol rises. Not only that, but menopause seems to alter the way HDL works, turning this normally protective substance into an artery hardener.

• **Stiffer arteries.** When arteries harden, the heart is forced to work harder to pump blood through the body. The harder the heart has to work, the more vulnerable it becomes. That stiffness accelerates in the year following a woman's last menstrual period, according to a 2020 study published in *Arteriosclerosis, Thrombosis, and Vascular Biology*. This is especially true for African-American women.

Elizabeth Poynor, MD, PhD, a gynecologic oncologist and advanced pelvic surgeon in private practice in Manhattan. Dr. Poynor is board certified in obstetrics and gynecology and gynecologic oncology; performs surgery at NYU Langone Medical Center and Northwell Health Lenox Hill Hospital; and is a clinical professor of obstetrics and gynecology at NYU Langone. Her practice is a blend of allopathic and integrative medicine. PoynorHealthNewYork.com/

• **A slowdown in metabolism.** Estrogen helps regulate metabolism and healthy weight. When it goes down, the scale moves in the opposite direction. Many women in perimenopause and menopause notice this weight gain, which is difficult to reverse even with exercise and diet. Complicating matters, menopausal weight gain tends to accumulate around the belly, the worst kind of fat for your heart as it raises levels of triglycerides, artery-clogging fat that increases the risk of heart attack and stroke.

Preliminary research presented at the 2021 American Heart Association conference suggested that hitting menopause by age 40 increases the lifetime risk of developing coronary disease by 40 percent compared with women who didn't go through early menopause. Coronary disease is a specific type of heart disease that occurs when plaque builds up in the arteries (atherosclerosis). This research did not include surgically induced menopause, but other research indicates that heart disease risk doubles for women who have their ovaries removed at a young age.

This adds up to the fact that once a woman enters menopause, her heart disease risk equals a man's. It is the number one cause of death for American women, responsible for one in every three female deaths.

Reduce Risk

Losing the cardioprotective effects of estrogen is a difficult, but not unbeatable, challenge. About 80 percent of heart disease cases can be avoided with strategic lifestyle changes.

• **Follow the Mediterranean diet.** This anti-inflammatory plant-based approach emphasizes produce, beans, whole grains, and heart-healthy fats like olive oil, nuts, seeds, and avocado. Small amounts of oily fish and chicken are included. Saturated fats are limited and trans fats are eliminated. Not only is the Mediterranean way of eating heart healthy, but it may also ease menopause symptoms such as hot flashes and night sweats.

• **Exercise regularly.** Aim for 30 to 60 minutes of aerobic exercise most days of the week, alternating moderate-intensity days

Revisiting Hormone Replacement

In 2002, the Women's Health Initiative (WHI) study dealt a major blow to hormone replacement therapy (HRT), which had long been routinely prescribed to menopausal women to manage symptoms and protect against heart disease. The WHI study concluded that HRT did not decrease heart disease risk but did increase the risk of blood clotting, stroke, and breast cancer. The medical community quickly responded by decreasing or stopping the practice of prescribing HRT.

More recently, it's been questioned whether the WHI findings pertain to all menopausal women, and how much the timing and type of HRT used might matter. Many studies have since been published showing that the benefit of introducing estrogen and other hormone therapies within a few years of menopause far outweighs the risks for many women. Ask your doctor about a more modern approach to hormone replacement, including natural forms of estrogens and progestins, such as estradiol and progesterone; other hormones produced by the ovary that decline with age, such as testosterone and DHEA; and even thyroid hormone.

—Dr. Elizabeth Poynor

with vigorous-intensity days. Add in two days of full-body strength training or resistance work a week and stretch whenever you can.

• **Ask your doctor about cholesterol medications.** You may be a candidate for a statin, a class of cholesterol-lowering drugs beneficial in people with coronary heart disease.

• **If you smoke, quit, especially if you're considering hormone replacement therapy.** Mixing the two significantly raises the risk of blood clots.

• **Be open with your doctor.** Since your current physician likely isn't the same one you had during your reproductive years, definitely share details of your pregnancy history, including whether you experienced high blood pressure (preeclampsia) or gestational diabetes. Both increase the risk of heart disease about 10 to 15 years after delivery. Let your doctor know if you experienced early menopause so he or she can help you create a plan for reducing various associated health risks.

Can Exercise Trigger a Heart Attack? Putting the Risk into Perspective

Barry A. Franklin, PhD, director of preventive cardiology/cardiac rehabilitation at Beaumont Health in Royal Oak, Michigan. He is a member of the *Bottom Line Health* advisory board. DrBarryFranklin.com

---

Regular physical activity offers a wide range of health benefits, including protection against the development of heart disease. *But in rare cases, it appears to have the opposite effect…*

Exercise-related acute cardiovascular events —and sudden cardiac deaths—have been reported in the medical literature and the lay press. In some people with underlying heart disease, exercise-related increases in heart rate and blood pressure can cause coronary plaque rupture, thrombosis, and lethal heart rhythm irregularities. The cause of exercise-related cardiovascular events largely depends on the exerciser's age. Coronary artery disease is the most frequent autopsy finding in individuals over the age of 40. In contrast, inherited structural cardiovascular abnormalities are a major cause of fatal heart rhythms during strenuous physical activity in younger athletes.

Risk in Perspective

The incidence of cardiovascular events during light- to moderate-intensity activities is extremely low and similar to that expected at rest. Unaccustomed vigorous physical exertion, however, especially in people with un-

derlying heart disease, appears to transiently increase the risk of acute cardiac events. Activities such as competitive squash/racquetball, basketball, cross-country skiing, water skiing, heavy weight-lifting, and high-intensity interval training may place undue stress on the heart and are not recommended for people with known or suspected heart disease. Arm work, straining, breath-holding, and exposure to cold and wind appear to heighten the risk of acute cardiac events as well.

Safer Workouts

There are several steps you can take to reduce your risk of experiencing a cardiovascular event when exercising.

•**If you are currently inactive, always start with a walking program.** An initial goal is to walk at a speed of at least three miles per hour on a level surface, without symptoms.

•**Warm up and cool down.** The best warm-up for any activity is performing that activity at a lower intensity.

•**Reduce the intensity of exercise** in hot, humid weather and when working at high altitudes.

•**Don't ignore symptoms** such as chest pain, dizziness, lightheadedness, heart palpitations (fast, slow, or irregular heartbeats), unusual fatigue, or shortness of breath. Many people who have experienced exercise-related cardiovascular complications had these symptoms in the days or weeks before the event. If you experience any of these symptoms while exercising or have pain or discomfort from your belly button up, stop exercise immediately and consult with your physician. Medical clearance is required before resuming your exercise regimen.

•**Exercise regularly.** The likelihood of cardiac events appears to be reduced by up to 50 percent in regular exercisers. For people who gradually progress to vigorous exercise, the more frequently vigorous exercise is performed, the lower the cardiac risk of each exercise bout. In other words, don't cram your vigorous exercise into just one or two bouts per week. When it comes to extremely strenuous exercise, being a "weekend warrior" (or even less frequently) can be hazardous to your health.

HIIT May Not Be Safe for People With Heart Disease

Study of 1,500 adults led by researchers at Norwegian University of Science and Technology, Trondheim, Norway, published in *BMJ Open*.

Recent finding: High-Intensity Interval Training (HIIT) is aerobic exercise such as jogging, swimming and cycling that alternates between short bursts of high heart rate and low heart rate intervals. While it is generally safe for most people, even older adults, it may be dangerous for people who have or are at risk for heart disease. Check with your health-care provider.

More Young Women Are Dying of Heart Disease

Study of mortality rates over a 19-year period led by researchers at The Johns Hopkins University School of Medicine, Baltimore, published in *European Heart Journal: Quality of Care & Clinical Outcomes*.

Heart disease is increasing as a cause of death for women under age 65. If trends continue, heart disease may overtake cancer as the leading cause of death for women in that age group. Researchers say one-third of women's heart problems occur before age 65, but they're often not warned about their risk until they've had a heart attack....and that too many women put the health and well-being of their families before their own. Women can substantially lower their risk by eating a healthy diet, not smoking and getting enough exercise.

Broken-Heart Syndrome: Stress Cardiomyopathy Can Mimic a Heart Attack

Gregory Chapman, MD, a University of Alabama at Birmingham cardiologist and professor of medicine. He is author of *A Strong and Steady Pulse: Stories from a Cardiologist*.

We all know that severe stress is bad for our health. Job loss, the death of a loved one, or the fallout from an auto accident, serious illness, or natural disaster can ruin our sleep, disrupt our diets, and cause pain throughout the body.

In some cases, extreme stress can even cause sudden, dramatic changes in our hearts, producing chest pain, shortness of breath, and something that feels very much like a heart attack. Doctors call the condition stress cardiomyopathy.

You may know it better as "broken heart syndrome," the name often used in news stories about people who fall ill and sometimes even die in the days after the death of a loved one. It's also been suspected when deaths rise suddenly after hurricanes and earthquakes.

The Role of the Pandemic

Now the condition has been tied to another big stressor: the COVID-19 pandemic. In the early months of the pandemic, researchers at the Cleveland Clinic found a clear uptick in cases among patients showing up with possible heart-attack symptoms. Before the pandemic, fewer than 2 percent of such patients turned out to have the disorder, but during the spring of 2020, that quadrupled. None of those patients had COVID-19 itself. Instead, researchers speculated that the stresses associated with the outbreak—everything from isolation to job loss to increased health worries—triggered the increase in stressed-out hearts. It's not clear if the increase in cases has continued, but the stresses of COVID-19 certainly have, so, it's a good time to learn a little more about this condition.

What Is Stress Cardiomyopathy?

In stress cardiomyopathy, the heart's left ventricle, the chamber responsible for pumping oxygen-rich blood to the rest of the body, becomes enlarged and weakened. The condition develops suddenly, typically within a few days of an especially stressful event. Usually, these are upsetting events, but even a happy surprise, such as winning a lottery, can be a trigger.

> The good news is that 95 percent of patients will recover. Within two to three months, the enlarged part of the heart will return to its normal size and function.

A leading theory is that stress hormones, such as adrenaline, surge into the heart tissue and disrupt normal functioning. It can happen in someone with no previous heart troubles or risk factors for heart disease. Women past menopause are at the highest risk, but doctors don't know why. Some increased risk also is seen in people with anxiety, depression, and schizophrenia.

Because typical signs and symptoms include chest pain, shortness of breath, and irregular heartbeat, patients who show up in emergency rooms are rightly treated as if they might be having classic heart attacks. That kind of heart attack is technically known as a myocardial infarction and is usually caused by a clot blocking blood flow to the heart, damaging or destroying the muscle.

Someone suffering from stress cardiomyopathy will have some test findings that match those of a person suffering a myocardial infarction, such as levels of certain cardiac enzymes, but a coronary angiogram, a kind of X-ray done to look for blocked arteries, will find no blockages. Instead, tests will reveal the distinctive enlarged left ventricle.

How Is It Treated?

Once someone is diagnosed with stress cardiomyopathy, they usually spend two to three days in the hospital for observation. Many will develop no further signs of trouble and will go home without needing additional treatment. However, in studies, between 12 and 45 percent of hospitalized patients with stress cardiomyopathy develop acute heart failure, meaning that their hearts fail to pump enough blood through their bodies. When that happens, doctors prescribe these patients the same medications used for other heart-failure patients, such as beta-blockers, angiotensin-converting enzyme (ACE) inhibitors, and diuretics.

A smaller number of patients develop cardiogenic shock, the most severe form of heart failure. Their hearts pump so weakly that far too little oxygen is delivered to the brain, kidneys, liver, and other organs, threatening permanent damage or death. This is the main cause of death for the 5 percent of patients who die from stress cardiomyopathy. Aggressive treatments, including the placement of a temporary device to help the heart pump, may be needed.

What's the Prognosis?

The good news is that 95 percent of patients will recover. Within two to three months, the enlarged part of the heart will return to its normal size and function. It is thought that this remodeling of the heart muscle is possible because the affected cells have been stunned, but not destroyed, by the onslaught of stress hormones. Some people will be advised to continue medications as their hearts heal, and some will suffer some lingering fatigue or other symptoms.

While survivors of broken heart syndrome can go on with their lives, they should know that they face some risk of recurrence, about 20 percent over 10 years, according to researchers. So, it's important to pay attention to suspicious symptoms and to always seek medical care for a possible cardiac emergency.

High Blood Pressure Alerts for Women

Women: Check Your BP Numbers

Women should have lower blood pressure than men. Current guidelines state a single "normal" range with 120 mmHg as the maximum systolic ("upper") number.

Recent finding: The maximum normal range for women is 110 mmHg systolic. Using 110 as the threshold for women could help prevent and treat cardiovascular disease, heart attack, stroke and heart failure.

Study of more than 27,000 people by researchers at Cedars-Sinai's Smidt Heart Institute, Los Angeles, published in *Circulation*.

High Blood Pressure in Women Often Is Dismissed as Menopause

When men have high blood pressure, it's usually treated as hypertension, but when it happens to women, health-care providers often attribute it to menopause due to an overlap of symptoms such as hot flashes and palpitations. Leaving the condition untreated puts women at greater risk for atrial fibrillation, heart failure and stroke and is harder to treat when identified later in life.

Study by researchers at Radboud University Medical Center, Nijmegen, Netherlands, published in *European Heart Journal*.

Different Blood Pressure Readings Between Arms Could Signal Risk

Study of nearly 54,000 people by researchers at University of Exeter, UK, published in *Hypertension*.

Consistently getting different blood pressure readings between your right and left arms is associated with greater risk for serious circulatory issues. Blood pressure readings are given in millimeters of mercury (mmHg). For every 1 mmHg of difference between the right and left arms, a patient's risk of developing angina, heart attack or stroke increases by one percent. Differences in blood pressure between the two extremities can be caused by stiffening of the arteries, a risk marker for these conditions. Ask health-care providers to take your blood pressure readings from both arms.

Abnormal Blood Pressure During Sleep Boosts Heart Disease Risk

Kazuomi Kario, MD, professor of cardiovascular medicine, Jichi Medical University, Tochigi, Japan, and lead author of a seven-year study of 6,300 people published in *Circulation*.

People whose blood pressure dropped or spiked abnormally during sleep were at significantly increased risk for cardiovascular disease events. Overnight systolic pressure (upper number) increases of 20 mmHg or more raised risk for heart disease and stroke by 18 percent and risk for heart failure by 25 percent. Blood pressure is normally about 10 percent to 20 percent lower during sleep… but overnight decreases greater than 20 percent were found to double risk for stroke. If you're concerned about your nighttime blood pressure level, ask your doctor about nocturnal monitoring and discuss strategies for managing blood pressure around the clock.

Yogurt Helps Manage Blood Pressure

Alexandra Wade, PhD, postdoctoral researcher at University of South Australia, Adelaide, and lead author of a study of 915 people, published in *International Dairy Journal*.

People with high blood pressure who ate a daily serving of yogurt had an average blood pressure reading seven points lower than people who never ate yogurt. Yogurt is high in calcium, magnesium and potassium—all of which help regulate blood pressure—and contains bacteria that produce proteins that have blood-pressure–lowering effects.

Best: Yogurt that contains live cultures and is low in sugar.

Sex and Heart Attacks: What's Safe?

Barry A. Franklin, PhD, director of preventive cardiology/cardiac rehabilitation at Beaumont Health in Royal Oak, Michigan. He is a member of the *Bottom Line Health* advisory board. DrBarryFranklin.com

---

You just had a mild heart attack and underwent emergency coronary angioplasty. Is it safe to resume sexual activity?

This question is commonly asked by middle-aged and older heart patients. Fortunately, numerous studies now provide reassurance to those who have such concerns.

Sexual activity is associated with a very light to moderate energy expenditure and associated transient increases in heart rate and blood pressure. I often counsel patients that

---

Try to Simplify Blood Pressure Medications

Increasing the dosage of blood pressure medication may be more effective than adding a second drug. While both approaches lower blood pressure, patients—especially older ones—are more likely to stick to a drug regimen with fewer medications.

Best: Personalizing treatment to bring down high blood pressure.

Lillian Min, MD, associate professor of geriatric and palliative medicine at University of Michigan, Ann Arbor, and senior author of a study published in *Annals of Internal Medicine*.

---

if they can exercise at a 3 METs workload, such as walking at 3 miles per hour (mph) on a level treadmill or walking at 2 mph on a 3.5 percent grade or higher without adverse signs or symptoms, they can safely resume sexual activity.

Studies show that sexual activity is a probable contributor to heart attacks in fewer than one percent of all cases. In the hour after sexual activity, the relative risk of a heart attack does increase two- to fourfold, but it rapidly returns to baseline. An intriguing finding from these studies is that regular physical activity reduces the risk of sex precipitating a heart attack. Individuals in the studies who exercise vigorously three or more times each week had no increased risk of having a heart attack triggered by sex.

Extramarital sex appears to be more demanding from a cardiovascular perspective for men with known or suspected heart disease. Most coital deaths occur with mistresses or prostitutes. Researchers believe that excess alcohol intake, cigarette smoking, and other stressors may further increase arousal and the demands on the heart.

When Standing Is Unbearable: Women During Child-Bearing Years Are at High Risk

Cyndya Shibao MD, MSCI, FAHA, FAAS, associate professor, department of medicine, division of clinical pharmacology, Vanderbilt Autonomic Dysfunction Center, Vanderbilt University Medical Center, Nashville, Tennessee.

Like everything else, your blood is subject to the laws of gravity. When you stand up, gravity pulls blood into your abdomen and legs.

To counteract this effect, your leg muscles help pump blood back to the heart, which speeds up slightly with the help of a boost of adrenaline. A burst of norepinephine constricts blood vessels to further guide blood back to the heart and, in turn, the brain. If you've ever had a rush of dizziness when standing too quickly, you've experienced a momentary delay in this normally elegant system. If you have postural orthostatic tachycardia syndrome (POTS), there's more than a delay: The mechanisms designed to avoid blood pooling into your abdomen and legs fail.

A Faulty System

The longer you stand, the more the blood pools. Your body still tries to correct the pooling by releasing norepinephrine and epinephrine, which cause your heart to beat faster, but the blood vessels don't constrict as they're supposed to. The pooled blood isn't returned to the heart, which creates a chain reaction where insufficient blood gets to the brain, causing symptoms such as lightheadedness, nausea, vomiting, dimmed vision, altered hearing, and fainting. The heart tries to compensate by beating faster, leading to an elevated heart rate (called *tachycardia*).

The reaction can be triggered by standing, sitting at a desk, standing in line, taking a shower, and seeing blood or gore. It can occur in people who overly restrict their salt intake or don't drink enough water—both of which help maintain healthy blood pressure by retaining fluid in blood vessels. Being overheated, scared, or anxious are triggering factors as well.

While there's not yet a cure for POTS, there are a variety of treatments and strategies that can minimize its effects on daily life.

Dietary Tips

Many women with POTS have low blood volume, which can often be rectified by increasing salt and fluid intake. At the Vanderbilt Autonomic Dysfunction Center, we recommend eating 6 to 9 grams of dietary salt and drinking 2 to 3 liters of water each day.

Follow a low-carbohydrate diet and avoid large meals that divert blood flow to digestive organs. Small, frequent meals are a bet-

Less Oxygen May Help Heart Failure

Controlled oxygen deprivation, used by athletes to boost performance, could help heart failure patients who suffer from severe shortness of breath because their weakened heart muscle cannot pump blood properly.

Simon Maybaum, MD, medical director and principal investigator of a pilot study at Montefiore-Einstein Center for Advanced Cardiac Therapy, reported at PumpingMarvellous.org, the website for the Pumping Marvellous Foundation, a UK charity led by heart-failure patients.

ter option. It's also wise to avoid alcohol, which causes veins to dilate.

Compression Clothing

While the corsets of yore caused an epidemic of fainting spells, a modern take on abdominal compression can decrease blood pooling. Abdominal binders or back braces that can be loosened when sitting and then tightened when standing are good options. Waist-high compression stockings can also help if they have at least 30 to 40 millimeters of mercury of compression, but they can be both difficult to put on and uncomfortable to wear.

Posture and Movement

When POTS symptoms strike, you may be able to move in ways that can help reduce blood pooling…

- **Stand on your toes,** cross your legs, or put one leg on a chair when standing.
- **Flex your leg and buttocks muscles.**
- **Sit in a low chair,** in a knee-chest position, or with your feet on a footstool.
- **Lean forward when sitting.**
- **Bend forward at the waist when walking** (such as when you're pushing a shopping cart).
- **Slightly elevate the head of your bed to retain fluid at night.**

• **If you feel faint,** grip one hand with the other and push your arms away while contracting your muscles for two minutes.

Exercise

While exercise can worsen POTS symptoms at first, a program that builds tolerance can yield dramatic benefits. Patients who could only tolerate a minute or two of activity have been able to build up to vigorous 45-minute workouts over time. The key is to start small and be patient.

Even if you are bedridden, you can start with simple exercises that can be done while reclining...

• **Put a pillow between your knees,** squeeze for 10 seconds, release, and repeat.

• **Repeat the same exercise with the pillow between your palms.**

• **Write your name in the air with your toes.** Over time, work on the whole alphabet.

• **Lie on your side,** lift your leg up sideways, and bring it back down without touching your legs together. Repeat.

• **Lie on your back,** lift your left leg up, and point your toe towards the ceiling. Switch legs and repeat.

• **Mildly stretch your whole body,** starting with your feet then moving to your legs, back, arms, and neck.

Add Challenge

For a more challenging workout, look to recumbent exercises, such as recumbent biking or rowing, that allow you to work harder without triggering the POTS response.

Swimming keeps you in a reclined position and builds strength in your legs, which itself can reduce orthostatic symptoms. Because the pressure from water helps prevent orthostatic symptoms, some people with POTS can even stand for lengthy periods in a pool.

Weight training increases strength and helps muscles more efficiently use oxygen and tolerate orthostatic stress. Start with light weights and use them in a reclined or seated position. Focus on the muscles in your legs and abdomen. Lifting your arms over your head can aggravate symptoms.

As your fitness increases, you may be able to work up to upright activities like walking, jogging, or biking. Avoid outdoor exercise when it is hot, and always warm up and cool down. Taking the medication *propranolol* may improve your exercise capacity.

Medications

If lifestyle strategies don't ease your symptoms, medications may help. Drugs like *fludrocortisone* (Florinef) and *midodrine* (Proamatine) can increase blood volume and blood vessel contraction, which can help return blood to the heart. Beta-blockers such as *metoprolol* (Toprol XL, Lopressor), *atenolol* (Tenormin), and *propranolol* (Inderal LA) can slow down the heart rate upon standing. If these medications fail, *verapamil* (Verelan, Calan SR) or *ivabradine* (Procoralan) can be added for additional heart rate control.

For patients who have symptoms such as flushing, excessive sweating, and jitters, medications such as *clonidine* (Catapres) and *guanfacine* (Intuniv ER) that reduce the release of or response to epinephrine and norepinephrine can help.

iPhone 12 Promax Warning If You Have a Pacemaker

Study led by researchers at Brown University, Providence, Rhode Island, published in *Journal of the American Heart Association*.

The FDA says cell phones do not put people with pacemakers or defibrillators at risk. But according to the American Heart Association (AHA), the MagSafe magnets in the iPhone 12 Pro Max may block an implanted defibrillator from responding to an arrhythmia and may cause abnormal pacing in pacemakers.

Caution: Having this phone lying over your pacemaker or defibrillator, such as in your breast pocket, could be dangerous.

A New Imaging Study Predicts Repeat Heart Attack Risk

Study titled "Identification of Vulnerable Plaques and Patients by Intracoronary Near-Infrared Spectroscopy and Ultrasound (PROSPECT II): A Prospective Natural History Study," by researchers at NewYork-Presbyterian/Columbia University Irving Medical Center, New York City, and Lund University, Sweden, et al., published in *The Lancet.*

They even sound dangerously unhealthy: fatty plaques. Forming inside artery walls, they are a main cause of heart attacks. When these plaques rupture, a blood clot can form and block blood supply to the heart muscle. The usual way to find these blocked coronary arteries is by angiogram, which is placing a thin tube called a catheter into the arteries of the heart, injecting a dye, and taking x-ray pictures. A blocked artery can then be opened by placing a stent to restore blood flow. This procedure is called a coronary angioplasty (also called percutaneous coronary intervention).

Non-Culprit Lesions...for Now

During the angiogram, other plaques may be present, but they have not ruptured and formed a clot. Doctors call these *non-culprit lesions.* These are also plaques, but they are not the cause of the heart attack. However, some of these lesions will go on to rupture and cause a future heart attack. Researchers at Lund University in Sweden wanted to find a better way to image these lesions and predict which ones were most likely to rupture over time. This could be a way to predict a future heart attack and prevent it with a stent.

NIRS/IVUS Shows More

The Lund University study used a more advanced type of imaging, known as near-infrared spectroscopy (NIRS) and intravascular ultrasound (IVUS). Unlike the x-ray angiogram that just shows an outline of a lesion, the NIRS/IVUS technique can show the amount of fat in the lesion.

The study recruited 898 patients who had a heart attack and stent placement in the previous four weeks. All the patients had NIRS/IVUS imaging.

Over an average of four years, slightly more than 13 percent of patients had another major adverse cardiac event (MACE) such as death, heart attack or symptoms of severe or progressive chest pain (angina). High-fat lesions increased the risk of a MACE significantly. Of the 898 patients, 112 had a MACE and 66 events were caused by 78 untreated non-culprit lesions. The results of the study are published in the medical journal *The Lancet.*

How to Stop a Major Adverse Cardiac Event

Now that these subtle culprits can be found, more studies are needed to determine how to treat these lesions. A preliminary study suggests that stenting these lesions could reduce MACEs by 50 percent.

Alcohol Quickly Boosts the Risk of Atrial Fibrillation (A-Fib)

European Heart Journal.

In a recent study, just one serving of an alcoholic beverage doubled the odds of an episode of A-fib occurring within four hours. Daily alcohol consumption increased the risk of A-fib by 16 percent (one drink per day) to 47 percent (four drinks per day).

Dairy Fat OK for Your Heart

Study titled "Biomarkers of Dairy Fat Intake, Incident Cardiovascular Disease, and All-Cause Mortality: A Cohort Study, Systematic Review, and Meta-Analysis," led by researchers at The George Institute for Global Health, Sydney, Australia, published in *PLOS Medicine*.

If you've been limiting yourself to low or no-fat dairy foods for heart health and sacrificing flavor in the process, here's some good news for your tastebuds: A growing number of studies are finding that not all dairy fats are bad for your heart. In fact, some dairy fat may actually reduce your risk of heart disease.

One country that tops the list of dairy lovers is Sweden. Researchers there wanted to investigate the effect of dairy fat on the heart health of Swedish citizens. Previous studies have relied on self-reported dairy food consumption. Because dairy is in so many types of foods, and relying on diet memory can be inaccurate, the researchers sought out a better way to track dairy fat in the diets of study participants.

Odd-Chain Fatty Acids Measure Dairy Fat Intake

The Swedish researchers measured a type of fatty acid called *odd-chain fatty acids*. Odd-chain fatty acids are found in the blood when dairy fat is digested. Two odd-chain fatty acids are *pentadecanoic acid*, also called fatty acid 15:0, and *heptadecanoic acid*, called fatty acid 17:0. The researchers used these as biomarkers for dairy fat in the diet.

How You Sleep and Work Affects Your Heart

Unconscious Wakefulness Doubles Women's Risk of Dying from Cardiovascular Disease

A study of 8,001 people found that women who experienced unconscious wakefulness most often and for longer periods of time had nearly double the risk of dying from cardiovascular disease than women in the general population. This normal part of the sleep cycle can be triggered by anything from noise or light to sleep apnea or pain. In men, a high number of what's also called cortical arousals had a smaller effect, increasing the risk of cardiovascular death by just over a quarter.

European Heart Journal

Working the Night Shift Elevates the Risk of Atrial Fibrillation

Data on 283,000 people showed that those who regularly worked the night shift had a 12 percent higher risk of A-fib than those who worked only during the day. The risk was 22 percent higher among people who worked an average of three-to-eight night shifts per month for 10 years or more.

European Heart Journal

Beware of On-the-Job Physical Exertion

High levels of leisure-time activity are associated with reduced risks for heart problems and death.

Recent finding: Lots of physical activity at work is linked to greater risk for heart attack, stroke and death.

Possible reasons: Leisure-time exercise may be more aerobic, while occupational activity is more likely to involve repetitive resistance exercise with little recovery time. Leisure-time exercise also typically involves 30 to 60 minutes of workouts several days a week, while occupational activity is often six to eight hours a day for many days in a row.

Ten-year study of more than 104,000 adults, ages 20 to 100, by researchers at National Research Center for the Working Environment, Copenhagen, Denmark, published in *JAMA*.

To track these fatty acid biomarkers, the researchers used a long-term study of Swedish adults called the Stockholm Cohort. The participants were 60-year-old men and women who had blood testing at the beginning of the study in 1997 and 1999—and then their health events were tracked through December 2014. During the years of tracking, any heart or blood vessel disease (cardiovascular disease) event was recorded. These events included heart attacks, strokes, and hospital admissions for chest pain (angina). Deaths from any cause were also included.

Higher Levels of Fatty Acids, Lower Risk of Heart Disease

The primary goals of the study were to compare cardiovascular events and deaths from any cause between people with high levels of dairy fat biomarkers to those with low levels. The results of the study are published in the journal *PLOS Medicine*. The study included more than 4,000 people in the Stockholm Cohort, and they also included 17 other studies from the United States, Denmark, and the UK. These other studies also had recorded blood levels of fatty acids of 15:0 and 17:0, as well as cardiovascular history and deaths. In total, the study included close to 43,000 people.

The key results of the study were that people in the top one-third for blood levels of fatty acids 15:0 and 17:0 had a significantly lower risk of cardiovascular disease events than people in the lower third of blood levels. For type 15:0, the risk was 12 percent less. For type 17:0, the risk was 14 percent less. People in the high-level fatty acid group did not have an increased risk of death.

More (Good) Fat May Mean More Nutrients

The researchers suspect that benefits from dairy fat may include anti-inflammatory elements as well as heart-health boosts from vitamin K and from probiotics in fermented dairy products like yogurt and cheese. They note that yogurt and cheese may be more beneficial than butter and milk. More research is needed, but the warning to avoid all full-fat dairy products for heart health needs to be reexamined. The researchers also noted that fats in fish, nuts, and vegetable oils may have greater benefits than dairy fats.

Pecans Reduce Risk for Cardiovascular Disease

Liana L. Guarneiri, PhD candidate in the department of nutritional sciences at University of Georgia, Athens, and first author of a study published in *The Journal of Nutrition*.

Recent finding: Participants at risk for cardiovascular disease who ate 2.4 ounces of pecans (about 470 calories) daily for eight weeks significantly lowered their total cholesterol by an average of 5 percent and LDL cholesterol by between 6 percent and 9 percent—whether they added the nuts to their diet or substituted them for other calories. Pecans are high in healthy fatty acids and fiber, which are linked with lowering cholesterol.

More Potassium—Not Less Sodium—Is Good for the Heart

Study by researchers at University of Porto, Portugal, published in *Nutrients*.

In a review of studies examining the relationship between cardiovascular disease and the consumption of sodium and potassium, reducing sodium intake did not significantly lower risk for disease. Instead, increasing potassium consumption to achieve a lower ratio of potassium to sodium appeared key to improving outcomes.

Best food sources of potassium: Bananas, oranges, spinach, broccoli, potatoes, and mushrooms.

Under-Used Blood Pressure Medicine Has Less Side Effects

Study titled "Comparative First-Line Effectiveness and Safety of ACE (Angiotensin-Converting Enzyme) Inhibitors and Angiotensin Receptor Blockers: A Multinational Cohort Study," published in the American Heart Association journal *Hypertension*.

There are several options available when starting a medication to treat high blood pressure. Two frontline recommendations are angiotensin-converting enzyme (ACE) inhibitors and angiotensin receptor blockers (ARBs). Angiotensin is a hormone that narrows blood vessels. ACE inhibitors block production of angiotensin. ARBs block the effects of angiotensin in blood vessels.

ACE inhibitors are prescribed more frequently than ARBs. Both medications lower blood pressure and they both have side effects, but few studies compare the two head-to-head. A new study by a team of international researchers compared the effectiveness and side effects of both medications in nearly three million people starting high blood pressure treatment with a single drug. Their study is published in the American Heart Association journal *Hypertension*.

Study Reviews Side Effects

The researchers used eight databases from the United States, Germany, and South Korea to gather data on effectiveness and side effects of the two drugs between 1996 and 2018. For effectiveness, the researchers compared the prevention of high blood pressure complications (called cardiovascular events). They included heart attack, heart failure, stroke or some combination of these complications. For safety, they looked at over 50 possible side effects.

ACEs Can Cost Less But with More Side Effects

Results of the study found that about three times as many patients were prescribed an ACE inhibitor as an ARB. This specific study did not determine why ACE inhibitors are preferred by physicians...but a possible reason is that ARBs can be more expensive. *Both medications were equally effective at preventing cardiovascular events, but the ACE inhibitor had significantly more side effects, including...*

• **Triple the risk for swelling of the skin and mucous membranes (angioedema)**

• **About 30 percent higher risk for persistent, dry cough**

• **About 30 percent higher risk for inflammation of the pancreas (pancreatitis)**

• **About 20 percent higher risk of bleeding in the gastrointestinal tract (GI bleeding).**

Doctors Should Favor ARBs

The researchers conclude that when starting a blood pressure medication, an ARB should be favored over an ACE inhibitor. The American Heart Association guidelines for starting high blood pressure medication are to use a diuretic, ACE inhibitor, ARB or a calcium channel blocker. All these medications can lower blood pressure and reduce cardiovascular events. The AHA recommends that these medications be used in conjunction with a heart-healthy diet and lifestyle.

For more information: To learn more about medications for hypertension, visit the American Heart Association online at Heart.org and search "high blood pressure medications."

Exercise Makes the Heart Resilient

Barry A. Franklin, PhD, director of preventive cardiology/cardiac rehabilitation at Beaumont Health in Royal Oak, Michigan. He is a past president of the American Association of Cardiovascular and Pulmonary Rehabilitation and the American College of Sports Medicine and a member of the *Bottom Line Health* advisory board.

Regular exercise and increased aerobic fitness are widely recommended by the American Heart Association, and for good reasons.

Moderate-to-vigorous physical activity improves the risk factor profile for heart disease, reduces the likelihood of inappropriate blood clotting, and, through autonomic nervous system adaptations, decreases the likelihood of inadequate blood flow to the heart muscle (ischemia) and threatening heart rhythm irregularities. Moreover, higher levels of aerobic fitness are strongly associated with a lower overall risk of acute cardiac events.

But it provides another and somewhat surprising benefit: Leisure-time or recreational physical activity can help you survive a heart attack.

What Is Preconditioning?

Decades ago, researchers found that regularly exercised dog hearts could be rendered largely resilient to major heart damage or life-threatening heart rhythm irregularities after experimentally induced heart attacks. Now, studies confirm that exercise preconditions the human heart in a similar way. A recent investigation of nearly 2,200 patients hospitalized for heart issues found that pre-admission physical activity habits reduced in-hospital death rates and improved cardiovascular outcomes one month after hospital discharge, even after adjusting for related outcome determinants.

Just one to three sessions of moderate-intensity physical activity corresponding to perceived exertion ratings of "somewhat hard," lasting from 20 to 30 minutes, provides

Even Moderate Alcohol Consumption Is Linked to Heart Trouble

Research has long shown that moderate drinkers enjoy a slightly reduced risk for heart failure compared with nondrinkers, but new research suggests that risk for atrial fibrillation—an irregular heartbeat that increases risk for stroke, heart failure and other heart-related complications—is a different story. In a 14-year study of nearly 108,000 people, those who averaged one drink per day had a 16 percent higher risk of developing atrial fibrillation than their teetotaling peers. The mechanism whereby moderate alcohol consumption increases atrial fibrillation risk is still unknown.

Study led by researchers at University Heart and Vascular Center Hamburg, Germany, published in European Heart Journal.

cardioprotective effects that persist for several days to more than a week after the last exercise session. Although the mechanisms responsible for the immediate cardioprotective benefits of the prior exercise remain unclear, researchers believe it may be due to transiently altered biochemical pathways or enhanced cardiac electrical stability. While moderate-intensity exercise provides robust protection against heart attacks, higher-intensity exercise does not bolster the magnitude of protection.

Practical Implications

Anyone with known or suspected heart disease should engage in multiple weekly bouts of exercise. If you don't think you have underlying heart disease, think again. Studies from the Cleveland Clinic suggest that approximately 85 percent of all Americans over the age of 50 have underlying atherosclerotic cardiovascular disease. Even if you're under 50, the American Heart Association recommends getting a total of 150 minutes of moderate physical activity over the course of the week.

Estimating Moderate Activity

What constitutes moderate activity differs for each person and depends largely on your current fitness level.

• **Talk test.** A quick way to estimate your exercise intensity is the talk test. At moderate intensity, you should be breathing harder than normal, but still be able to converse in brief sentences. If you can't say more than a few words without having to catch your breath, you've crossed into vigorous activity.

• **Heart rate.** You can also monitor your heart rate to estimate your workload. First, calculate your maximum heart rate (MHR) by subtracting your age from 220. Multiply your MHR by 0.5 and then by 0.7. That is the American Heart Association's recommended target range for moderate activity: 50 to 70 percent of maximum work. Wearing a heart rate monitor is an easy way to track your heart rate as you exercise, but you can also periodically check your pulse.

Whether you invest 20 minutes each day or an hour a few days a week, activities like brisk walking, water aerobics, dancing, biking, or playing doubles tennis can provide valuable heart benefits.

Safe, Simple Surgery May Help A-fib Patients

Richard Whitlock, MD, professor of surgery at McMaster University, Ontario, Canada, and leader of a study published in *The New England Journal of Medicine.*

Atrial fibrillation (A-fib) causes strokes when blood pools in a heart chamber and causes clots.

Recent finding: Removing the left atrial appendage, an extraneous sac where most pooling occurs, reduces stroke risk by more than one-third. If you have A-fib and are scheduled for heart surgery, discuss with your doctor about also having this procedure.

Common Medications Cause Blood Pressure Spikes

John Vitarello, MD, clinical fellow in medicine at Beth Israel Deaconess Medical Center, Boston, and leader of a study of more than 27,000 people, presented at the annual meeting of the American College of Cardiology.

One in five patients with hypertension take drugs that cause blood pressure to increase…including antidepressants, NSAIDs such as ibuprofen, and steroids for conditions such as rheumatoid arthritis. Ask your doctor if any prescription and/or over-the-counter medications you take could raise blood pressure. If any do, ask about alternatives that don't have that effect.

Is a Beta-Blocker Right for You?

Samuel J. Mann, MD, professor of clinical medicine in the division of nephrology and hypertension at New York Presbyterian/Weill Cornell Medical Center, New York City. He is author of several books, including *Hypertension and You: Old Drugs, New Drugs, and the Right Drugs for Your High Blood Pressure.*

If you have high blood pressure or coronary artery disease, your doctor may have prescribed a beta-blocker. These drugs block the effects of stress hormones, such as *epinephrine* (adrenaline) and *norepinephrine*, on the heart and arteries. As a result, your heart rate slows…your heart beats with less force…and your blood pressure gets lower.

Problem: Beta-blockers, also called *beta-adrenergic blocking agents*, are linked to a range of commonly known side effects—fatigue, weight gain and more. But some types of beta-blockers can cause other more significant problems that most patients—and even their doctors—are not aware of.

Even worse: Many people taking these drugs don't actually need to be taking them at all.

We asked hypertension specialist Samuel J. Mann, MD, about the side effects of beta-blockers and how to determine if you are taking the right one—or if you even need one...

The Truth About Beta-Blockers

Beta-blockers can be roughly categorized into two types...

• **Lipophilic (lipid-soluble),** including the most widely prescribed beta-blockers—*metoprolol* (Toprol) and *carvedilol* (Coreg)—as well as *propranolol* (Inderal).

• **Hydrophilic (water-soluble),** including *bisoprolol* (Zebeta), *nadolol* (Corgard), *atenolol* (Tenormin) and *betaxolol* (Kerlone).

Problem: The blood level achieved by a dose of a lipophilic beta-blocker differs greatly from patient to patient depending on how fast or slow the liver metabolizes the drug. A "rapid metabolizer" will end up with a very low, and therefore ineffective, blood level. A "slow metabolizer" will end up with a very high blood level and likely will suffer more side effects.

There's no easy test to determine whether you are a fast or a slow metabolizer, but the difference in blood levels can be tremendous—slow metabolizers may have 10 to 20 times higher levels of the drug in their bloodstream than fast metabolizers who are taking the same dosage. And the amount of the medication that reaches the bloodstream will determine whether or not you will suffer the following side effects and how severely.

• **Fatigue.** Many people taking beta-blockers—either lipophilic or hydrophilic—who feel less energetic assume that they're experiencing age-related fatigue. But there is a direct connection between beta-blockers and fatigue—both types of beta-blockers reduce heart rate and cardiac output, so the heart doesn't pump as much as it would

without the medication, causing the person to feel tired.

• **Weight gain.** Research shows that many people taking beta-blockers gain a few pounds, but a small percentage gain a significant amount of weight, likely related to the reduced energy caused by the beta-blocker.

Other side effects include cold fingers and/or toes, erectile dysfunction, and thinning hair.

What Your Doctor May Not Know

Unlike hydrophilic beta-blockers, lipophilic beta-blockers penetrate the blood-brain barrier and enter brain tissue, and that can cause the following more troubling side effects...

• **Mental dullness.** In addition to fatigue, lipophilic beta-blockers can cause subtle or not-so-subtle mental dullness or, as some patients describe it, "brain fog." This side effect impacts perhaps 10 percent to 20 percent of patients and might be more pronounced in those who have preexisting cognitive impairment. Many patients taking beta-blockers tolerate these side effects for years without suspecting that their medication is the cause.

• **Depression.** Doctors have long suspected a link between beta-blockers and depression, but research now indicates that the medication itself does not seem to be the direct cause.

New finding: In a 2021 meta-analysis published in the American Heart Association journal *Hypertension*, researchers examined data from more than 50,000 individuals collected in 258 studies involving beta-blockers. They found that while depression was the most frequently reported mental health side effect, it did not happen more often during treatment with beta-blockers than during treatment with a placebo.

Exception: Propranolol specifically has been linked to increased risk for depression and nightmares.

Fish-Oil Supplements: Proceed with Caution

Fish Oil May Increase Heart-Rhythm Problems

Omega-3 fatty acids have long been considered heart-protective. But new research associates fish oil with 37 percent higher risk for atrial fibrillation (dangerously irregular heartbeat) among people with high cardiovascular disease risk and triglyceride levels.

If you are at risk: Do not take fish oil until more research has been done.

Thomas Marshall, PhD, professor of public health at University of Birmingham, Birmingham, UK, commenting on an analysis of five placebo studies led by researchers at Virginia Commonwealth University in Richmond published in *European Heart Journal*.

Omega-3 Supplements May Not Be Heart-Healthy

Doctors have long recommended omega-3 fatty acid supplements, which contain *eicosapentaenoic acid* (EPA) and *docosahexaenoic acid* (DHA), to protect the heart. New research suggests that while EPA reduces major cardiovascular events, DHA may cancel the benefits of EPA.

Viet Le, PA-C, cardiovascular physician assistant at Intermountain Heart Institute, Salt Lake City, and leader of a study presented at the 2021 conference of the American College of Cardiology.

A Better Approach

No one should have to tolerate these side effects. Fortunately, there are effective and readily available alternatives. In many cases, the patient's condition can be treated without a beta-blocker or with one that is less likely to cause these side effects. *Steps to take…*

•**Ask your doctor about alternative treatments for your condition.** When treating hypertension, many physicians are quick to write prescriptions for beta-blockers, but in most situations, other drugs—ACE inhibitors, angiotensin receptor antagonists (ARBs), calcium channel blockers or diuretics—are more appropriate and usually cause fewer side effects.

Exception: Hypertension driven by the sympathetic nervous system is better treated with a beta-blocker. This type of high blood pressure often has a mind-body component and may be accompanied by anxiety and/or rapid heart rate. Your doctor may want you to take both a beta-blocker and an alpha-blocker. Like beta-blockers, alpha-blockers block the effects of stress hormones on the body, but they also cause the blood vessels to dilate (vasodilate), which can mitigate the cold hands and feet that beta-blockers sometimes cause. The most widely prescribed alpha-blocker is *doxazosin* (Cardura). This combination is highly effective and underutilized. A beta-blocker *nebivolol* (Bystolic) also has vasodilating effects.

Caution: The beta-blocker *carvedilol* (Coreg) includes an alpha-blocker, but it is lipophilic and so crosses into the brain, where it can cause the associated side effects.

•**If you must continue to take a beta-blocker,** ask your doctor if you can switch to a hydrophilic beta-blocker, which doesn't cross the blood-brain barrier.

Examples: *Bisoprolol* (Zebeta), *nadolol* (Corgard), *atenolol* (Tenormin) and *betaxolol* (Kerlone). Blood levels of these beta-blockers are more predictable, and the side effects are fewer.

You also can inquire about taking a lower dose.

Example: Bisoprolol comes in a standard five-milligram pill, but half a pill often is sufficient to treat high blood pressure.

•**If you have had cardiac bypass surgery, angioplasty, or stenting,** ask your doctor how long you have to continue taking a beta-blocker after the procedure. There is no clear evidence that beta-blockers need to be continued beyond the first year in patients who have undergone these procedures. Yet many of these patients continue taking a beta-blocker indefinitely.

New Treatment for Recurrent Pericarditis

Allan Klein, MD, is director of Center for the Diagnosis and Treatment of Pericardial Diseases, Cleveland Clinic. ClevelandClinic.org

Pericarditis is a painful condition involving inflammation of the lining around the heart. Treatment with NSAIDs, colchicine and steroids is effective but comes with side effects, and there's a 15 percent to 30 percent chance of recurrent flare-ups. The FDA has approved *rilonacept* (Arcalyst), injected weekly, a biologic that treats acute flare-ups, allowing patients to taper off other drugs while reducing recurrence risk by 96 percent.

Diagnosis May Also Be Treatment for DVT

Study titled "Ultrasound-Responsive Nanopeptisomes Enable Synchronous Spatial Imaging and Inhibition of Clot Growth in Deep Vein Thrombosis," by researchers at Penn State College of Engineering, University Park, published in *Advanced Healthcare Materials.*

Health diagnostic tests pinpoint the cause of illness and determine the best treatment. But can a test be a treatment? Researchers from Penn State recently investigated this possibility with a dangerous condition known as deep vein thrombosis (DVT).

Why Worry About DVT

DVT is a blood clot in a vein, usually in the leg. It can cause warmth, redness, and swelling over the vein, or occasionally no symptoms at all. DVTs are dangerous because they can break free and travel back to the heart and lungs causing a life-threatening condition called a pulmonary embolism. A new study from the Penn State Department of Engineering has found a new way to diagnose DVTs that may be more accurate than traditional methods. While doing the study, they also found that their new technique stops blood clot formation, making it both diagnostic and therapeutic. Researchers call this a theranostic study.

Study details: Current diagnosis of DVTs uses sound wave imaging, called ultrasound. Ultrasound imaging does not give a precise image of a DVT in real time. To improve imaging of DVTs, the research team used microscopic particles they have developed called *nanopeptisomes* (NPeps). NPeps are droplets of fluorine-based oil surrounded by a capsule that binds to the surface of a blood clot. The research is published in the journal *Advanced Healthcare Materials.*

Binders Breakdown Blood Clots

After injecting the NPeps, ultrasound waves cause the oil in the NPeps to vaporize into a gas bubble. These bubbles show up precisely during ultrasound imaging, indicating the exact location of the clot. The research team was surprised to find that when a DVT was seen on ultrasound, it began to break up within about 15 minutes. They suspect that the NPeps may saturate the surface of the DVT, preventing a blood clotting protein called *fibrinogen* from binding to the clots. Fibrinogen is a natural protein that blood clots need to keep growing. The vaporization of the NPeps under ultrasound may also help break up the clots.

More studies are needed to learn exactly how NPeps break up or inhibit DVTs. So far, researchers have only tested this technique on cattle (bovine) veins.

Safer treatment: Current treatment for DVTs is medication to break up a clot, which may cause internal bleeding…or removing the clot with a catheter threaded into the vein. Catheter removal can also cause bleeding or infection. This theranostic study offers a safer and more accurate way to find and treat DVTs.

How You Can Spot Heart Trouble...In Your Parents

Bobbi Bogaev, MD, board-certified specialist in cardiovascular diseases, advanced heart failure and internal medicine. Currently she is medical director, heart failure, at Abiomed, maker of Impella, a heart pump for patients with severe coronary artery disease.

Thanks to the far-reaching effects of the COVID-19 pandemic, the American Heart Association predicts that rates of heart disease, already the number-one cause of death in the US, will rise. These risks increase with age, leaving the elderly most vulnerable.

Many of us may be unaware of our older loved ones' new heart-related symptoms. It's important to take a closer look and see if parents or other older relatives may be showing signs of heart disease.

Easy-to-Miss Warning Signs

When most people hear the words "heart disease," they think of chest pain, labored breathing, high blood pressure and rapid heartbeat. And those certainly are indicators of heart disease, a heart attack or heart failure. (Contrary to how it sounds, heart failure doesn't mean that the heart has stopped but rather that it can't pump enough blood to keep up with the body's demands.)

But did you know that your 80-year-old father quitting his golf game...your 90-year-old mother no longer wearing her trademark lipstick...extra pillows on your parents' bed...or a switch from them cooking to eating frozen meals all could be signs of failing heart health?

Heart Disease Signs

Recognizing often-disguised heart-health warning signs could mean the difference between life and death for your aging loved ones. *The next time you see them, ask yourself...*

• **Are they no longer doing the things they used to love?** Fatigue is one of the most common symptoms of heart failure, a symptom of heart disease and the leading cause of hospitalization in people over age 65. If your parent used to love playing golf several times a week but has stopped...or no longer gardens even though it gave him/her great joy, that could be a tip-off that heart failure–related fatigue is keeping them from their usual passions.

Depression and heart disease often go hand in hand. Depression can increase risk for heart attack and/or heart disease by increasing inflammation or causing platelets—cells that help with blood clotting—to become too sticky, clogging arteries in the process...or heart disease can fuel depression when one feels too tired to engage in favorite pastimes and begins to feel hopeless or worthless. At least one in five people with heart failure develops depression.

• **Are they cooking meals...or stocking premade and frozen foods?** Cooking requires a surprising amount of mental and physical energy, from recipe planning to grocery shopping to meal preparation. That's a lot of effort for someone who feels exhausted. Check your parents' kitchen for evidence of cooking. Is the olive oil bottle full? Is the fridge produce drawer full of fresh vegetables—or worse, produce past its prime? Or is it relatively bare and the freezer full of frozen dinners? Complicating matters, premade, frozen, and shelf-stable meals are notoriously high in sodium, which can aggravate existing heart issues.

• **Do you notice puffy weight gain?** Heart failure can cause people to accumulate fluid around the liver and the ankles. It may appear to have developed out of nowhere and is more likely to happen if high-sodium foods are being consumed. A parent may report that it's suddenly hard to button his pants.

Don't mistake excess body fat for fluid—25 percent of adults over age 76 reported weight gain as a result of the pandemic, according to a 2021 Harris Poll conducted for the American Psychological Association. This type of weight gain tends to be all over the body, while fluid accumulation due to heart failure is localized around the middle and in the legs and ankles. It also feels different—when a physician thumps the belly of a patient with fluid buildup, it has a dull sound, like tapping a watermelon.

Other signs: Swollen ankles...a visibly pulsing jugular vein in the neck...and tenderness under the right ribcage (from fluid accumulating in the liver).

• **How many pillows are they using?** Heart failure can cause fluid to accumulate in the lungs, leading to shortness of breath, especially when lying flat. Patients often say that it feels like they're suffocating when they lie down, so they prop themselves up to avoid that feeling. Some people take to sleeping in a recliner. Patients also may awaken from sleep with shortness of breath.

• **Does Mom pass "The Lipstick Test"?** It's always reassuring when an older patient reports to a doctor's appointment wearing lipstick. It shows that she has the energy to keep up her normal routine. This is the type of clue you may not have noticed if you haven't seen your parents in person in several months. Is mom still putting on lipstick? Is dad still shaving? If parents seem to be letting themselves go, it can be a tip-off to start asking more questions.

Other signs: Is mail piling up that didn't used to? Did they not decorate for the holidays even though they've been hanging Christmas lights for decades? These are similar red flags of low energy.

• **Are there bottles of antacid everywhere?** If you spot antacids in the medicine cabinet, on the kitchen island and on their bedside table, ask about episodes of heartburn. Chest pain (angina) often masquerades as heartburn, especially chest pain that worsens with exertion, such as during a brisk walk. It even can be a symptom of a heart attack. The acid indigestion–like feeling can be accompanied by shortness of breath or fatigue. Although this "angina equivalent" can feel like heartburn caused by reflux, it has everything to do with the heart. Women are especially likely to experience atypical heart attack symptoms such as heartburn-like pain, fatigue and shortness of breath, as opposed to classic symptoms such as crushing chest pain.

• **Can they walk for six minutes straight ...or sit and stand five times in a row?** If your loved one gets winded from navigating stairs or struggles to get up from a chair, suggest taking a walk together. If he can't walk for six minutes without stopping, he may have heart disease. Pay attention to whether he tries to make excuses to stop during the walk, such as chatting or tying his shoes.

You also can suggest they try the "5 Times Sit-to-Stand Test." This is a simple way to look for a heart disease symptom called frailty. Frailty is an age-related syndrome involving deteriorations in several body systems, including stamina, strength, weight, and fitness.

How to do it: Have your loved one sit in a standard-height chair with his back against the back of the chair. Using a timer, ask him to stand up straight as quickly as he safely can, five times in a row without stopping, his arms remaining folded across his chest. Stop timing him when he stands for the fifth time. Someone age 70 to 79 ideally will finish in 12.6 seconds or less...someone age 80 to 89, 14.8 seconds or less.

Recent finding: A 2021 *BMC Geriatrics* meta-analysis concluded that frailty is an increasingly common heart disease symptom in older adults, affecting nearly one-fifth of heart disease patients.

Next Steps

If you recognize any of these symptoms, encourage your parent to schedule a visit with his primary care physician. If you can't attend the visit, help make a list of concerns to show the doctor. (This is especially helpful for adults with memory issues.) With a little investigative work, you can help get Mom or Dad back to playing golf, gardening and feeling engaged with life.

Chapter 9

INFECTIOUS DISEASE

Enhancing Your Immune System

Since the pandemic struck in early 2020, there has been an unprecedented amount of talk about the immune system—in the press, with our health-care providers and even among family and friends. But other than a vague notion that our bodies have a goal of keeping us healthy, the immune system remains largely a mystery for many of us. *We asked naturopathic physician Laurie Steelsmith, ND, LAc, to explain how the immune system works to fight off all kinds of infections…*

Immune System 101

Every day, our bodies are exposed to thousands of viruses, bacteria, parasites and other pathogens. Our immune system—the body's natural defense against infection and illness—keeps those bugs from taking up residence and making us sick. This complex biological system includes two main branches that work in tandem—the *innate* immune system, which we are born with…and the *adaptive* immune system, which builds up as we move through life, developing defenses against germs.

A healthy immune system includes millions of white blood cells that defend against and disable foreign invaders and abnormal cells. Your bone marrow produces these cells, as does your thymus gland. Some types of white blood cells, including *phagocytes*, literally consume bacteria and other germs.

Other immune system cells create antibodies, proteins formed after initial exposure to a virus or bacteria that protect you the next time you encounter the same bug. This is why someone who contracts and recovers from COVID-19 has some protection against repeat infections. It's also why many healthy people feel fine after their first shot of a two-part COVID-19 vaccine but temporarily develop fever, chills, and body aches after the second shot—the immune system recognizes COVID and starts to attack it.

Lymph nodes are the watchdogs of the lymphatic system, an immune-supporting

Laurie Steelsmith, ND, LAc, licensed naturopathic physician, licensed acupuncturist and coauthor of the best-seller *Natural Choices for Women's Health*, the critically acclaimed *Great Sex, Naturally* and her latest, *Growing Younger Every Day*. A leading advocate for natural medicine, Dr. Steelsmith is medical director of Steelsmith Natural Health Center in Honolulu and associate clinical professor at Bastyr University, a leading center for the study of natural medicine. DrSteelsmith.com

network of organs, tissues and vessels that circulate a fluid called *lymph* (which contains everything from proteins and minerals to precancerous cells and bacteria). The reason your lymph nodes sometimes grow swollen or tender is because they're packed with white blood cells and act as filters for foreign invaders, preventing them from reaching the rest of the body. Lymph nodes near the area of infection typically will swell up because they are hosting white cells in their war against the foreign substance—bacteria or viruses, for example. There are lymph nodes all over the body, but clusters exist in the armpits, groin and neck, and they can easily be felt when you have an infection. If swollen lymph nodes are accompanied by other signs of illness—fever, sore throat and/or congestion—a foreign invader that was able to sneak by the immune system has been recognized, and the immune system is mounting an attack.

The skin also serves as a physical barrier to keep harmful toxins out of the body. Another filter—the spleen—strains pathogens and abnormal cells from the blood. You can live without your spleen, but when someone loses this organ—due to an illness or accident, for example—he/she is considered immunocompromised and is susceptible to everyday germs that most people can easily fight off. Mucus is yet another immune system player. The slimy substance that lines the inside of the nose traps bacteria and viruses as they try to sneak into the body.

The Immune System Hub

A huge amount of your immune potential lives in the gut—70 percent to 80 percent of the body's immune cells, in fact. Deep in the bowels of your body, a vast ecosystem of trillions of microorganisms and good and bad bacteria—known collectively as the gut microbiome—exists.

Among the gut microbiome's varied jobs: Engaging in a constant dialogue with the immune system…helping to detect foreign invaders…and mounting a proper defense when pathogens are detected.

Interesting: A 2021 *Gut* study looking at microbiome data from 27 recovering COVID-19 patients found that, compared with healthy individuals, those with COVID-19 infection lacked certain strains of good gut bacteria, suggesting that microbiome health may influence the severity of COVID-19 infection.

Enhance Your Immune System

Here are ways to help fortify your body's natural defense system…

• **Eat a whole-foods diet.** *The foods you eat hold incredible sway over your ability to stave off infections…*

• Shoot for organic, whole foods, such as fresh fruits and vegetables, unprocessed grains, and nuts.

• Avoid red and processed meat. They cause inflammation, thanks to their high saturated-fat content. Inflammation is good when you need to fight off a bug, but unrelenting inflammation contributes to a dysregulated immune system and potential autoimmune disease, allergies, chronic pain, and tissue dysfunction.

• Eat a serving or two of probiotic- and prebiotic-rich foods a day. Probiotics are good-for-you bacteria—kefir, yogurt, sauerkraut, kimchee, miso, tempeh and Kombucha all are probiotic. Prebiotics are a type of indigestible fiber that serve as food for the probiotics—garlic, onions, leeks, Jerusalem artichokes, barley, bananas, and flaxseeds.

• Fiber is your friend…sugar is not. The former bumps up the immune system's responsiveness, while too much of the latter suppresses it.

• **Move your body.** Exercise can help flush bacteria out of the lungs, reducing the chances that you will develop a cold, flu, or other respiratory illness, and it helps distribute white blood cells and antibodies throughout your body, boosting your immune system's ability to identify and fight intruders. Also, by temporarily increasing body temperature, exercise may function similarly to a fever, helping the body fight any lurking infections.

Recent finding: A 2021 *Sports Medicine* meta-analysis found that higher levels of regular exercise are associated with a 31 percent lower risk of acquiring an infectious disease. Aim for 150 minutes per week of moderate-intensity aerobic exercise, including walking, running, cycling, or dancing.

•**Work with your immune system…not against it.** It's common for people to use decongestants and fever reducers when they have a stuffy nose or other cold symptoms, but those symptoms mean that your immune system is doing its job. Decongestants dry up the mucous membranes, preventing them from flushing the virus from your body. Fever reducers—*ibuprofen* (Motrin, Advil), *acetaminophen* (Tylenol) and aspirin—inactivate the work being done by your immune system to raise your body temperature.

If you're feeling unwell and your fever is below 104°F, support your body's natural ability to fight off infection by feeding it warm liquids (tea, soup)…holding your head over a bowl of steaming water and eucalyptus oil for five minutes several times a day (put one or two drops of eucalyptus oil into a bowl with four cups of boiling water, then create a tent over your head with a towel while you inhale)…and taking immune-enhancing supplements and herbs such as zinc (15 mg/day)…vitamin E (40 IU/day)…vitamin C (1,000 mg/day)…and quercetin (500 mg/day).

Note: For temperatures of 104°F or above, seek medical attention.

•**Try dry brushing.** Using a soft shower brush or loofah, lightly stroke your dry skin, always brushing toward the heart. This encourages the healthy flow of blood and lymph throughout the body, stimulates detoxification and removes dead skin cells for overall skin health. Try this technique once a day. Afterward, rub your skin with three drops of essential oil of cedar wood diluted in one tablespoon of jojoba oil.

•**Use antibiotics judiciously and only for bacterial infections.** They don't work on viral infections and can do more harm than good.

Coffee and Vegetables Help Prevent COVID-19

Researchers examined data on 37,988 people and found that those who drank at least one cup of coffee or ate at least 0.67 servings of vegetables per day had a slightly lower risk of COVID-19 infection (about 10 percent). Conversely, eating just about one ounce of processed meat elevated risk. Nutrition affects immunity and immunity plays a key role in a person's susceptibility and response to infectious diseases.

Marilyn Cornelis, PhD, associate professor of preventive medicine (nutrition), Feinberg School of Medicine, Northwestern University, Chicago.

Pollen May Increase COVID-19 Risk

Study by researchers at Rutgers University, New Brunswick, New Jersey, published in *Proceedings of the National Academy of Sciences*.

When there is more pollen in the air, immunity against seasonal respiratory viruses and COVID-19 decreases in people who are allergic or otherwise susceptible to pollen. A recent study showed that rates of infection increased after high pollen-count days and a strict lockdown cut infection rates by half. High-risk individuals should wear the strongest possible masks during times of high pollen concentration—especially in the spring.

Hand-Washing Mistake

Study of 190 adults by researchers at the School of Nursing, Tung Wah College, Hong Kong, published in *Journal of Environmental and Public Health*.

About half of adults don't wash their fingertips…and nearly one-third neglect the backs of their hands.

Best: Cover your whole hands with soap and water—fingertips, thumbs, fronts, and backs, and between each finger. Singing "Happy Birthday" or "Yankee Doodle" ensures that you scrub long enough.

Omicron Has Been More Contagious—But Less Deadly

William Schaffner, MD, is professor of preventive medicine at Vanderbilt University, Nashville, and medical director of the National Foundation for Infectious Diseases, Bethesda, Maryland.

O micron is adept at invading cells in the membranes in the throat and behind the nose, where it rapidly multiplies. When a sick person exhales, they blow out a viral cloud that easily infects others. But Omicron is not nearly as good at attacking cells in the bronchial tubes and lungs, which makes it less deadly than previous COVID variants.

The Many Variants of Omicron

Pia MacDonald, PhD, MPH, CPH, is an infectious disease epidemiologist at RTI International in Research Triangle Park, North Carolina.

W hile we had hoped that Omicron was COVID's last hurrah, the virus has consistently surprised us with more variants. How transmissible and/or virulent those variants might be—and how much protection existing vaccines and prior infections will offer—can't be predicted.

Good news: With each variant, we learn more about the virus and develop better tools for managing it. Expect rollouts of mRNA vaccines and boosters targeting new strains.

Possible Reactions to the COVID Vaccine

COVID Shots Can Affect Your Period

Many women reported early, unexpected, or heavy bleeding within days after the injection. This is usually not cause for alarm. An ibuprofen with each meal can reduce heavy flow up to 40 percent. Postmenopausal women who get unexpected post-injection flow should talk to their physicians about endometrial cancer risk—more likely revealed by the injection than caused by it.

Jerilynn C. Prior, MD, professor of endocrinology and scientific director of The Centre for Menstrual Cycle and Ovulation Research, University of British Columbia, Vancouver.

Post-Vaccine Lymph Swelling Mimics Cancer Symptoms

Some women receiving COVID-19 vaccines have noticed swollen lymph nodes, especially in the armpit on the side where they were vaccinated. Some have mistaken the swelling for breast lumps and been concerned about cancer. Any swollen lymph nodes can show up on a mammogram even if women can't feel them, triggering a false-positive reading. To avoid unnecessary worry, doctors say women should postpone mammography until at least four weeks after their final COVID-19 shot.

Roundup of breast cancer specialists reported at WebMD.com.

New Antiviral Drug Saves COVID Patients

Joseph Feuerstein, MD, assistant professor of clinical medicine at Columbia University, New York City, commenting on a study of 10,000 patients led by researchers at University of Oxford, UK.

H ospitalized immunocompromised COVID patients are significantly more likely to die from COVID.

Recent finding: Patients such as these who received the drug REGEN-COV, a combination of two monoclonal antibodies that bind to COVID spike protein receptor sites, had one-fifth lower chance of dying than similar patients who received the usual care.

Headed to the Hospital? Protect Yourself from an Infection

David Sherer, MD, retired American physician, author, and inventor. He is the lead author of *Hospital Survival Guide: The Patient Handbook to Getting Better and Getting Out* and *What Your Doctor Won't Tell You.* His current focus is on patient education, patient advocacy and writing. DrDavidSherer.com

The hospital is the place we go to get well and feel better. But far too often, patients seek medical attention at the hospital for one issue…and end up sick with something entirely different—and more dangerous.

Shocking statistic: Every year, nearly two million patients contract infections in a health-care setting such as a hospital, long-term rehab facility or dialysis center. Nearly 100,000 of them die as a result.

Hospital-acquired infections, now known as healthcare-associated infections (HAIs) or nosocomial infections, can enter the body

New Tampons Can Detect Urinary Tract Infections

Researchers are designing tampons and sanitary pads that change color in the presence of the bacteria that cause urinary-tract infections.

Study by researchers at Manipal Institute of Technology, India, published in *ACS Omega.*

through the nose, mouth, lungs, skin, blood and urinary tract. They can be bacterial, viral or fungal and include surgical-site infections, catheter-associated urinary tract infections, pneumonia and more.

Why the Uptick in Infections

For years, HAI rates were dropping steadily, thanks to enhanced infection-prevention and control strategies. But the COVID-19 pandemic, which dramatically increased the number of hospitalized patients requiring more frequent and longer use of catheters and ventilators, has led to increases in several common HAIs. And staff and supply shortages haven't helped matters.

According to a new Centers for Disease Control and Prevention analysis published in *Infection Control & Hospital Epidemiology,* rates of ventilator-associated events, central line-associated bloodstream infections, catheter-associated urinary tract infections and antibiotic-resistant staph infections (such as *methicillin-resistant Staphylococcus aureus —MRSA*) increased 45 percent, 47 percent, 19 percent and 33.8 percent, respectively, from 2019 to 2020—especially during the fourth quarter of the year. Interestingly, surgical-site infection rates did not increase, perhaps because there were fewer elective surgeries.

Anyone can contract an HAI, but certain factors increase risk, including older age, longer hospital stays (or any type of ICU stay), a suppressed immune system, comorbidities such as diabetes, obesity or heart disease and more.

Most Common HAIs

Most HAIs are related to surgical procedures or the insertion of an invasive device. *They include…*

●**Catheter-associated urinary tract infection (CAUTI).** Between 15 percent and 25 percent of hospitalized patients receive a urinary catheter, a thin tube inserted through the urethra to drain urine from the bladder during their stay. Prolonged catheter use is a risk factor for a urinary tract infection (UTI), an infection in any part of the urinary system, including the urethra, bladder or kidneys. Catheter use is associated with 75 percent of hospital-acquired UTIs. Symptoms include fever, pain or burning in the lower abdomen, and/or bloody urine. The mortality rate is about 2 percent.

• **Central line-associated bloodstream infection (CLABSI).** A central line is used to deliver medicine, fluids and/or nutrients into a vein near or inside the heart. CLABSI causes a fever and red, sore skin around the entry point of the central line. Another *Infection Control & Hospital Epidemiology* study found that COVID-19 patients experienced more than five times the number of CLABSIs as those who did not have COVID.

Possible reason: Hospitalized COVID patients often receive intravenous antibiotics as well as the steroid *dexamethasone* to tame the inflammatory response to COVID infection, both of which can be delivered through a central line. Between 12 percent and 25 percent of CLABSI patients die from their infections.

• **Ventilator-associated pneumonia (VAP).** A patient may need to be intubated for treatment of respiratory failure or ventilated during a surgery that requires anesthesia. That means a breathing tube is placed into his/her trachea (windpipe), forcing oxygen-enriched gas into the lungs. If germs enter the tube, pneumonia or another infection can develop.

New finding: A 2021 *Critical Care* study found that COVID-19 patients are significantly more likely to develop VAP than patients without COVID, partly but not entirely due to increased duration of ventilation. Symptoms of VAP include fever, faster heart rate, pus in lung secretions and low blood oxygen levels. It has a mortality rate of close to 50 percent.

• **Surgical-site infection (SSI).** Any type of surgery—from a coronary bypass to a spinal fusion—provides a prime opportunity for germs to sneak into the body. Surgical-site infections often are caused by *Staphylococcus aureus* or MRSA, an especially dangerous type of staph that is resistant to antibiotics.

Symptoms include redness, tenderness and warmth at the site of the surgical incision, fever and delayed healing. When staph or MRSA enters the body, it can spread almost anywhere—to the blood (where it can cause life-threatening sepsis)…lungs (where it can cause pneumonia)…and heart (where it can cause endocarditis, an infection of the heart valves). About 3 percent of SSI patients die.

Note: Bedsores and kidney dialysis also are risk factors for acquiring an SSI.

• ***Clostridioides difficile* infections (CDI).** Also known as *C. diff,* this bacteria causes sometimes life-threatening diarrhea, along with fever, abdominal cramping, nausea and appetite loss. Infections usually occur after a patient has been treated with an antibiotic that alters the types of bacteria—good and bad—living in his/her gut, allowing *C. diff* to flourish. One in 11 people over age 65 diagnosed with this HAI will die within a month.

Interesting: While other HAIs have been increasing in prevalence in the age of COVID, *C. diff* infections have been decreasing, despite a rise in antibiotic use. This may be attributed to infection-mitigation measures, such as masking and hand hygiene.

COVID-19: A New HAI?

Early in the pandemic, COVID-19 became a type of HAI, with hospitals becoming "an important setting for viral transmission," per a study in the American Medical Association's journal *JAMA*. In China, it's estimated that 44 percent of 179 early COVID infections were caught in the hospital, and a July 2020 outbreak in a Massachusetts teaching medical center was attributed to staff removing their masks in a break room.

Thanks to improvements in masking, personal protective equipment (PPE) and hygiene practices, those numbers have dropped significantly…but the risk isn't gone. A 2021 *International Journal of Environmental Research and Public Health* study estimates the hospital-acquired COVID-19 rate is 12 percent to 15 percent.

How to Protect Yourself or a Loved One

Fortunately, you can influence your care in a way that can keep you from becoming the one in 31 hospital patients with at least one HAI. *Here's how...*

•**If you need a catheter, request it be removed as soon as it is safe to do so.** Using a catheter for longer than six days is a risk factor for a CAUTI. Ask your doctor to remove it as early as possible. Always clean your hands before and after touching your catheter, and make sure your urine bag hangs below the level of your bladder to prevent urine from flowing back into your bladder, where it could cause an infection.

•**Make sure you're receiving only necessary medications.** Antibiotics are notoriously overprescribed, fueling growth of superbugs such as MRSA, which can cause infections at surgical sites, in catheters and other places. Antibiotics also can cause *C. difficile*. Ask if your antibiotic is absolutely necessary.

Important: Whether you are in the hospital or at home, let your health-care provider know if you have three or more episodes of diarrhea within 24 hours while taking antibiotics. This could be a sign of *C. difficile*.

Narcotics are problematic, too. They make it harder for older adults, especially men, to urinate, increasing the likelihood of a catheter needing to be inserted.

•**Ask all visitors to wash their hands before entering your hospital room.** This will limit your exposure to staph and other bacteria. About 30 percent of people have staph living on their skin or in their nose at any given time. They may not get sick from it, but they can spread it to other people.

•**Research the hospital's infection rates**—if you can choose where you will be treated—by visiting Medicare.gov/hospitalcompare (search for hospitals, rehab facilities or nursing homes). Many will list infection rates (under "Complications & Deaths") including how they compare to national benchmarks.

C. Auris Is Not a Threat to Healthy People

Candida auris (C. auris), a fungus more resistant to drugs than other species, causes severe illness if it spreads to the bloodstream. Recently cases resistant to all commonly used drugs have been found—including at two facilities in Texas and one in Washington, DC. While *C. auris* often spreads in health-care settings, the risk of acquiring *C. auris* is low in healthy people.

Meghan Lyman, MD, medical officer in the Mycotic Diseases Branch of the Centers for Disease Control and Prevention, Atlanta, and coauthor of a report on *Candida auris*.

Note: If you belong to a Medicare Advantage Plan, this link won't provide information about whether your care will be covered in a certain hospital, so check with your plan.

•**Address major medical risk factors to stay out of the hospital.** You won't die from an HAI if you're not in the hospital.

•**Lose weight if you are overweight or have obesity.** Being overweight makes it harder to clear your airway, and excess skin folds are a perfect hiding spot for bacteria looking to cause an infection.

•**Quit smoking.** You've heard it before—smokers are more prone to infection.

•**Get vaccinated against COVID-19.** Patients hospitalized with COVID-19 are at a much higher risk of developing a number of HAIs.

Shingles 101: Prevention Beats Intervention

Jeffrey Brown, DO, assistant professor at Cleveland Clinic Learner College of Medicine and Heritage College of Osteopathic Medicine, Cleveland, Ohio.

For a condition as common as shingles—one in three people, more women than men, will get it at some point—there's a surprising lack of awareness about symptoms, transmissibility, and prevention. There's even a false news report circulating that links the virus with one of the COVID-19 vaccines. *Let's take a few moments to demystify this condition...*

Signs and Symptoms

Most commonly, shingles is a painful rash that occurs in people who have had chickenpox. It's more common in people over age 50. Hormonal changes with menopause put women at high risk.

Typically, the first sign is a burning, stabbing, or aching pain on one side of the chest, abdomen, back, or waist. The degree of discomfort and people's response to it runs the gamut from mild achiness for a week to unrelenting months-long intensive pain that makes even wearing a shirt difficult because the touch of fabric triggers a nerve-based response. In some people, it only itches.

Two or three days after the pain begins, about 75 percent of people develop a bumpy red rash that turns into blisters over the affected area. In some cases, the rash comes first, or both symptoms appear at once.

Under the Surface

Shingles isn't a new infection. Rather, it's the reactivation of one you had in childhood: chickenpox. When you get chickenpox, your body fights off the varicella-zoster virus (VZV) that causes it, but it doesn't vanquish the virus. Instead, VZV goes into hiding just outside of your spinal cord at the base of a nerve. There, it stays quietly hidden until a trigger causes it to reactivate and travel along a nerve path, causing the telltale band of pain and rash.

Women are more likely to get shingles than men, and Caucasians get shingles in greater numbers than African Americans. People with a weakened immune system have a higher risk of developing the condition and of experiencing severe symptoms and complications. This includes people who have cancer or HIV or who are being treated with immune-suppressing medications. Organ transplants, chemotherapy, rheumatologic conditions, and stress all increase the risk as well.

So while it behooves everyone to be aware of the signs and symptoms, if you are a white woman over 50 who is navigating a stressful life event or being treated with a drug that suppresses your immune system, you might want to be on high alert.

Contagious for Only Some People

People with no history of chickenpox or shingles vaccination can catch the VZV virus by being in close contact with an infected person. Transmission occurs through airborne droplets or direct contact with open blisters. Instead of developing shingles, though, they would develop chickenpox.

If you've already had chickenpox, you can't catch shingles from someone else: The VZV virus is already in you and may or may not reactivate. Likewise, you can't spread shingles to someone who has had chickenpox.

Treatment

Shingles treatment is tricky because, although there are antiviral medications that can minimize the pain and the rash, *valacyclovir* and *acyclovir*, the drugs are effective only if they are administered within 72 hours of the initial onset of symptoms.

Other treatments are used to strictly treat the symptoms: Ibuprofen helps reduce pain, and cold compresses and oatmeal baths help soothe the rash and blisters. Some prescription pain medicines can help reduce discomfort, but even these are not guaranteed to provide relief.

The pain and rash usually subside within three to five weeks, but about 10 to 15 percent of people who get shingles have long-lasting pain, called postherpetic neuralgia (PHN), that can continue for three to six months or more. PHN is often likened to the sensation of an electric shock, but it can also feel numb.

COVID-19 Confusion

Shingles was in the news recently when headlines insinuated a correlation between the virus and the Pfizer COVID-19 vaccine. The articles and subsequent discourse were based on a study conducted in Israel in April that found that out of about 500 participants, six women with autoimmune inflammatory rheumatic diseases experienced mild shingles symptoms for the first time after receiving their first dose of the Pfizer COVID-19 vaccine. All six women were taking immunosuppressant drugs and none had received the shingles or chickenpox vaccine. The study authors did not find any evidence that the vaccine caused the shingles cases, which could have been coincidental, especially considering that immunosuppressant drugs increase the risk for developing shingles. There have been no reports of an increase in shingles cases after COVID-19 vaccination in the United States.

—Dr. Jeffrey Brown

Prevention

If you're age 50 or older, you can likely avoid shingles with a vaccine called Shingrix, which is 91 to 97 percent effective at preventing shingles and PHN for at least four years. You should get the vaccine even if you are not sure if you had chickenpox, previously received the Zostavax shingles vaccine, or have already had shingles. (About 20 percent of people get it more than once.) There is no specific length of time that you need to wait after having shingles before you can receive Shingrix, but generally you should make sure the shingles rash has gone away and any pain has resolved before getting vaccinated.

The shingles vaccine is different from the chickenpox shot, even though both conditions are caused by VZV. The chickenpox vaccine is a live attenuated virus, meaning it stuns the live virus to make it non-infectious. If you have a severely suppressed immune system and get the chickenpox vaccine, you can get chickenpox, so it's given only to healthy children who generally have robust immune systems. Shingrix, however, is not a live virus, so it is safe in people who have suppressed immune systems.

Gum Disease Linked to Higher Risk of Illness

University of Birmingham

Researchers analyzed data on 64,379 patients and found that people with a history of gingivitis or periodontitis have a 37 percent higher risk of developing mental ill-health compared with people without gum disease. Further, gum disease was linked to a 33 percent higher risk of developing autoimmune disease, an 18 percent higher risk of developing cardiovascular disease, and a 26 percent higher risk of developing Type 2 diabetes.

Lyme Lessons

John Aucott, MD, director of the Johns Hopkins Lyme Disease Clinical Research Center, associate professor of medicine, and former chair of the tick-borne diseases working group at the U.S. Department of Health and Human Services. For more information, visit HopkinsLyme.org.

A tiny tick can cause big problems. Here's how to stay safe this summer.

We've been hearing a lot about long-haulers: the people who experience fatigue, body aches, and difficulty concentrating for many months after a COVID-19 infection. This isn't the first time we've seen this phenomenon: COVID-19 long-haulers bear a striking resemblance to people who are living with post-treatment Lyme disease (PTLD).

Lyme disease comes from the bite of a tick that carries the bacteria *Borrelia burgdorferi*.

211

In the early stages, it can cause joint pain, weakness, and flu-like symptoms, often (but not always) in association with a round, red lesion at the site of the tick bite.

If the infection is quickly diagnosed, a course of antibiotics will knock it out in two to four weeks for 80 percent of people, with no long-lasting complications. But for the 20 percent of people with PTLD, fatigue, difficulty concentrating, and joint pain can continue for months or even years after treatment.

Like the COVID long-haulers, people with post-treatment Lyme disease experience these symptoms long after the initial pathogen is no longer detectable.

Potentially Devastating

PTLD isn't just like having chronic allergies; It can steal people's lives out from under them. One sufferer, Amanda (named changed to protect privacy), described it this way: "Imagine the worst flu you've ever had and then imagine having it day after day, year after year, interspersed with times of health when you think, 'Finally it's over, I've got my life back,' only to get sick again over and over for 40 years."

For five years, Amanda had extreme joint and muscle pain, severe fatigue, gastrointestinal issues, and skin rashes. She had no explanation for her symptoms, but at age 30, she experienced something of a recovery. Instead of being sick every day, she felt well for weeks at a time, experiencing bouts of illness about every six weeks—for 18 years. But at 48 years old, she was diagnosed with cancer. After nine months of cancer treatment, her mysterious illness returned, and it was worse than before. To her, "cancer and chemotherapy paled next to the despair of knowing I was facing this terrible dark place again. With cancer, I could still live life, even though I might be facing death. But this illness was a living death, one no one knew how to help me with."

It took Amanda close to 25 years to even get a diagnosis, but even when she knew what she was facing, her physicians were limited in what they could do: Clinically proven treatments are limited. There are anecdotal and speculative treatment possibilities, but they aren't yet supported by clinical trials, so it's unclear if they're effective.

Prevention

For that reason, prevention and early diagnosis are the most powerful tools we currently have available to fight Lyme disease. *Follow these tips…*

• **Stick to the path.** Ticks live in leaf litter and grassy, brushy, or wooded areas. Stay on paths, trails, and the mowed part of your lawn.

• **Cover up.** Wear long pants with socks that fully cover your ankles. Spray your clothing and shoes with 0.5 percent permethrin to repel ticks.

• **Do a tick check.** When you get home, first check your clothing. Then undress and run your clothes through a hot dryer for 10 minutes while you take a shower. The water can help wash off unattached ticks while you check your hair, the backs of your knees, your groin and underarms, and in and around your ears.

If You Are Bitten

• **If you find an attached tick,** hold tweezers as close to your skin as possible and pull upward to remove it. Try not to separate the mouth from the body, and don't squeeze the abdomen. Wash the area and your hands with soap and water.

• **You may want to tape the tick to an index card and note the date** so if you later develop symptoms, the tick can be identified and potentially tested for tick-transmitted infections (Lyme disease is one of at least 15 infections).

• **Pay attention to symptoms.** If you develop any kind of illness a week or two after outdoor activities, consider the possibility of Lyme disease. Look over your body for a round, oval, red rash (possibly a bullseye shape). If you find one, take a picture in case it goes away before your doctor's visit. But

The Psychological Consequences of Lyme Disease

As many as 1,200 suicides may be attributed to Lyme disease each year, according to a study published in the journal *Neuropsychiatric Disease and Treatment*. On the surface, this could be explained by the unrelenting symptoms and their devastating effect on quality of life, but there's more to the story.

Lyme encephalopathy is brain dysfunction that causes problems with cognition, emotions, attention, memory, and mood. Studies have linked late-stage Lyme disease to the development of major depression in up to 66 percent of patients, as well as aggression, explosive anger, mood swings, paranoia, panic disorder, bipolar disorder, social anxiety disorder, substance abuse, generalized anxiety disorder, dementia, schizophrenia, anorexia nervosa, and obsessive-compulsive disorder.

In his book, *Conquering Lyme Disease*, Dr. Brian Fallon, director of Columbia University's Lyme and Tick-Borne Diseases Research Center, explains that he believes a subgroup of patients with Lyme disease have altered brain chemistry or brain neuro-circuits that will not respond to standard antibiotic treatment of the infection.

To address that brain dysfunction, then, you need to look beyond Lyme treatment. Antidepressant or anti-anxiety medication can improve mood and may help reduce pain. Studies show that meditation and yoga can improve cognition, decrease pain, lower inflammatory cytokine levels, and boost energy. Dr. Fallon reports that he has had patients find pain and mood improvements with transcranial magnetic stimulation (TMS), a noninvasive treatment that uses magnets, but he stresses that no clinical trials have yet been done on TMS.

remember that only 20 percent of people get the rash, and even those who do can't always see it, so the absence of a rash does not exclude the possibility of Lyme disease.

•**Don't ignore it.** *Lyme disease isn't like a cold:* If you don't treat it, it doesn't go away. Rather, it can progress and cause arthritis, facial palsy, neuropathy, cognitive impairment, and heart damage. Take the possibility seriously and demand that your doctor does, too.

Two New Ways to Prevent Lyme Disease on the Horizon

Richard Horowitz, MD, is medical director of Hudson Valley Healing Arts Center in Hyde Park, New York.

Pfizer plans to start phase III clinical trials in late 2022 with a three-dose vaccine that produces an immune response against the bacteria that cause Lyme. And University of Massachusetts researchers have begun human trials on a seasonal shot that uses a monoclonal antibody that disables the bacteria. The treatment was 100 percent effective in animal trials.

A Common Virus May Cause Multiple Sclerosis

Study titled "Longitudinal Analysis Reveals High Prevalence of Epstein-Barr Virus Associated with Multiple Sclerosis," by researchers at Harvard T.H. Chan School of Public Health, Boston, published in Science.

Multiple sclerosis (MS) is one of the most common disabling neurological diseases that primarily affects young adults. According to the National Multiple Sclerosis Society, women are three times more likely than men to develop it. The complete cause is unknown, but one theory involves a common viral infection. Researchers at the Harvard T.H. Chan School of Public Health have uncovered Epstein Barr-Virus (EBV) as a trigger for MS. In fact, their recent study, published in *Science*, points to EBV as the leading cause of this debilitating disease.

EBV is so common that by adulthood about 95 percent of individuals have been infected. EBV is a member of the herpes virus family and the cause of mononucleosis in children and young adults. Although most people have been infected with EBV, few adults develop mono. They may have mild cold symptoms or no symptoms. However, once EBV is in your system, it remains dormant and can be reactivated in times of physical or emotional stress. A prior EBV infection can be diagnosed by a blood test for EBV antibodies that develop in response to the infection.

How EBV Triggers MS

The researchers suspect that repeated reactivation of EBV virus affects a person's immune system in a way that triggers MS. Once a person has MS, their immune system mistakenly attacks the nerves of the brain and spinal cord, typical of an autoimmune disease. Reactivation of EBV has also been linked to several types of cancer.

Study details: In the study, millions of young adults in the U.S. Armed Forces were tested for antibodies to EBV twice every year and then followed for about 20 years for indications of MS. The researchers eventually identified 801 service members who developed the disease. Only one person had not tested positive for EBV antibodies before coming down with MS. The researchers also tested for other common viral infections, but only EBV predicted future MS.

Compared to service members who did not test positive for EBV, the EBV-positive service members were 32 times more likely to develop MS. Although few people who have EBV get MS, the study suggests that EBV is a necessary step in developing MS, since almost all people who get MS have EBV. Genes that are passed down through families may increase the risk of MS, and there may be other causes that contribute to MS, but EBV is the leading cause or trigger for the disease, concludes the research team.

No treatment for EBV: At this time there is no treatment to prevent EBV infection or to keep EBV from remaining in the immune system. There is also no vaccine to prevent EBV. There are effective treatments for MS, but there is no cure. The researchers say that finding an antiviral drug to treat EBV or a vaccine to prevent EBV could ultimately cure or prevent MS.

Vaccine for EBV on the Horizon

Because mononucleosis can be a serious infection, and EBV-associated cancers account for 150,000 deaths worldwide each year, a vaccine for EBV has been in development for over 30 years. Other herpes viruses such as chickenpox and shingles have successful vaccines…and recent advances in immunology and vaccine technology are encouraging, so a vaccine for EBV may be licensed in the near future.

Poison Ivy Alert

Laura Ferris, MD, PhD, an associate professor of dermatology at the University of Pittsburgh.

Long walks in nature, trips to the local forest preserve, and destination hikes are all excellent exercise options in the warm weather, but danger could be lurking in that low-lying shrub or bush featuring clusters of three glossy leaves.

Poison ivy contains an oily resin called *urushiol* that causes an allergic reaction in about 80 to 90 percent of people.

Urushiol is extremely potent: Just 50 micrograms, less than a grain of salt, is enough to cause an itchy, blistery rash that usually has a streaky or patchy appearance.

Myth Buster: The Poison Ivy Rash Is Not Contagious

There is a common misconception that touching a poison ivy rash can spread it to other parts of your body or to other people. This is a myth. Unlike impetigo, the rash is not contagious and there is no "poison" or urushiol inside the blisters.

Urushiol is absorbed at different speeds on different parts of the body, so new areas of the rash can continue to appear over several days. That doesn't mean the rash is spreading—only that it's still developing. For example, you might have walked through a patch of low-lying plants and exposed your legs, then reached down to tie your shoe, transferring the oil to your hands. If you then pick up a backpack and transfer the oil to the straps, you can easily get it on your shoulders and have another affected area.

The resin can survive for years on clothing, gardening gloves, and tools, and you can reinfect yourself by touching them. But once the oil is removed, the risk is gone.

The rash appears a day or two after exposure to the oil.

The exception is your very first exposure, which rarely causes a reaction. It primes the immune system to respond to subsequent urushiol exposures in a way that's similar to how a vaccine trains your body to attack a certain virus.

Know What to Avoid

Start with the simple adage, "Leaves of three, let it be." Poison ivy always has a trio of three pointed leaves that may be smooth-edged or jagged, shiny, or dull. They start out red in the spring and turn yellow, red, or orange in the fall. White berries or greenish-white flowers may be present. The roots of the plant often climb trees and look like thick, hairy vines. Every part of the poison ivy plant, from the leaves to the roots, contains urushiol, even when dead.

If you're not sure whether you'll be near the toxic plant, wear long sleeves and pants, taking care to tuck them into your socks. When gardening or doing yard work, wear heavy-duty gloves and wash them, your clothes, and your tools afterward. Dogs and cats aren't allergic to poison ivy, but the resin can live on their fur, so if you think that the two of you have been exposed, give your pet a bath, wearing rubber gloves to protect yourself.

Prevention

If you do brush against the plant, wash up as quickly as possible. Getting the oil off your skin as soon as you've been exposed can prevent the rash from ever developing. You can use regular soap and water, but a recent article published in the *Journal of the American Academy of Dermatology* reported that dishwashing soap may be a smarter choice, thanks to its ability to break down oil.

Use a washcloth and forcefully rub any affected areas in one direction only, rather than back and forth, using hot water. Rubbing alcohol can also work. Consider carrying alcohol wipes with you on walks.

Treatments

If you don't get the oil off quickly enough to prevent the rash, you're looking at about a week or two of itching. For mild cases, do-it-yourself treatments like soothing oatmeal baths and cool, wet compresses applied to affected areas three to four times a day for 20 minutes may be enough to ease the itch. Over-the-counter topical treatments such as hydrocortisone cream or calamine lotion may help, as can non-sedating oral antihistamines such as *loratadine* (Claritin) *fexofenadine* (Allegra), or *cetirizine* (Zyrtec) during the day or *diphenhydramine* (Benadryl) at bedtime. More severe cases and rashes around the eyes may require a course of prescription oral steroids, sometimes lasting for up to three weeks. Your primary care physician or dermatologist can prescribe these. Some doctors may be tempted to prescribe a quick five-day course of oral steroids, but poison ivy cases have been known to rebound with too short of a course.

Resist the Itch

Some scratching is inevitable, but do your best to avoid it as much as you can, especially if you have blisters. While the poison ivy rash is not contagious (see box on page 215), bacteria on your hands could cause an infection called impetigo that is. Impetigo shows up as itchy red sores that break open, releasing a thick yellow fluid that forms a honey-colored crust. If you notice this happening, see your doctor, as you may need a topical or oral antibiotic.

If you can't control the scratching and a blister does break open, keep the area clean and apply an ointment like petroleum jelly to protect the skin. Do not apply an over-the-counter antibiotic ointment, which itself can cause contact dermatitis.

Poison Oak and Poison Sumac

Urushiol is also found in poison oak and sumac. The leaves-of-three adage doesn't work with these plants. Poison oak's hairy leaves can also be in groups of five or seven, while poison sumac leaves grow in clusters of seven to 13 leaves. Urushiol is in cashew shells and mangoes, too. In fact, previous exposure to poison ivy can predispose a person to developing an allergic reaction called mango dermatitis, characterized by tingling, redness, and itching in and around the mouth.

There's a New Weapon Against Drug-Resistant Bacteria

Study by researchers at Wistar Institute, Philadelphia, published in *Nature*.

The antibiotic in development attacks bacteria in two ways instead of one. Bacteria can and do mutate to develop drug resistance to single-attack antibiotics, but it is harder for them to develop two forms of resistance at the same time.

Newly Approved HIV Treatment Can Be Given Monthly

John Farley, MD, director of the Office of Infectious Diseases, FDA Center for Drug Evaluation and Research, Silver Spring, Maryland.

To avoid complications, HIV-infected people must take pills daily. *Cabotegravir* (Cabenuva), an FDA-approved extended-release injection given monthly, was shown to be as effective at maintaining viral suppression in HIV-infected adults.

Chapter 10

KIDNEY, BLADDER, AND LIVER HEALTH

How to Be a Living Organ Donor

Hundreds of millions of people have registered to serve as organ donors when they die. But not everyone will get the chance. In fact, only three out of 1,000 people die in a way that allows their organs to be used, meaning that the demand for life-saving transplants far outpaces the number of viable organs.

Enter living donation: A living donor gives a kidney...part of his/her liver...or another type of tissue to a loved one, acquaintance or even a stranger who needs it. Unlike hearts and lungs, which come only from deceased donors, kidneys and livers lend themselves well to living donation. A person needs only one of his/her two kidneys to live...and the liver regenerates, or grows back, so a donor can give a portion of his liver to a recipient, and both their livers will grow to full size. (Donating a portion of your pancreas, intestines or lung is possible but very rare.)

Addressing a Growing Need

Organs from living donors have several advantages over organs from deceased donors.

The recipients often spend less time waiting for an organ because they have actively sought out a live donor. And in many cases, expenses for the donor are picked up by the recipient's insurance (see page 219 for details). The surgery can be scheduled in advance, giving all parties enough time to prepare. And because the donor organ is working up until mere moments before transplantation, long-term outcomes are improved and recovery times shortened for the recipient. Living donors often are related to the patient, and the increased likelihood of genetic matching (versus an organ from a deceased stranger) may reduce the odds of organ rejection. Additionally, every time a live donation occurs, a different candidate on the organ-transplant waiting list moves up. More than 106,000 Americans currently are on the list, with someone new added every nine minutes.

Most patients needing a kidney are in kidney failure related to diabetes and/or high blood pressure. Common ailments that can be treated with a new liver include nonalco-

---

Abhinav Humar, MD, clinical director of the Thomas E. Starzl Transplantation Institute and chief of the division of abdominal transplantation surgery at University of Pittsburgh Medical Center. He is a professor in the department of surgery at University of Pittsburgh School of Medicine and a staff physician at Pittsburgh VA Medical Healthcare System. MedSchool.Pitt.edu

holic steatohepatitis (NASH, or liver inflammation caused by fat buildup in the liver), liver cancer and autoimmune liver diseases such as primary biliary cholangitis and primary sclerosing cholangitis. Hepatitis C used to be a common cause for liver transplants, but today's effective antiviral treatments mean that far fewer people with hepatitis C require transplants.

Organ recipients typically take immunosuppressive drugs indefinitely to prevent their bodies from rejecting the new organ.

The donor reaps many rewards as well, not the least of which is the knowledge that he/she has saved another person's life. As one donor wrote on the National Kidney Foundation blog, "To see a loved one who's been pale, weak, and often listless for many months or years gradually become their old self again is pretty powerful. Seeing [my son's] smile when he came into my hospital room the day after the transplant was unforgettable."

Many Ways to Give

There are several ways to donate…

• **Directed donation.** You give your organ to a relative, spouse, friend, colleague or unrelated person in need. You must be a match for the recipient, meaning that your blood type and tissue type are compatible.

• **Paired donation (organ exchange).** This involves two or more pairs of living donor/recipients "swapping" donor organs.

Example: Jean wants to donate a kidney to her friend Jerry but isn't a match. Another pair—Lisa and her mother, Judy—are incompatible with each other as well, preventing Judy from receiving Lisa's kidney. But Jean and Judy are a match, and Lisa and Jerry are a match. Transplant centers connect incompatible pairs, ensuring that each recipient receives a compatible organ.

• **Nondirected donation.** Some individuals (called altruistic donors or Good Samaritan donors) donate to a medically compatible stranger.

• **Never-Ending Altruistic Donor (NEAD) kidney chain.** A person gives an organ to a stranger who already has an incompatible

donor. In exchange for that kidney, the recipient's incompatible donor donates to another stranger in need of a kidney, and the cycle continues. The nation's longest NEAD kidney chain, still happening at the University of Alabama at Birmingham, has seen 114 people receive kidneys from strangers.

How Living Donation Works

Innovations in transplant surgery have made donating easier and more effective.

• **Kidneys.** Laparoscopic surgery allows kidney removal via several tiny incisions during a three-to-five-hour surgery, reducing the average hospital stay to a day or two. This shortens overall recovery time, reduces post-op pain and lowers the risk for complications. Donors usually are able to return to work in two to four weeks and are back to normal in four to six weeks.

• **Livers.** Liver donation is a bigger endeavor. Anywhere from 25 percent to 65 percent of the liver is removed via incision in a four-to-six-hour surgery. Pain following donation is significant, but improvements in post-op pain control have shortened the average hospital stay from seven to five days, and donors often are back to work in four to six weeks and resume normal activities in 10 to 12 weeks.

Both surgeries require general anesthesia. Besides pain, risks include surgical complications such as infection…blood loss or blood clots…and injury to surrounding tissue.

Potential long-term risks of kidney donation may include high blood pressure, reduced kidney function or hernia, but these risks are rare. The risk of dying from the surgery is extremely low, about one in 5,000 cases (0.02 percent).

Possible risks for liver donors include future bile duct problems, hernia, and organ failure. Again, these complications are relatively uncommon. The risk of dying from this surgery is higher than that for kidney donation—about one in 500 cases (0.2 percent)—but is still quite low.

Some donors experience psychological difficulties afterward, including worrying about their future health or symptoms of anxiety or depression. But most donors report a profound sense of fulfillment and a strong bond with the recipient (if they know each other). According to the American Society of Transplantation, nearly 98 percent of live donors say that they'd donate again if they could.

Starting the Process

Living donors must be at least 18 years old and usually no older than 60 to 65 (kidney) or 55 to 60 (liver). Race and ethnicity don't matter—matches frequently occur between people of different backgrounds. Donors undergo extensive physical and mental health evaluations to rule out underlying medical issues such as heart disease, diabetes, and depression. Certain well-controlled conditions, such as mild high blood pressure, may be permitted. Many transplant centers require donors and recipients to be vaccinated for COVID-19.

During an informed-consent process, doctors ensure that you fully understand the risks and benefits…are not being coerced into volunteering…and understand how your personal, work, emotional and social life may be impacted in the months following donation.

Ready for the Next Step

For a directed donation, contact the transplant center your friend or family member is working with. For a nondirected donation, contact any center you want. The US Department of Health & Human Services' Organ Procurement and Transplantation Network (OPTN. transplant.hrsa.gov/about/search-member ship) lists programs nationwide.

The recipient's insurance usually will cover the donor's medical expenses, including evaluation, surgery, and follow-up testing. (Medicare covers the cost of care for donors.) That said, complications related to donation may not be covered, and some donors experience difficulty obtaining or keeping insurance coverage. Check with your insurance provider or ask your transplant center if it offers medical and disability insurance for donors. Recently introduced legislation,

the Living Donor Protection Act, would protect living donors from excessive insurance premiums and help guarantee time off from work to recover. The National Living Donor Assistance Center (LivingDonorAssistance. org) may be able to help cover nonmedical expenses such as travel and housing.

The Future of Organ Donation

Researchers in the field of regenerative medicine are actively exploring the possibility of growing human-compatible organs in pigs, as well as using specialized 3-D printers filled with a patient's own stem cells instead of ink to create human tissues and organs. Both would address—and perhaps end—the donor-organ shortage while avoiding organ rejection. (In the case of pig organs, the animal's genes would be edited to avoid attack by the human immune system.) Exciting progress has been made—skin, urethras, and other tissues have been built by hand using patients' cells and successfully implanted into people—but engineering or growing solid organs such as kidneys and livers has proven more challenging. In October 2021, surgeons at NYU Langone Health in New York City connected a gene-edited pig kidney to a brain-dead patient with malfunctioning kidneys, resulting in swift improvements in kidney function. (The patient's family consented to the experiment.) Widespread use of these procedures isn't in the near future, but they could be game changers if they come to pass.

Kidney-Stone Prevention Plan

David S. Goldfarb, MD, a professor of medicine at New York University Grossman School of Medicine. He is chief of nephrology at New York Harbor VA Healthcare System and the cofounder of Moonstone Nutrition.

Kidney stones, made from chemicals in urine, tend to make their presence known in the warmest months of the year. One likely reason is that people sweat more, don't drink enough to make up for it, and end up with more concentrated urine, allowing crystals to form and grow into stones. In places where it's fairly warm year-round, such as the southern United States, kidney stones are more common than in colder climes. And according to recent surveys, women (especially younger women) are experiencing an increase at an alarming rate.

In fact, around the world, the incidence of kidney stones is rising in all populations. In the United States, the lifetime risk of having at least one kidney stone is now about 10 percent, up from 3.8 percent in the 1970s, according to the National Kidney Foundation.

Among possible reasons: the warming climate and the migration of people to warmer urban areas. But heat isn't the whole story. The way we eat and drink and the rise of obesity and diabetes likely play roles, too.

From Unnoticed to Unbearable

Typical stones may be as small as a grain of sand or as large as a chickpea. More rarely, they can be as large as golf balls. A small stone may sit in your kidney unnoticed for months or years before it gets big enough or starts moving enough to cause trouble. Often, that happens when a stone moves from a kidney to a ureter, one of the tubes leading to the bladder. The stone may get stuck there, blocking urine flow, or causing irritation as it makes its way through the ureter and bladder and out through the urethra. *Once a stone becomes problematic, symptoms can start suddenly...*

- **Intermittent mild to severe pain** in the side, back, or groin for five to 15 minutes
- **Stomach pain, nausea, and vomiting**
- **Blood in the urine**
- **Fever, chills, and bad-smelling or cloudy urine**
- **Kidney damage that may linger.**

Diagnosis and Treatment

If you show up in an emergency room or doctor's office with a possible kidney stone,

---

Four Kinds of Kidney Stones

Not all kidney stones have the same causes. Knowing which type you're prone to can help you tailor your prevention plan.

- **Calcium oxalate.** Most kidney stones form when calcium in urine combines with oxalate, a salt. Calcium oxalate stones make up as many as 85 percent of cases. They are linked to inadequate fluid intake and diets that are high in oxalates and salt but, paradoxically, low in calcium.
- **Uric acid.** These stones are linked with conditions including type 2 diabetes, obesity, and gout and with diets high in animal protein.
- **Struvite.** These stones occur mostly in women with chronic urinary tract infections. That's because some bacteria secrete enzymes that make urine less acidic, allowing stones to form.
- **Cystine.** These rare stones are found only in people with a genetic disorder called cystinuria that causes the kidneys to excrete excessive amino acids. They tend to recur.

—Dr. David Goldfarb

---

expect to get a CT scan, an ultrasound, or an x-ray to confirm the stone as well as its size and location. You also will get blood and urine tests to check for kidney function, levels of stone-forming substances, and infection.

Unless the stone is quite large or causing unmanageable pain or other complications, your doctor is likely to send you home to see if the stone will pass, which will happen within a few weeks in 80 percent of cases in which stones are no larger than 4 millimeters. Larger stones are less likely to pass. While some people will need prescription painkillers to get through the process, others will do fine with an over-the-counter anti-inflammatory painkiller. *Naproxen* (Aleve) is a good choice. Anything that helps you relax, even a warm bath, can help. You may also get medication to relax the ureter or change the acidity of your urine.

8 Steps to Prevent Stones

1. Drink up. Staying hydrated is important for everyone, but especially for people prone to kidney stones. Aim for 12 cups of fluid (96 ounces) every day. Water is better than sodas or tea. If you are sweating a lot, drink more.

2. Get enough calcium. Even though the most common stones contain calcium, a calcium-rich diet helps prevent them. That's because calcium in food binds with oxalates in your digestive tract, preventing these minerals from reaching high concentrations in your kidneys. Good sources include low-fat milk, cheese, and yogurt, sardines, and fortified cereals and juices. Calcium supplements may increase stone risk, but you can blunt that risk by choosing calcium citrate rather than calcium carbonate products. Taking them with food helps, too.

3. Limit sodium to 2,000 milligrams per day. Excessive sodium leaches calcium from the bones and concentrates it in the urine. Watch out for the salt hidden in restaurant meals and processed foods, such as soups, bread, and sandwich meats.

4. Limit foods that are high in oxalates. If you are prone to stones containing oxalate (see sidebar on page 220), your doctor may suggest that you limit foods such as strawberries, spinach, beets, nuts, organ meats, chocolate, tea, coffee, and cola.

5. Limit animal protein to about 80 grams per day. Diets heavy in meat and seafood are linked with both calcium and uric acid stones (see sidebar on page 220).

6. Watch out for sweeteners. High-fructose corn syrup, found in many foods and drinks, is linked with uric acid stones.

7. Talk to your doctors about medications and supplements that might help prevent your type of stone. These can include pills or drinks containing citrate and medication to reduce uric acid levels. Some medications can increase your risk of kidney stones. Talk to your doctor or pharmacist to review all of the medications that you take.

8. You can also try a home remedy to reduce your risk. Mix one-half cup of lemon juice with two quarts of water and drink throughout the day.

—Dr. David Goldfarb

Contrary to popular belief, studies have not found that drinking extra fluids after a stone forms helps it to pass, though extra fluids can help prevent future stones.

Advanced Interventions

When stones appear unlikely to pass unaided or are causing complications, the next step is a procedure to remove or destroy them. *There are several options...*

• **Ureteroscopy.** A small instrument, called a ureteroscope, is inserted through your urethra and bladder to reach the stone. Then, in most cases, a laser is used to break up the stone so it can be easily expelled.

• **Shockwave lithotripsy.** For this procedure, you lie on a surgical table or in a tub of water while shockwaves are aimed at the stone to break it apart.

• **Percutaneous nephrolithotomy.** This less-common procedure is used for large or irregularly shaped stones or in other special circumstances. A surgeon makes a small incision on the back, uses instruments to see and break up stones, then suctions out the fragments.

What Can You Do?

Anyone who's ever suffered through a kidney stone shares one fervent wish: They never want to do it again. Yet, half will develop another stone within a few years. Those who've had two or more stones are at even higher risk.

One reassuring fact: Most kidney stones can be prevented, no matter the season. See the box above to learn how.

Artificial Kidney Works Without Drugs

Shuvo Roy, PhD, technical director, The Kidney Project, University of California San Francisco Schools of Pharmacy and Medicine.

A prototype of an artificial kidney has been successfully implanted. The smartphone-sized device combines a filter that removes waste products and toxins from the blood and a bioreactor that replicates other kidney functions, such as balancing electrolytes. The unit is powered by blood pressure and does not require the use of immunosuppressant drugs. The researchers will now move on to more rigorous preclinical testing, and, ultimately, clinical trials.

Menopause: When Incontinence Hits Women the Hardest

Study titled "Prevalence and Factors Associated with Overactive Bladder and Stress Urinary Incontinence in the Japan Nurses' Health Study," by researchers at Gunma University, Maebashi, Japan, published in *Menopause*.

TV commercials for incontinence products attempt to be discreet and sometimes make light of shopping for adult diapers. But incontinence is no laughing matter. It's an embarrassing condition for millions of women.

An overactive bladder can happen to a woman at any time in life, especially during pregnancy. But there's a certain span of life when incontinence hits women the hardest, according to a recent study out of Japan.

The study found that women between the ages of 45 to 54 were more likely to have an overactive bladder...the time when menopause is most likely to occur. The researchers also found that being overweight and having multiple childbirths were the most

significant risk factors for overactive bladder and stress incontinence. This was the largest study ever conducted to learn about the frequency and risk factors associated with overactive bladder and stress incontinence in women. It was recently published in the journal of The North American Menopause Society, *Menopause*.

Two Kinds of Incontinence

Unwanted loss of urine (incontinence) is a sign of overactive bladder, along with more frequent urination and a frequent urge to pass urine. It is a major quality-of-life issue for many women. There are two types of incontinence associated with overactive bladder. Stress incontinence is the most common type in women. This involuntary loss of urine occurs when the bladder is stressed by increased pressure (the dreaded "oops" leakage that occurs when you sneeze, cough, or laugh). The other type of incontinence is urge incontinence, which is loss of urine due to an uncontrollable need to urinate...even if the bladder is not full (such as during a urinary tract infection).

Other studies have found that women are more likely to have overactive bladder and urinary incontinence around the time of menopause, and that incontinence increases with age. In the U.S., about 17 percent of women have incontinence after age 20. After age 60, close to 40 percent of women have incontinence.

What the Japanese Study Found

The new study documented symptoms of overactive bladder in more than 12,000 Japanese women. The women's ages ranged from 27 to 82. The researchers also looked for risk factors that might contribute to incontinence such as weight, age, and number of births.

The study found that there was a significant association between overactive bladder in postmenopausal women between the ages of 45 to 54. *Other key findings included...*

•**One out of five women in the study reported overactive bladder or stress incontinence.**

• Just over 18 percent of women between the ages of 50 to 54 were affected by stress incontinence.

• There was a significant association between postmenopausal status and overactive bladder in women between ages 45 and 54.

• Stress incontinence symptoms decreased in the years after menopause.

• Stress incontinence increased in women who were overweight and had multiple childbirths.

Blame Estrogen (Again)

The probable cause of incontinence during menopause is a falling level of estrogen that causes the pelvic floor muscles that control urination to become weaker. Bladder leakage is one of the many manifestations of perimenopause and menopause, along with hot flashes, night sweats, and mood swings. The average age of menopause for women in the U.S. is 51.

The researchers conclude that women between the ages of 45 and 54 who are postmenopausal should be questioned about symptoms of overactive bladder, especially women who are overweight and have had multiple pregnancies with childbirth. The researchers recommend further studies to learn about overactive bladder symptoms in the time after menopause and in the time around menopause, called perimenopause.

There are two possibilities for nighttime incontinence: One is that this is a normal part of aging that can be addressed with some simple diet and lifestyle changes. The other possibility, which is less likely, is that there is something wrong.

As we get older, our bladders can become less elastic and let us know sooner that it's time to use the bathroom. If you find yourself too busy during the day to empty your bladder very often, or if you drink most of your fluid later in the day, your bladder will inevitably wake you up at night and disturb your sleep. Although it is normal to wake up approximately one to two times per night as we get older (and even increase into our later years), this symptom can be improved with a few simple adjustments.

Our bodies need to empty a certain amount of urine throughout a 24-hour period, so one tip would be to try and adjust your fluid intake more during the first part of the day and much less after dinner. Also, try and space out your fluid intake throughout the day so that you're not drinking more than 6 to 8 ounces at any one time.

Going to the bathroom regularly throughout the day (approximately every two to four hours) is generally recommended. Sometimes, it is hard to stop and do this, but remember that we aren't camels.

If these strategies don't work for you, it might be time to see a doctor and make sure that everything is working as it should.

If Your Bladder Keeps You Up at Night...

Jill Maura Rabin, MD, a professor of obstetrics and gynecology at Zucker School of Medicine at Hofstra Northwell in Hempstead, New York. Dr. Rabin, a nationally recognized authority on urogynecology and female pelvic medicine, is the co-author of *Mind Over Bladder: A Step-By-Step Guide to Achieving Continence.*

D o you wake up multiple times at night to use the bathroom? Don't settle for a poor night's sleep. *Why this happens and what to do...*

Overcome Fatty Liver Disease

Arun J. Sanyal, MD, a professor in the division of gastroenterology, hepatology, and nutrition at the Virginia Commonwealth University School of Medicine, current chair of the Liver Study Section at the National Institutes of Health, and the 2017 recipient of the Distinguished Scientific Award Winner from the American Liver Foundation.

T he liver is a three-pound, rubbery organ that sits on the right side of your abdomen, below the diaphragm and above the stomach, and it's very good at multitasking.

It filters blood; manufactures proteins, including those that help clot the blood; detoxifies chemicals and drugs; stores and regulates cellular fuel; produces the bile that helps digest fat; metabolizes and stores several nutrients, like iron and vitamin D; and helps respond to and destroy viruses and other germs. In other words, the liver is crucial to your health and well-being. But a lot of our livers aren't doing very well.

An astounding one out of every three Americans—more than 80 million people—have a fatty liver: Their liver cells are filled with excess fat, in the form of triglycerides. Most people with fatty liver have a relatively innocuous form that doctors call nonalcoholic fatty liver (NAFL), but about 20 to 25 percent have a more active form of the disease called *nonalcoholic steatohepatitis* (NASH). Together, they are called nonalcoholic fatty liver disease (NAFLD).

High-Risk NASH

In NASH, fat-engorged liver cells weaken, balloon, and die in greater numbers than normal, leaving the liver inflamed and scarred (a condition called fibrosis). NASH increases your risk of colon cancer and death from a heart attack, heart failure, or stroke. It doubles the risk of liver cancer, and it can lead to cirrhosis, or extensive and life-threatening scarring of the liver. NASH is the fastest-growing cause of cirrhosis-related liver transplants.

And the situation is only getting worse. Research shows that by the end of this decade, more than 100 million Americans will develop NAFLD, with the number of deaths from NAFLD expected to double.

Here is perhaps the most daunting statistic of all: Nine out of 10 people who have NAFLD don't know they have the problem, because it doesn't usually cause symptoms.

Risk Factors

Here's how to determine if you're at risk for NAFLD and what to do about it.

You're more likely to have NAFLD if you are overweight or obese, have high blood pressure, and/or have type 2 diabetes. If you have all three of those risk factors, the odds are 75 percent that you have NASH.

If you have any or all of the three main risk factors for NAFLD, talk to your primary care physician about monitoring the health of your liver. An easy way to do that is with a measurement called Fibrosis-4, or FIB-4. This uses two blood tests: a liver panel, which measures liver enzymes, and a platelet count, which is part of a standard blood test called a complete blood count (CBC) test. A formula using two liver enzymes, platelet count, and your age produces a measurement that correlates to the amount of fibrosis in the liver. (Your doctor can find a FIB-4 calculator at Hepatitisc.uw.edu/page/clinical-calculators/fib-4.)

If your score is 1.3 or lower, there is a low probability that you have liver scarring.

If your score is between 1.4 and 2.5, you may want to see a hepatologist for additional testing to determine your risk of cirrhosis, such as a special ultrasound test of your liver called Fibroscan.

If your score is 2.6 or higher, there is a high probability that you have significant scarring. You should see a liver specialist (hepatologist) to determine your treatment options, with the goal of preventing cirrhosis or diagnosing cirrhosis that may already be present.

The FIB-4 test should be repeated every year. An increasing score is a strong indication that the condition of your liver is worsening and treatment is needed.

Weight Loss

The first and most important lifestyle treatment is decreasing fat in the liver—in other words, losing weight. But you don't have to lose a lot of weight: Losing just 5 to 10 percent of your total body weight will generate dramatic improvement in your risk for NAFLD. For example, if you weigh 200 pounds, losing 10 pounds is significant.

Don't try to lose it all at once. First, stop weight gain, and then start to lose weight at a reasonable, achievable pace of about one pound per month. *The best way to lose weight is also the simplest...*

• **Generate a mildly negative caloric balance so you burn more calories than you consume.**

• **Limit your intake of refined carbohydrates** (such as white flour and white sugar) and other processed foods, and favor whole foods, such as lean meat, fish, low-fat dairy products, fruits, vegetables, beans, whole grains, nuts, and seeds.

• **Limit your consumption of high-fructose corn syrup,** a sweetener that has been linked to liver inflammation and fibrosis.

• **Increase your intake of omega-3 fatty acids,** which are found in fatty fish such as salmon and sardines.

• **Drink more coffee,** which may protect against fibrosis.

Improve Fitness

Any type of aerobic exercise is good for reducing the level of triglycerides in the liver. Walk, bicycle, swim, dance, or do any activity that makes your heart beat faster for 30 minutes at least five days a week. Pick an aerobic exercise you like and will do regularly. For many people, that's walking.

Regular resistance exercise and/or high-intensity intermittent training are also effective. Talk to your doctor before starting an exercise program.

Sleep Better

Scientific findings show that lack of sleep is linked to insulin resistance and stress, both of which lead to more fat in the liver.

To improve your sleep, follow the principles of good sleep hygiene...

• **Go to bed and wake up at the same time every day.** If you need to change your sleep time, do it gradually.

• **Follow a nightly routine.** Give yourself 30 minutes before bed to wind down.

• **Avoid blue light from televisions and computers 30 to 60 minutes before bed.**

• **Use your bed only for sleep and sex.**

• **Keep your bedroom dark, quiet, and cool.**

Medical Treatments

There are several medications for NASH in clinical trials—such as *obeticholic acid*, which reduces inflammation and balances blood sugar—but none have yet been approved by the U.S. Food and Drug Administration.

In the interim, some physicians treat NASH with off-label (not FDA approved) medications. They include the diabetes drug *pioglitazone* (Actos), which improves insulin resistance, and the weight loss drug *semaglutide* (Ozempic). There is also evidence that high-dose vitamin E (800 international units daily)—a prescriptive dose that should be used only with the approval and supervision of a physician—may help control NASH. The American Association for the Study of Liver Diseases recommends both pioglitazone and vitamin E for most people with proven NASH.

Bariatric surgery for weight loss is also an important consideration for people with obesity. In one study, NASH was completely resolved in 84 percent of those who had the surgery.

A "Green" Mediterranean Diet Cuts Common Liver Disease in Half

Study titled "Effect of green-Mediterranean diet on intrahepatic fat: the DIRECT PLUS randomized controlled trial," by researchers at Ben-Gurion University of the Negev, New York City, published in *Gut*.

Non-alcoholic fatty liver disease (NAFLD) affects 25 percent to 30 percent of people in the United States and Europe. Having it increases the risk of several

Cinnamon Warning

Cinnamon supplements and spice may contain the liver toxin and potential carcinogen *coumarin*. More so in cassia cinnamon, the most common type, than Ceylon cinnamon. When tested, samples of the spice and the supplements, which are taken to moderate blood sugar levels, contained more than half the tolerable daily intake for adults and exceeded it for children. Oregon's Wild Harvest and Swanson Cinnulin PF Cinnamon Extract supplements had the least coumarin...as did the spice FGO Organic. Consuming cassia cinnamon occasionally is safe.

Tod Cooperman, MD, is president and editor-in-chief at ConsumerLab.com. His report was published on ConsumerLab.com.

health problems, including type 2 diabetes and cardiovascular disease. Weight loss is the most widely recommended solution to combat intrahepatic fat (fat in the liver), so doctors often recommend change in diet when it comes to beating NAFLD.

Recent development: Now a research team from Ben-Gurion University of the Negev has found that following a green Mediterranean diet reduced intrahepatic fat more than other diets and cut the presence of NAFLD by 50 percent after 18 months.

Meet the Enhanced Mediterranean Diet

The modified green Mediterranean diet used in this recent research is rich in vegetables, walnuts and less processed meat and red meat, while the "green" portion features high-polyphenol foods such as green tea and a Mankai (a tiny green plant also known as duckweed that is packed with nutrients) shake daily. Research shows that polyphenols keep blood vessels flexible and strong, which reduces the risk for heart disease. Polyphenols have also been shown to lower blood sugar levels, reducing risk for type 2 diabetes.

The Mediterranean diet has long been accepted as a healthy lifestyle choice, but lead researcher Iris Shai, PhD, an epidemiologist in the BGU School of Public Health and adjunct professor at the Harvard T.H. Chan School of Public Health, asserts that she has 20 years of research to prove that it's the healthiest of all...with additional refinements.

Study details: Beginning in 2017, the international research team led by Dr. Shai developed and tested a modified green Mediterranean diet over the course of 18 months. Study participants included 294 individuals in their fifties, all with abdominal obesity, a common trait in people with NAFLD. They were randomly divided into three groups to participate in either a healthy dietary regimen, traditional Mediterranean diet, or "green" Mediterranean diet.

In addition, all participants were given a physical exercise regimen and free gym membership. Participants underwent MRI scans both before and after the trial to assess any change in the proportion of excess intrahepatic fat. While each diet led to liver fat reduction, the green Mediterranean diet resulted in the greatest change, 39 percent less, compared to the traditional Mediterranean diet, which reduced fat by 20 percent, and the healthy dietary guidelines, which reduced it by only 12 percent.

The green Mediterranean diet also significantly reduced the instance of NAFLD in participants, who at baseline showed about 62 percent prevalence. The green Mediterranean diet reduced this to 35 percent, while the traditional Mediterranean diet brought NAFLD prevalence down to 47.9 percent and the healthy-habits diet reduced it to 54.8 percent.

An Added Boost for Liver Health

The research suggests that the addition of walnuts and Mankai to the Mediterranean diet, and the reduction of processed meat and red meat, may have been the most helpful modifications to reduce liver fat, potentially due to the higher levels of polyphenol.

"Addressing this common liver disease by targeted lifestyle intervention might promote a more effective nutritional strategy," says Anat Yaskolka-Meir, MD, one of the study authors and member of the BGU School of Public Health. "This clinical trial demonstrates an effective nutritional tool for NAFLD beyond weight loss."

Cholesterol Can Be Good for Your Liver

Study by researchers at Washington University School of Medicine in St. Louis, published in *Science*.

HDL3, a specific type of high-density lipoprotein—the so-called "good" HDL cholesterol—has recently been found to block certain gut bacteria signals that trigger inflammation and can lead to liver damage.

Cocoa May Help Fight Obesity and Fatty Liver Disease

Study titled "Dietary Cocoa Ameliorates Non-alcoholic Fatty Liver Disease and Increases Markers of Antioxidant Response and Mitochondrial Biogenesis in High-Fat-Fed Mice," by researchers at Penn State College of Agriculture Sciences, University Park, published in *The Journal of Nutritional Biochemistry*.

You've probably heard that a little bit of dark chocolate daily can chase away the blues and may help your heart. And it's true that several studies suggest that cocoa's antioxidants and other nutrients may have beneficial effects that reduce the risk of type 2 diabetes, heart disease and stroke. Cocoa powder used to make chocolate or hot cocoa drinks has important nutrients like fiber, iron, and phytochemical antioxidants. Antioxidants prevent cell DNA damage.

Excess Sugar Hurts Your Liver

Eating added sugar doubles fat production in the liver. Study subjects received a daily drink sweetened with fructose, glucose, or sucrose and then analyzed the effect of the sugary drinks on lipid metabolism. They found that the body's fat production in the liver was twice as high in the fructose group as in the glucose group or the control group, even 12 hours later. Sucrose boosted fat synthesis even more. Increased fat production in the liver can lead to fatty liver and type 2 diabetes.

Philipp Gerber, MD, MSC, department of endocrinology, diabetology and clinical nutrition, University of Zurich, Switzerland.

Can Cocoa Help a Fatty Liver?

Armed with the knowledge that chocolate can be healthy, researchers at Penn State College of Agriculture Sciences wanted to see if cocoa powder could help eradicate a condition called non-alcoholic fatty liver disease (NAFLD). NAFLD is common in obese individuals. It can lead to scarring of the liver (cirrhosis) and liver cancer.

Study details: To discover the possible healing powers of cocoa, the researchers worked with obese mice with fatty livers. These mice are fed high-fat diets and used in many laboratory obesity and diet studies...a step before research is moved into human trials. If cocoa worked its antioxidants in obese mice and reversed NAFLD, it could mean that humans would benefit from this tasty, plant-based ingredient.

The mice were fed the human equivalent of about 10 tablespoons of cocoa powder per day over 10 weeks. At the end of the 10 weeks, the mice were evaluated for weight, liver fats called hepatic triacylglycerols and DNA cell damage from oxidative stress. The results are published in *The Journal of Nutritional Biochemistry*.

Compared to high-fat-fed obese mice that were not given cocoa supplements, the cocoa-fed mice gained weight at a 21 percent lower rate, had 28 percent less fat in their livers, and 75 percent less DNA damage from oxidative stress.

Possible Reason Why Cocoa Curbs Obesity

Why cocoa offers healing benefits for obesity and fatty liver disease is not completely understood, but some studies suggest that cocoa blocks the digestion of fat and carbohydrates. This means that less fat and sugar from foods are absorbed into the digestive system.

Takeaway: It's too soon to say that cocoa can prevent or reduce obesity and fatty liver disease in humans, but the researchers suggest replacing a few daily "treats" in an otherwise heart- (and liver-) healthy diet with a cup or two of hot cocoa (preferably home-made with pure cocoa and little to no sugar).

Tylenol Could Be Toxic If You're Low on This Nutrient

Study titled "Selenium Status in Diet Affects Acetaminophen-Induced Hepatotoxicity via Interruption of Redox Environment," by researchers at University of Bath, United Kingdom and College of Pharmaceutical Sciences of Southwest University, China, published in *Antioxidants & Redox Signaling.*

Over-the-counter *acetaminophen* (Tylenol) is taken by millions of people around the world to relieve pain and fever. It's a safe drug at proper doses. But too much acetaminophen is a major cause of liver failure.

Recent finding: A study done with mice serves as a warning that people who are deficient in the common mineral selenium could experience liver toxicity at a much lower amount of acetaminophen, possibly within the range of the recommended maximum dose.

Acetaminophen is broken down (metabolized) in the liver and usually eliminated from the body, but at very high doses, ac-

etaminophen becomes toxic. The maximum recommended dose for an adult is two 500 mg tablets four times per day, or 4,000 mg per day.

The Role of Selenium

People usually get selenium from their diet. The mineral plays an important role in liver health because it works as a powerful antioxidant. Too much or too little selenium can cause oxidative stress on liver cells and liver damage. This damage may slow down the metabolism of acetaminophen, allowing it to build up in the liver. Over time, this can lead to liver failure.

Unfortunately, selenium deficiency is fairly common. It occurs in about one out of seven people worldwide. People at highest risk are older, malnourished and/or in poor health. The study on selenium's relationship to acetaminophen is a collaboration between researchers at Bath University in the United Kingdom and the University of Chongqing in China. Their research was published in the journal *Antioxidants & Redox Signaling.*

The Selenium Balance

Selenium is one of the many nutrients that cannot be manufactured by the body, so it needs to be supplied by an outside source. The researchers advise against using supplements because too much selenium can be as dangerous as too little. The best source of selenium is a balanced diet. Fortunately, selenium is common in several foods. The richest sources include Brazil nuts, meat, fatty fish, eggs, brown rice, lentils, mushrooms, and sunflower seeds.

Takeaway: Watch your intake of acetaminophen. The researchers suggest that people who are frail, elderly or have chronic conditions associated with malabsorption should avoid acetaminophen at the maximum recommended dose, especially if they take it on a regular basis. Eat a balanced diet and discuss your intake of pain relievers with your doctor.

Chapter 11

NATURAL REMEDIES AND SUPPLEMENTS

How Food Fights COVID

COVID-19 first appeared in the United States in early 2020, and as of mid-2022, scientists—and a weary public—are still debating the whys and wherefores of the pandemic.

While scientists and citizens argue over vaccines, treatments, masks, and testing, one fact is clear to all: COVID-19 isn't going away. Given that ongoing reality, many of us remain determined to minimize our risk of catching COVID-19 and to minimize the severity of the disease if we get it. One tool is as close as your kitchen.

The Role of Metabolic Health

Anyone with poor metabolic health has an elevated risk of disease. When metabolic processes, such as the absorption of nutrients and the regulation of blood sugar, are not working normally, your immune system is weakened, and it's easier for microbes like viruses and bacteria to infect you. People with obesity, type 2 diabetes, heart disease, and cancer have impaired metabolism—and it's scientifically established that they're more likely to catch COVID-19 and to have severe or deadly disease. Data show that a 10 per-

cent reduction in obesity, diabetes, and heart disease in the U.S. population would have prevented 11 percent of the hospitalizations from COVID-19 that have occurred since November 2020.

It's also scientifically established that diet plays a role in metabolic illnesses like obesity, diabetes, and heart disease.

So an international team of 29 scientists and I conducted a study to answer this important question: Could the quality of a person's diet affect the risk and severity of COVID-19—not just for people with poor metabolic health, but for everyone?

Our Study

To answer that question, we used data from the smartphone-based COVID-19 Symptom Study, in which nearly 600,000 participants in the United States and the United Kingdom volunteered to provide information about COVID-19 symptoms and infections. The participants also provided information about their diet and lifestyle habits, including their

Jordi Merino, PhD, a research associate at the Diabetes Unit and Center for Genomic Medicine at Massachusetts General Hospital, and an instructor in medicine at Harvard Medical School. He is one of the lead authors of the scientific study featured in this article: "Diet quality and risk and severity of COVID-19."

consumption of plant-based foods (whole grains, fruits, vegetables, nuts, and legumes) as well as processed or non-plant foods (potato chips, white bread, soda, sweets, fried eggs, and red meat).

The results, published in the medical journal *Gut* in October 2021, were interesting. We found that the people eating the healthiest foods were 9 percent less likely to get COVID-19 than those who ate the least healthy foods. If the healthy eaters did get the disease, they were 41 percent less likely to develop severe symptoms of COVID-19.

Diet didn't have to be perfectly healthy to be protective. That is, protection didn't come from eating only plant-based foods. Rather, small changes in diet—adding another serving of whole grains one day, or an additional serving of vegetables the next—was enough to generate a protective effect.

However, there was one confounding factor: People with "socioeconomic deprivation" who live in areas where healthy foods aren't as affordable or available are more likely to get COVID-19 or suffer severe symptoms than people who don't live in such areas. Yes, poor diet was a big contributor to excess risk for COVID-19, but so was deprivation.

All in all, if people ate a healthy diet and didn't have socioeconomic deprivation, 33 percent of the cases of COVID-19 could have been prevented.

It's also important to note that our observational study didn't *prove* that a good diet was protective against COVID-19: It showed a possible *association* between a good diet and protection against the disease and its symptoms. But these results strongly suggest there may be a direct correlation between what you eat and how your body responds to the novel coronavirus.

More Research

Researchers from Stanford University, Columbia University, Johns Hopkins University, and the Cedars-Sinai Medical Center also studied the link between diet and COVID-19, publishing their results in the June 2021 issue of *BMJ Nutrition, Prevention, and Health*.

In a study of nearly 3,000 people from the United States and Europe, the researchers found that people who followed a plant-based diet had a 73 percent lower risk of moderate-to-severe COVID-19 than people who didn't eat a plant-based diet.

They also found that people eating a pescatarian diet (plant-based foods plus fish and seafood) had a 59 percent lower risk. People who followed a "low-carbohydrate, high-protein diet" had a nearly four times higher risk of moderate-to-severe COVID-19.

HELPFUL FOODS, HARMFUL FOODS

In our study, the following foods were either helpful or harmful in protecting against COVID-19 and severe symptoms from the disease.

HELPFUL	HARMFUL	
Whole grains	Refined grains	Dairy
Vegetables	Potatoes	Eggs
Fruits	Fruit juice and sugar-sweetened beverages	Meat
Legumes		Fast food
Nuts	Sweets and desserts	

Nutritional Supplements

Nutritional supplements may also play a protective role. When researchers from King's College London looked at health data from more than 400,000 women, they found that those who took a nutritional supplement were less likely to be infected with the coronavirus…

- **14 percent less for those taking probiotics**
- **12 percent less for those taking omega-3 fatty acids**
- **13 percent less for those taking multivitamins**
- **9 percent less for those taking vitamin D.**

Why a Healthy Diet Is Protective

Good nutrition and good immunity go hand in hand. *There are many nutrients linked to stronger immunity…*

- **Trace elements.** Zinc, iron, and selenium
- **Vitamins.** A, B6, B12, C, D, and E

•**Polyphenols,** antioxidants found in plant foods.

Whole foods like vegetables, fruits, whole grains, and legumes are excellent sources of all these nutrients. Nutrients and nutritional compounds work in many ways to boost immunity—including supporting antiviral defenses that protect against a respiratory infection like COVID-19 and its severe symptoms.

While healthy diet and supplements can't replace vaccines, masking, and social distancing, they can make those efforts more effective.

How to Make Fire Cider

Fire cider is a traditional mix of apple cider vinegar and herbs that has been used to boost health and ward off colds.

To prevent colds: Drink one tablespoon per day…add it to tea or juice.

For a scratchy throat: Use as a gargle. You also can sprinkle it on salads and add it to vegetables, soups, chilis and cocktails.

Recipe: In a one-quart jar, combine one-third cup of grated-together horseradish and ginger, one-quarter cup peeled and diced turmeric (or two tablespoons of dried turmeric powder), six cloves of minced garlic, one-half cup peeled and diced onion, one or two habanero chiles cut in half (or one-half teaspoon cayenne pepper), one large lemon sliced including the rind, two tablespoons each of fresh chopped rosemary and thyme (or one teaspoon each of dried), one-half cup parsley, one cinnamon stick, a few allspice berries, a few cloves and one teaspoon of black peppercorns. Then add enough raw unfiltered apple cider vinegar to cover the ingredients by an inch or so (about four cups). Shake well, and let it sit for a few weeks in a cool dark place, shaking the mixture daily. Next, strain and add honey to taste. Store it in the refrigerator and use within one year.

The Old Farmer's Almanac. Almanac.com

Diet Changes Can Lower Your Risk for Gout

Chris Iliades, MD, retired ear, nose, throat, head, and neck surgeon who now dedicates his time to educating patients through his medical writing.

When gout strikes your toes, feet, ankles, or knees, the pain can be so intense that a bedsheet on your skin can be unbearable. Redness, swelling, and pain intensify for the first 24 hours and then linger for a week or more. Over time, untreated gout can destroy joint tissue, causing long-term pain, disability, and deformity.

Under the Surface

Gout starts with a basic molecule called a purine. Humans need purines to build DNA. You make some purines naturally and get more from your diet. After your body uses purines, they are broken down into uric acid. Normally, this acid is removed by your kidneys and causes no problems. But in some people, such as those with kidney disease or overconsumption of high-purine foods, the uric acid level can get too high and forms crystals that resemble microscopic needles. Those crystals can get trapped inside a joint, where they cause a sudden and severe attack of inflammation and pain.

People at Risk

Not everyone with high levels of uric acid forms these crystals. In fact, researchers have discovered that several inherited genes may be to blame for those who do. If you have a family history of gout, you'll want to be extra careful to reduce other modifiable risk factors. You can't do anything about your age (the risk of gout increases as you grow older) or your sex (it's more common in men but women during and after menopause are also at high risk), but you can control your diet. *There are three diet changes to help reduce gout…*

231

- Limit your calories and get adequate exercise to prevent obesity.
- Avoid purines in your diet.
- Follow the Dietary Approaches to Stop Hypertension (DASH) diet to lower your risk of gout, even if you have gout genes.

Avoiding Purines

Avoiding purine-rich foods can lower your risk of developing gout and, if you already have it, help manage the condition.

Avoid alcohol, especially beer. Having two or more beers per day more than doubles your gout risk. If you want to drink, the safest choice is a glass of wine.

Avoid sugar-sweetened beverages and anything sweetened with fructose to decrease your gout risk by about 80 percent.

Avoid eating shellfish and ocean fish, which increase gout risk by about 50 percent.

Avoid red meat, especially wild and organ meat to reduce risk by about 40 percent.

You may be able to lower gout risk by about 50 percent by eating more low-fat dairy products and foods high in vitamin C and drinking six or more cups of black coffee every day.

The DASH Diet

At the 2021 meeting of the European Congress of Rheumatology, researchers presented a study that showed that the typical American diet, which is rich in red meat, saturated fat, processed foods, refined grains, and sugar-sweetened beverages, was associated with a higher risk of gout than the DASH plan, even in people who had a genetic risk for gout. The DASH diet was originally developed to reduce high blood pressure and the risk of heart disease, but studies published in 2016 and 2017 found that it also lowers uric acid levels.

This diet limits calories to an average of 2,000 per day and outlines a target number of servings by food group…

- Six to eight servings of whole grains
- Four to five servings of fruits and vegetables
- Two to three servings of low or fat-free dairy foods
- Six or fewer servings of lean meat, poultry, and fish
- Two to three servings of fats and oils, but no trans fats
- No more than 2,300 milligrams of sodium

The diet also limits nuts, seeds, dry beans, peas, and sweets to five or fewer servings per week. (See below for examples of serving sizes.)

Not only can the DASH diet help prevent and control gout, but it can help you maintain a healthy blood pressure and body weight, too.

WHAT'S IN A SERVING?	
Whole grains	one slice of bread, 1 ounce of dry cereal, ½ cup of cooked rice or pasta
Vegetables	1 cup of raw leafy greens, ½ cup of raw vegetables
Fruits	One medium piece of fruit, ¼ cup of dried fruit
Low or fat-free dairy foods	1 cup of milk or yogurt, 1½ ounces of cheese
Lean meat, poultry, or fish	1 ounce of meat, poultry, or fish, 1 egg
Fats and oils	1 teaspoon of soft margarine or vegetable oil, 1 tablespoon (Tbsp) of mayonnaise
Nuts and seeds	⅓ cup of nuts, 2 Tbsp peanut butter or seeds
Beans and peas	½ cup cooked legumes
Sweets	1 Tbsp sugar, 1 Tbsp jelly or jam, or 1 cup of lemonade

Irritable Bowel Syndrome? Try the FODMAP Diet

Janet Bond Brill, PhD, RDN, FAND, registered dietitian nutritionist and author of *Intermittent Fasting for Dummies, Blood Pressure DOWN, Cholesterol DOWN,* and *Prevent a Second Heart Attack*. DrJanet.com

You may have heard the term FODMAP circulating in the nutrition world. FODMAP stands for fermentable oligosaccharides, disaccharides, monosaccharides, and polyols—scientific terms describing short-chain fermentable carbohydrates (sugars) that the small intestine absorbs poorly. Some people—especially those with diagnosed irritable bowel syndrome (IBS)—experience digestive distress after eating them, including bloating, flatulence, cramping, indigestion, and diarrhea. Stomach pain and bloating are the most common symptoms.

• **Oligosaccharides** (many sugar molecules) include wheat products such as bread, cereals, and crackers; beans, peas, and lentils (legumes); and vegetables such as garlic, onions, artichokes, Brussels sprouts, and asparagus.

• **Disaccharides** (two linked sugar molecules) include dairy products such as milk, yogurt, ice cream, and cheese. Lactose, the main carbohydrate in dairy, is often the culprit for dairy-sensitive people.

• **Monosaccharides** (single sugar molecule) include many types of fruit. Fructose is the main culprit for people sensitive to monosaccharide-laden foods. Stone fruits, which get their name from the pit or stone in their center, are especially problematic, including peaches, nectarines, plums, cherries, apricots, dates, mangoes, and lychees. Honey and agave nectar are also high in monosaccharides.

• **Polyols** (sugar alcohols) are found in blackberries, lychees, chewing gums, mints, and diabetic products.

Low-FODMAP diet

Studies have proven that the diet appears to improve digestive symptoms in most adults with IBS. *The foods that trigger symptoms vary from person to person, so start with a three-step elimination diet…*

• **Step 1** is the most restrictive phase. Eliminate all FODMAP foods for a test period of two to four weeks. *Base your meals around these proven low-FODMAP foods…*

  • Beef, pork, chicken, fish, eggs, and tofu

  • Cheese: Brie, Camembert, cheddar, and feta

• Almond and rice milk

• Grains: rice, quinoa, oats, gluten-free bread, and pasta

• Vegetables: bell peppers, carrots, green beans, eggplant, potatoes, tomatoes, cucumbers, and zucchini

• Fruits: oranges, grapes, melon, kiwi, strawberries, blueberries, and pineapple

• Nuts: almonds, pine nuts, and peanuts.

• **Step 2.** Slowly add back one FODMAP food at a time and chart which foods trigger symptoms.

• **Step 3.** Once you identify the problematic foods, avoid or limit them while enjoying everything else worry-free.

Natural Relief for Gas and Bloating

Jamison Starbuck, ND, a naturopathic physician in family practice in Missoula, Montana., and producer of *Dr. Starbuck's Health Tips for Kids*, a weekly program on Montana Public Radio, MTPR.org.

"I feel like I'm six months pregnant! It's so embarrassing and my doctor says nothing is wrong!"

This is a frequent refrain at my office. I see many patients who are miserable with gas and bloating shortly after meals but have normal lab tests, scans, colonoscopies, and endoscopies. Suggestions from conventional medical providers are often limited to antacids, weight loss, and sometimes antidepressants. I have a different approach.

If you have gas and bloating after meals daily, something is wrong. It's entirely appropriate to get a physical exam and tests to rule out serious conditions such as Crohn's disease, ulcerative colitis, and even cancers of the digestive tract. But if all of those are normal, your solution may lie in naturopathic medicine. *Consider these possibilities…*

• **Digestive deficiency.** Gas and bloating happen when foods are not thoroughly broken down inside the digestive tract. The first step in digestion is chewing and mixing food with saliva. As it moves to the stomach, food is bathed in hydrochloric acid and dissolved from solid into liquid form. Partially digested food then moves to the small intestine, where it is coated with pancreatic enzymes and bile released from the gallbladder. As food moves through the intestines, nutrients are absorbed and the remaining waste is eliminated via stool.

When any step in this process is deficient—if you don't chew your food thoroughly, don't make adequate saliva, or don't secrete enough hydrochloric acid, bile, or pancreatic enzymes to digest your food—gas and abdominal distention occurs. A naturopathic physician can assess the specific nature of your digestive deficiency and help you choose the most effective natural medicine to correct your problem.

Over-the-counter gas remedies, such as charcoal capsules, chewable papaya tablets, peppermint, and chamomile tea are very safe and surprisingly effective. But readily available digestive enzymes and gut "cleansing" formulas can make things worse. It's best to consult with a physician before tinkering with your digestive health, especially if you have a history of an ulcer or gut inflammation.

•**Food allergy.** I have many patients whose digestion is just fine as long as they avoid their food allergens. If they eat even a little bit of whatever they are allergic to, they know it pretty quickly. The top three food allergens are dairy, wheat, and eggs. The next tier includes peanuts, almonds, citrus, coffee, and sugar. You can determine food allergens by a process of elimination and reintroduction or by undergoing food allergy blood testing.

•**Excessive dietary sulfur.** Sulfur is an essential nutrient that is abundant in our foods. It plays an important role in protein metabolism, DNA formation, and the repair and protection of our cells. But too much sulfur causes gas: the stinky kind. If that's your trouble, try eliminating high-sulfur foods, such as garlic, onions, meat, peanuts, legumes, horseradish, and mustard, for one week. If your

gas subsides, reintroduce these foods slowly, and in small quantities. Most folks tolerate them, but only in reduced doses.

Grow a Home-Remedy Garden

Elizabeth Millard, co-owner of Bossy Acres, an organic farm in Minnesota, and author of *Backyard Pharmacy*, which details how to grow and use dozens of herbs.

It's easy to create your very own home-remedy garden with herbs, flowers and more.

Herbs to Start With

People tend to think "exotic" when it comes to healing herbs, but many of the culinary ones that you already reach for have medicinal properties, so they're a great place to start. You can find out about other medicinal herbs at the National Library of Medicine's website, NLM.nih.gov/about/herbgarden/index.html, or consult my book, *Backyard Pharmacy*. *Here are some of the most popular and easiest-to-grow medicinal plants…*

•**Basil.** Chewing on basil leaves can freshen breath and even ease cold symptoms. There are dozens of varieties of basil, but holy basil is the variety most often used for medicinal purposes including reducing inflammation and fighting aging caused by free radicals. It is widely available in garden centers and supermarkets in small starter plants that grow very well when planted in your garden. Pluck larger leaves at the bottom and leave tiny ones at the top to help the plant regenerate. Snip off flowers as they appear in order to prolong growth.

Ideal conditions: Six to eight hours of sun daily and well-drained, loosened soil.

•**Cayenne peppers** are rich in *capsaicin* and have antibacterial and anti-inflammatory properties. They are easy to dry and grind for year-round use. They're a great anti-cold remedy all winter long, particularly when mixed with warm water, honey, and crushed garlic. Buy small plants at garden centers in mid-spring.

Ideal conditions: Eight to 10 hours of full sun daily and well-drained, loosened soil.

• **Chamomile's dried flowers** make a great infusion for easing anxiety and helping you get to sleep. I recommend German chamomile over the more common Roman. It tends to have more flowers, and that's what you will be using for remedies.

Ideal conditions: Eight to 10 hours of sun daily and well-drained soil.

• **Echinacea's dried flowers** support the immune system and can ease cold symptoms. The flowers of both echinacea and its cousin chamomile will add beauty and attract birds and butterflies to your garden.

Ideal conditions: Six to eight hours of sun daily and loamy soil.

• **Garlic,** important for boosting heart health and relief from colds and flu, is surprisingly easy to grow. In a shallow trench and spacing them about eight inches apart, plant the largest individual cloves from one or more heads (buy those grown specifically for propagation)—root-side down, pointy end up. If you love garlic, set aside an eight-foot-by-three-foot patch for your trenches to be able to harvest at least a three-month supply.

Garlic should be planted in fall, left to develop root structure over the winter, and harvested in summer. Stored in a cool dark cabinet, the heads will last for months.

Ideal conditions: Six to eight hours of sun daily and well-drained, loosened soil.

• **Lemon balm** has been used for centuries as a calming agent, including to ease a queasy tummy, and it also can help manage seasonal allergies. It thrives in cool weather so you can get a head start on it in early spring. It also makes a great addition to hot and iced teas or other beverages and even can be used as a flavoring for desserts.

Ideal conditions: Six to eight hours of sun daily and well-drained, loosened soil.

• **Mint** provides an energy boost and can soothe stomach issues. Chew on the leaves or brew them into a tea. Mints of all varieties are hardy and easy to grow from seed. It can be invasive so you might want to keep it in pots or place it in the garden where it has plenty of room to grow.

Ideal conditions: Full sun or partial shade and well-drained, loosened soil.

• **Oregano's dried leaves** make a wonderful tea that is high in antioxidants and is used to treat digestive complaints. Fresh leaves can be turned into a poultice to soothe itchy skin. It is best to plant oregano at the margins of your garden because its low-lying branches spread easily between vegetables. It gets bushy, so you'll need to thin it every few years.

Ideal conditions: Full sun and well-drained, loosened soil.

Seed or Starter Plant?

Plants that you start from seed may take hold better outdoors because they develop in the local environment, but there are no guarantees! Seeds usually are less expensive than starter plants, even when you buy organic, which I recommend. How many starter plants to buy depends on your needs and uses and available space. But two or three of each should be a good start. Avoid buying large transplants, such as those in six-inch or larger containers. Small ones are less likely to experience shock when you replant them. Look for two- or four-inch starters.

If you're buying seeds: Good seed sellers include Johnny's Selected Seeds...Seeds of Change...Strictly Medicinal Seeds...and Hudson Valley Seed Company.

Hint: Once you have started growing your seeds and transplanted them outside, make your own planting notes right on the packets and store the packets in a dedicated bin as you would recipe cards.

If you're buying starter plants: Small transplants from a local nursery, state fair or farmers' market are a great option if you're getting a late start...are less experienced...or you want to try an herb you've never grown before. Ask the seller for tips about what grows best in your local area and soil and how much space it will need.

Enjoying Your Herbs

There's nothing quite like plucking fresh herbs for a relaxing afternoon tea or to enhance home cooking. But if you don't use them frequently, regularly trim the plants back to encourage new growth, and dry the cuttings for future use.

At the end of your growing season, harvest your herbs. You can cut fresh herbs, chop them and put them in ice cube trays with a little olive oil and water, then freeze and transfer to freezer bags for storage. You also can dry them on a mesh screen or in bundles by tying the stems together and hanging them, stem end up, to dry. Or freeze the fresh or dried herb in a plastic bag in the freezer.

Store dried herbs in airtight glass jars and keep them out of the light. Enjoy them as teas…or as tinctures, made by putting the herb in a container of two-thirds alcohol such as vodka and one-third water for at least two weeks. Or make balms or salves by placing your herbs in a jar of olive oil for a period of weeks to create an essential oil, then heating the oil with beeswax or coconut oil (once cool, it solidifies). Always do your research before using herbs to be sure they're safe for you.

Oats: Good Food and Medicine

Jamison Starbuck, ND, a naturopathic physician in family practice in Missoula, Montana., and producer of *Dr. Starbuck's Health Tips for Kids*, a weekly program on Montana Public Radio, MTPR.org.

When patients ask me what the best breakfast food is, I invariably say oatmeal. Many people are sur-prised by this response because they don't know that this ancient grain is packed with nutrition, including 6 grams of protein per cup of dry oats. Botanically known as *Avena sativa*, oats have been used as food and medicine for thousands of years. While modern "paleo" diets eschew all things grain, scientists, and archeologists have found remnants of wild oat starch on stones used by Paleolithic people to grind wild oats to form porridge and flour.

Healthy Food

Oats are a great source of vitamins B1 and B5, zinc, folate, and magnesium. They are rich in antioxidants and are a great source of beta-glucan fiber, a polysaccharide that can help lower cholesterol, stabilize blood sugar, improve bowel regularity and help with weight loss.

The mature oat seed is the part used as food. It is milled in a variety of ways, most commonly steel-cut, chopped (known as Scottish oats), rolled, and cooked. The nutritional value is fairly similar in most types of oats, but rolled and instant oats are steamed, softened, and, in the case of instant oats, partially cooked before being packaged for sale. Their flavor is blander than steel-cut or Scottish oats, and some nutrition is lost in the processing.

People often avoid the most nutritious raw oats because they think they don't have enough time to cook them in the morning before work. If that's you, try this trick: Mix one cup of steel-cut or Scottish oats with one cup of cow, soy, rice, or nut milk and refrigerate overnight. In the morning, add fresh or dried fruit, yogurt, nuts, and cinnamon, and eat warm or cold.

Natural Medicine

Oats are also good medicine. The fresh, immature milky seeds can be crushed and used immediately in a tea or made into a tincture.

• **Insomnia and anxiety.** Fresh, young oat seeds have a mild sedative effect. I almost always include *Avena sativa* in herbal tincture formulas I make for patients with insomnia or anxiety. Oat seed tincture is generally safe for children and useful for kids struggling with sleep or night terrors, but dosing must be adjusted for age and weight, so check with your pediatrician. Oats can be combined with other herbs that calm the nerves, such as skullcap, passionflower, and hops.

• **Addiction.** Oat seed tea or tincture can also be used for conquering addictions particularly to nicotine and caffeine. When used alone, for insomnia, addiction, or anxiety, a common daily dose of oat-seed tincture is 60 drops in 2 ounces of water, four times a day, away from meals.

• **Itchy skin.** To ease an itch, simply run hot water from your bathtub faucet through a sock stuffed with rolled or steel-cut oats. Soak in the tub for 10 to 20 minutes several times a day.

Note: Oats do not contain gluten, but they may be milled in facilities that also grind wheat and other gluten-containing grains. Read labels carefully when purchasing oats if you are gluten sensitive.

Breakthrough: Support This Enzyme to Shape Your Health

Russell Dahl, PhD, and Brunde Broady, MBA. Dr. Dahl was a professor of neuroscience and medicinal chemistry at the Chicago Medical School of Rosalind Franklin University before he founded Neurodon, a biopharmaceutical company that develops therapeutics that modulate sarco/endoplasmic reticulum calcium ATPase. Ms. Broady is a director at Neurodon and author of *The Calcium Connection: The Little-Known Enzyme at the Root of Your Cellular Health.*

While we most often think of calcium in terms of bone health, that's only one part of what it does in the human body.

A tiny fraction of the body's calcium (less than one percent) resides not in bones, but in and around every cell, where it plays a role in everything from contracting muscles to releasing neurotransmitters. That calcium relies on an enzyme called calcium ATPase (CA) to maintain a perfect balance of the mineral inside and outside the cell. When CA levels are deficient, there can be body-wide effects. *Researchers in multiple fields have linked low CA levels to a wide variety of illnesses...*

• **Cancer.** CA affects the growth and differentiation of cancer cells, contributing to cancer's progression. Reduced CA is directly associated with breast, lung, colon, thyroid, skin, and blood cancers, Johns Hopkins School of Medicine researchers reported in 2016.

• **Hypertension.** Reduced CA makes it harder for the arteries to relax, which results in constriction or narrowing and high blood pressure, according to research published in the *New England Journal of Medicine*, the *Chinese Medical Journal*, and the *American Journal of Hypertension*.

• **Inflammation.** Reduced CA triggers the release of inflammatory substances such as histamine, interleukin, and TNF-alpha. It can mimic an allergic response, even if there is no allergen present, or magnify the body's response to allergens, creating unnecessary inflammation, University of Kansas Medical Center researchers reported in *Frontiers in Immunology*.

• **Heart disease.** Intracellular calcium levels regulate the relaxation and contraction of the heart muscle. Decades of research show that reduced CA is associated with heart failure, atrial fibrillation, and a higher risk of heart attack and stroke.

• **Sleep.** When there is a reduction in CA, melatonin production drops and sleep quality deteriorates, the American Sleep Association notes. Reduced CA can also cause pineal cells to gradually degenerate and die, resulting in reduced melatonin production and poorer sleep.

• **Cognition.** In the brain, intracellular calcium levels affect the release of neurotransmitters, learning and memory formation, and neuroplasticity. If there isn't enough CA to restore calcium levels, though, too many neurotransmitters are released, which can cause cell death in the neural pathways we use most often, researchers from Purdue University discovered.

Dietary Support

As we age, CA levels naturally decline, but we can slow that decline with easily modifiable lifestyle choices. *To start, add more of these protective nutrients to your diet...*

• **Vitamin E** has positive effects on CA in the brain, liver, kidney, skeletal muscles, and heart. Food sources include almonds, olive oil, sunflower seeds, avocado, palm oil, sweet potato, butternut squash, peanuts, tomatoes, hazelnuts, pine nuts, turnip greens, mango, spinach, and wheat germ.

• **Ellagic acid** stimulates CA in the heart and normalizes levels in the kidneys after exposure to chemical toxins. Good sources include blackberries, raspberries, chestnuts, cranberries, green tea, strawberries, pecans, pomegranate juice, red wine, red grapes, and walnuts.

• **Green tea.** A compound in green tea, epigallocatechin gallate (EGCG), helps to maintain CA levels in the heart, maintains platelet CA levels, protects CA activity from drug-induced kidney damage, and increases CA levels after exhaustive exercise. An 8-ounce cup contains about 50 to 100 milligrams (mg) of EGCG. You can also take 300 mg of a green tea extract with EGCG.

• **Luteolin,** a bioflavonoid, increases levels of CA during heart failure and after a heart attack. Good sources include artichoke, radicchio, broccoli, red leaf lettuce, celery, rosemary, chicory greens, spinach, chili, green peppers, green bell peppers, parsley, yellow bell peppers, pumpkin, and thyme.

• **Lycopene,** a carotenoid, protects brain cells from the damaging effects of environ-

---

Exercise to Support Calcium ATPase

Regular exercise can increase CA levels in both your skeletal muscle and heart at any age. Aim for 30 minutes of high-intensity interval training three to five times per week and strength training three times per week.

—Dr. Russell Dahl

---

mental toxins. Good sources include asparagus, red cabbage, goji berry, red peppers, papaya, tomatoes, pink grapefruit, and watermelon.

• **Resveratrol** protects CA levels during cardiac trauma, protects CA levels in the heart from bacterial endotoxins' harmful effects related to sepsis, and counteracts some of the adverse effects pancreatitis has on CA in the pancreas and lungs. Food sources include cocoa powder/dark chocolate, red grapes, peanuts/peanut butter, red wine, pistachios, strawberries, and red grape juice.

Avoiding Toxins

Adding protective foods is just half of the equation. It's also important to reduce exposure to toxins. Choosing whole, fresh foods is a great place to start.

• **Read labels.** If you use packaged foods, read the labels so you can avoid chemicals, dyes, and preservatives that inhibit CA. Skip anything that contains potassium bromate or bromated flour; the preservatives tertiary butylhydroquinone (TBHQ), butylated hydroxyanisole (BHAQ), and butylated hydroxytoluene (BHT); and red dye #3 or #40, yellow #5 or #6, and blue #1.

• **Choose organic foods when possible.** Studies from the Environmental Working Group (EWG) have found organophosphate and pyrethroid pesticides, both of which inhibit CA, in up to 70 percent of analyzed urine samples. Choosing organic foods can lower those urinary levels in as little as one week, EWG researchers report.

• **Drink clean water.** Both tap and bottled water can contain lead, mercury, cadmium, chlorine, atrazine, fluoride, bisphenol, nonylphenol, and a variety of other toxins and pesticides that are linked to CA disruption. A reverse osmosis filter (countertop or whole house) removes most of these substances.

Calcium ATPase-Supporting Supplements

While whole, organic foods are almost always the best source of nutrients, it can sometimes be difficult to get a therapeutic dose through diet alone. *Alpha-lipoic acid and taurine are two such nutrients...*

● **Alpha-lipoic acid** protects CA activity in red blood cells during hyperglycemia and protects CA levels in the brain from toxins such as mercury and lead. Natural sources include organ and red meat, spinach, broccoli, tomatoes, and brussels sprouts. If you don't think you're getting enough from your diet, consider a supplement with a dosage of 600 to 1,800 mg daily.

● **Taurine** maintains red blood cell calcium levels in high glucose states and is heart protective. Taurine is found in animal products like fish, seafood, meat, poultry, eggs, and dairy products. Research has shown that taurine supplementation of 500 to 1,000 mg per day can have some profoundly positive health benefits in addition to its role in CA metabolism.

Before starting any supplement, it's imperative that you talk to your health-care team and buy from a reputable source. Look for third-party certification from a source like ConsumerLab.com.

—Dr. Russell Dahl

● **Avoid seafood with high mercury levels.** Good choices include salmon, trout, herring, shrimp, cod, catfish, crab, scallops, pollock, tilapia, whitefish, perch, flounder, and sole.

● **Avoid aluminum in cookware and cans.** Look for aluminum-free baking powders, and skip foods that contain the additive aluminosilicate, often used in soup mixes and nondairy creamers. Many antacids, such as Maalox, Mylanta, and Gaviscon, contain aluminum hydroxide. Aluminum foil, if used to cook acidic ingredients like tomatoes, citrus, and barbeque sauce, can seep aluminum into your food. Personal care products, such as cosmetics and antiperspirants, can be a source of aluminum, too.

● **Take care when grilling.** When fat from your food drips onto the coals and burns, it creates benzo(a)pyrenes, which have a negative effect on CA in the brain, red blood cells, and lungs. Reduce risk by putting the cooking surface as high as it will go and avoiding flareups.

● **Choose sunscreen and personal care products carefully.** Avoid products that include oxybenzone, avobenzone, octisalate, octocrylene, homosalate, and octinoxate. Avoid all sunscreen sprays. Instead, choose non-nanoparticle titanium dioxide and zinc oxide. Avoid nanoparticle titanium dioxide.

● **Clear the air.** Keep toxins out of your air as much as possible by upgrading your furnace and cooling system filters with electrostatic filters. Consider buying a HEPA stand-alone air filter, and use a vacuum with a HEPA filter and wet-mop floors once or twice a week.

Revive Cellular Energy With Coenzyme Q10

Jacob Teitelbaum, MD, cofounder of Kona Research Center, a nonprofit research organization that studies overlooked low-cost treatment options. He is the author of numerous books, including *Real Cause, Real Cure; From Fatigued to Fantastic!* and *Beat Sugar Addiction NOW!* Vitality101.com

You already know that organs are unique bodily structures, like your heart and lungs, that have specific and indispensable functions.

But you may not have heard of *organelles*, a word that means "little organs." Organelles are the organs of the cell—the microscopic structures that control cellular function, like the cell wall and the DNA-containing nucleus. One key organelle is the *mitochondria*, which numbers about 200 to 5,000 per cell.

Mitochondria are essential to cellular life because they produce energy. Most of that energy is generated in the form of adenosine triphosphate (ATP). ATP is to a cell what fuel is to a car.

ATP is manufactured in a molecular assembly line called the "electron transport chain"—and that process depends on the antioxidant coenzyme Q10 (CoQ10). Without CoQ10, your cells would run out of gas—and you'd run out of life. As a powerful antioxidant, CoQ10 protects cell membranes from oxidation, the internal rust that is a primary cause of aging and many chronic diseases. It also helps other antioxidants, like vitamins C and E, do their jobs. It cools chronic inflammation, another cause of chronic disease, and it helps regulate genes that control cellular growth and maintenance.

Given its importance to human health, it's no surprise that the body produces its own supply of CoQ10. Small amounts are also found in meat, chicken, and fish, but not enough to boost levels in the body. That's a potential problem because the cellular production of CoQ10 declines with age—an average 10 percent decrease every 10 years. In fact, many age-related diseases—including heart disease, diabetes, and Parkinson's disease—could benefit from supplementation with CoQ10, according to scientific studies.

Here's what you need to know to use CoQ10 to protect and improve your health.

High Blood Pressure

In one study, 10 weeks of treatment with CoQ10 (50 milligrams [mg], twice a day) decreased systolic blood pressure from 164.5 millimeters of mercury (mmHg) to 146.7 mmHg, and diastolic blood pressure from 98.1 mmHg to 86.1 mmHg.

Angina

In a small study by Japanese researchers, which was published in the *American Journal of Cardiology*, people with angina took either 150 mg of CoQ10 or a placebo for four weeks. Those taking the antioxidant had significantly increased exercise tolerance (time before angina pain) on a treadmill, a 53 per-cent reduction in angina episodes, and a 54 percent reduction in the number of nitroglycerin tablets needed to control pain.

Diabetes

Diabetes is a disease of chronically high blood sugar, affecting more than 37 million Americans. Another 95 million have prediabetes. High blood sugar increases the risk of heart disease, kidney failure, nerve damage, and Alzheimer's disease.

In a study published in the journal *BioFactors*, four months of daily treatment with 200 mg of CoQ10 lowered A1C (a measurement of long-term blood sugar levels) from 7.1 to 6.8—a significant drop. The researchers also found that CoQ10 helped control prediabetes.

Parkinson's Disease

In this disease, dopamine-producing cells of the brain shut down, causing muscular difficulties such as tremor, stiffness, slowed movement, and postural problems. In a meta-analysis of data from several studies, researchers found that taking high, therapeutic doses of CoQ10 (1,200 mg daily) improved the ability to walk normally and maintain a normal posture.

Migraines

This type of debilitating headache afflicts one in six Americans. In a study published in the journal *Neurology*, CoQ10 was three times more effective than a placebo in reducing the frequency of attacks, the average number of days people suffered with a migraine, and nausea (a common symptom).

In another study, people who took 150 to 200 mg of CoQ10 daily had a decrease in the average number of migraine attacks per month from 4.8 to 2.8.

Fibromyalgia

Afflicting about 4 million Americans, this disease causes widespread pain, tenderness, and sensitivity to touch. Most people with the illness—which strikes many more women than men—also have sleep problems and daytime fatigue. Research shows that people with fibromyalgia have low levels of CoQ10. In a small study, people with fibromyalgia who took 300 mg of CoQ10 daily had a significant reduction in pain.

The problem in fibromyalgia is not lack of effective treatment—it's a lack of effective physician education.

Mitochondrial Disorders

These are genetic disorders caused by the failure of the mitochondria to produce enough cellular energy. They afflict one in 4,300 Americans and can affect almost any part of the body, including the brain, heart, liver, kidneys, nerves, muscles, eyes, or ears.

In a study published in the journal *Muscle and Nerve*, researchers gave 30 patients with a mitochondrial disorder 1,200 mg of CoQ10 daily for 60 days. The treatment helped regulate biochemical imbalances in muscles and the brain.

Male Infertility

Oxidative damage of sperm cells is a likely cause for male infertility, and treatment with CoQ10 is a possible way to stop and reverse the damage. In a review of CoQ10 and male infertility in the journal *Antioxidants*, researchers found that supplementing with CoQ10 can improve the number of sperm (density), sperm movement (motility), the structural integrity of sperm (morphology), and increase the pregnancy rate.

Supplementation

CoQ10 comes in several forms: ubiquinol, ubiquinone, and semiquinone. By itself, a good form for supplementation is ubiquinol, which is absorbed three to four times better than ubiquinone.

For prevention and treatment, Dr. Teitelbaum typically recommends taking 200 mg daily with a meal that has some fat or oil in it to maximize absorption. For people with high blood pressure, heart problems, or di-

abetes (which raises the risk of cardiovascular disease), he usually recommends 400 mg daily for six weeks, and then 200 mg daily.

But new advances have changed his approach. A natural substance called *gamma-cyclodextrin* can increase the absorption of CoQ10 (and other nutrients) about eightfold. A CoQ10 supplement of 100 mg that includes gamma-cyclodextrin supplies the equivalent of 800 mg, with no worries about taking it with food for increased absorption

Is Vitamin D Spray as Good as a Capsule?

Pamela Magee, PhD, senior lecturer of human nutrition, Ulster University, Coleraine, Northern Ireland, UK.

A study comparing vitamin D3 capsules with an oral spray solution found that both were equally effective in raising levels of vitamin D in the blood. An oral spray may be better absorbed than capsules or chewable tablets. Other research suggests that sprays are good for people with digestive issues, since the vitamin is absorbed from the oral cavity directly into the bloodstream.

Do You Really Need That Supplement?

Renee Miranda, MD, DABMA, ETSU Health provider, assistant professor of family medicine, integrative medicine and medical acupuncture at East Tennessee State University, Johnson City, Tennessee.

According to the Centers for Disease Control and Prevention (CDC), 58 percent of US adults report taking a dietary supplement in the past 30 days...and one-quarter of people age 60 and older take four or more daily. In fact, Americans spent nearly $60 billion on dietary supplements in 2020 alone.

There was a time when swallowing handfuls of supplements was seen among older adults as evidence of their dedication to a healthy lifestyle. But we now know that people who consume a balanced diet and are in good health are likely getting all the nutrients they need.

Still, some supplements can fill in nutritional gaps for people who have food allergies…eat lots of junk food and eschew healthy produce…or avoid entire categories of food—picky eaters, vegans or people who skip, say, soy or dairy products because they fear they're unhealthy (they're not).

We asked integrative medicine specialist Renee Miranda, MD, who should be taking supplements…and which ones.

Do You Need a Supplement?

When a patient asks me about supplementation, my first two questions are, "What does your diet look like?" and "What is your goal?"

What does your diet look like? A varied diet rich in whole foods such as fruits, vegetables, beans and legumes, grains, dairy and protein provides all the required nutrients, so theoretically the only people who need supplementation are those with gaps in their diets.

To evaluate your diet: Keep a food log for three consecutive days, including at least one weekend day. Note portion sizes and preparation methods. This log can give you and your doctor an idea of any nutrient gaps.

To improve your diet, a good place to start is the American Heart Association recommendations (Heart.org). I recommend six to nine servings of fruits and vegetables daily…two to three servings of quality protein mainly from plant sources such as legumes (if you prefer animal products, lean toward unprocessed meats)…one to three servings of whole grains…and an occasional serving of nuts and seeds.

What is your goal? Some people want to improve their heart health, and they have read that a supplement might help…or they have been told that multivitamins boost overall wellness. New research is constantly emerging about whether certain supplements live up to the hype. Oftentimes, they don't.

A 2018 meta-analysis in *Journal of the American College of Cardiology* determined that supplementing with a multivitamin, vitamin D, calcium or vitamin C does not significantly reduce risk for heart attack or stroke or of dying from any cause. Also, supplementing with large amounts of certain antioxidants—found naturally in fruits and vegetables—may work *against* your goals by increasing risk for certain types of cancer or chronic diseases. This may be because some fat-soluble vitamins—such as A, D, E and K—are stored in the body for long periods and can accumulate to toxic levels when taken in large doses. And new research suggests that high doses of supplemental antioxidants may even *protect* cancer cells from the body's natural cancer-fighting process.

There are, however, instances when supplements make sense.

Example: Many older adults are deficient in vitamin B-12, especially those who regularly take acid-suppressing medication, such as *esomeprazole* (Nexium), *omeprazole* (Prilosec) and *lansoprazole* (Prevacid). Vitamin B-12 is critical for healthy functioning of the brain and nervous system.

Which Supplements Should You Take?

Here are the supplements that I recommend for certain patients and why…and how to get the most out of them…

•**Vitamin D** does everything from boost calcium absorption from foods (crucial for bone strength) to strengthen the immune system. Yet nearly one-half of Americans are deficient.

Reasons: Vitamin D isn't found in many foods besides oily fish such as salmon, fortified milk and juice, and UV-B-light–boosted mushrooms…we spend so much time indoors (depriving our skin of sunlight, which the body needs to produce vitamin D)…and when we are outside, we use sunscreen.

Also: Older adults, people with obesity, darker-skinned individuals and people living in colder, grayer climates are at increased risk for deficiency.

What to do: Ask your health-care provider for a blood test to assess your vitamin D level. If it is low, the doctor may recommend 400 international units (IU) to 600 IU daily... or a 50,000-IU pill weekly for four weeks. If your level is around 40 ng/mL—the lower end of normal—and you feel tired, that also suggests supplementation may be useful.

Encouraging: New research shows that older people in China who maintain healthy vitamin D levels had less cognitive impairment and healthier lipid levels than their deficient counterparts.

Note: Vitamin D is fat-soluble—it needs to be combined with a little fat to be absorbed. Swallow the supplement with a plant-based source of fat such as avocado or some almonds, walnuts or other nuts and seeds. Vitamin D also needs magnesium to be activated, so get enough of this mineral.

•**Vitamin B-12.** As you age, the stomach produces less and less *hydrochloric acid*, a compound needed to absorb B-12 from food. For the same reason, people taking acid-reducing medications may have lower levels of B-12.

Vegans (people who eat no animal products) and some vegetarians (people who don't eat meat) may need supplemental B-12 because B-12 is available only in animal products or fortified foods such as breakfast cereal and nutritional yeast. Individuals with celiac disease or Crohn's disease also may be deficient because their gut doesn't absorb the nutrient efficiently from food.

The average adult needs 2.4 micrograms (mcg) of vitamin B-12 a day. Supplements contain about 1,000 mcg to 2,000 mcg—so you'll need to supplement only a few times a week. Any excess will be excreted in your urine. Ask your doctor for guidance.

•**Magnesium.** About half the US population is magnesium-deficient, yet this mineral has a hand in dozens of bodily systems. It promotes regular bowel movements, calms anxiety, promotes sleep and more. Magnesium also converts food into energy, so low levels can cause fatigue.

Foods high in magnesium: Nuts, seeds, beans, whole grains, leafy green veggies and some fortified foods.

Adults absorb less magnesium as they grow older. People with type 2 diabetes lose magnesium in their urine, and certain medications can reduce magnesium levels. These include bisphosphonates such as *alendronate* (Fosamax) for osteoporosis...loop diuretics such as *furosemide* (Lasix) for high blood pressure...and prescription proton pump inhibitors such as *esomeprazole* (Nexium).

A blood test can check for magnesium deficiency, but there's little risk from supplementing. These supplements come in different forms, including *magnesium citrate* (recommended for constipation) and *magnesium chloride* (better suited for sleep and anxiety). Start with 200 mg a day, and see if symptoms improve. You can slowly move up to 400 mg/day. Toxicity symptoms at higher doses or due to inability to eliminate excess magnesium (common among people with kidney disease) include gastrointestinal upset, flushing, weakness and palpitations.

Warning: Start low, and go slow—magnesium citrate supplements can have a laxative effect. If you take any of the previously mentioned medications, space them several hours apart from your supplement.

Miraculous Magnesium

Lina Velikova, MD, PhD, medical advisor for Supplements101.net. She is an assistant professor at Sofia University St. Kliment Ohridski, Sofia, Bulgaria, and is a member of the editorial board of the *World Journal of Immunology*.

An essential mineral, magnesium is involved in blood glucose control, blood pressure regulation, muscle and nerve function, and protein synthesis.

When a person is deficient—as an estimated 50 percent of Americans are—the effects can be widespread, causing symptoms as varied as fatigue, loss of appetite, seizures, abnormal heart rhythms, and even personality changes. *Even if someone isn't deficient, low levels of magnesium can affect a variety of bodily systems...*

• **Sleep.** Magnesium regulates the nervous system, particularly the neurotransmitters that pass information back and forth from the body to the brain. It promotes relaxation, which improves the ability to fall asleep faster and obtain better sleep quality.

• **Asthma.** By relaxing the bronchial muscles and widening the airways, magnesium can alleviate asthma symptoms. It is not a first-line treatment but adding a magnesium supplement to traditional asthma medications can help prevent acute asthma attacks.

• **Anxiety and depression.** Magnesium has a vital role in the healthy functioning of the brain. There's a link between low magnesium levels and anxiety, which suggests that taking a supplement may ease anxiety. A cross-sectional study of close to 20,000 people published in 2019 reported that people who had more magnesium in their diets had lower rates of depression.

• **Type 2 diabetes.** Magnesium is essential for insulin metabolism and glucose control. Research has shown that most diabetics suffer from magnesium insufficiency and that magnesium helps manage the disease by improving insulin sensitivity. A meta-analysis published in the *Journal of Internal Medicine* in 2007 found that a 100 milligram (mg) per day increase in total magnesium intake decreased the risk of diabetes by 15 percent.

• **Blood pressure.** Adequate daily magnesium intake from food or supplements can decrease systolic and diastolic blood pressure in people who have both high blood pressure and magnesium deficiency. When blood vessels are narrowed or constricted, blood pressure rises, but magnesium reduces that constriction, allowing the blood to flow more freely. One meta-analysis of 22 studies concluded that magnesium supplementation decreased systolic blood pressure by 3 to 4

mmHg and diastolic blood pressure by 2 to 3 mmHg.

That may be why researchers found that people with serum magnesium levels in the highest quartile of normal (at least 0.88 millimoles per liter [mmol/L]) had a 38 percent lower risk of sudden cardiac death than people with levels in the lowest quartile (0.75 mmol/L or less).

• **Osteoporosis.** The National Institutes of Health reports that women with osteopenia and osteoporosis have lower serum magnesium levels than women without those conditions, suggesting that magnesium deficiency might be a risk factor for osteoporosis. Furthermore, several studies suggest a positive correlation between magnesium intake and bone mineral density in both men and women.

• **Migraine headaches.** A review of three placebo-controlled studies found that 600 mg per day of supplemental magnesium led to a small reduction in migraine frequency. The American Headache Society and the American Academy of Neurology note that magnesium supplementation should be considered for migraine prevention because evidence suggests that it is "probably effective."

The strongest evidence has been found in people who experience migraine auras and in women who have menstrual-related migraines.

Boosting Magnesium

The recommended dietary allowance for magnesium depends on age and sex. Women need about 310 mg each day when they are between 19 and 30 years old, and 320 mg after age 31. Men should aim for 400 mg through age 30, then bump up to 420 mg. A wide variety of foods are excellent sources of magnesium. (See page 245.)

You can also take a supplement. Magnesium supplements come in different forms, and absorption and bioavailability vary by type. Opt for magnesium citrate when available. If not, look for magnesium lactate and magnesium chloride, both of which are absorbed better than magnesium oxide and magnesium sulfate.

Prolonged soaking in Epsom salts may also increase magnesium levels in the blood.

Side Effects

The most common side effect of magnesium supplementation is diarrhea. In fact, magnesium can also be used as a treatment for constipation. High doses can cause nausea and abdominal cramping. Very large doses (more than 5,000 mg/day) have been associated with magnesium toxicity, which can cause hypotension, nausea, vomiting, flushing, urine retention, depression, muscle weakness, difficulty breathing, irregular heartbeat, and cardiac arrest.

Medication Complications

Before taking a magnesium supplement, talk to your doctor about potential medication interactions. Magnesium can decrease the absorption of oral bisphosphonates, such as *alendronate* (Fosamax), so they should be taken at least two hours apart. Similarly, if you're taking a tetracycline antibiotic, such as *demeclocycline* (Declomycin) and *doxycycline* (Vibramycin), or a quinolone antibiotic, such as *ciprofloxacin* (Cipro) and *levofloxacin* (Levaquin), take the magnesium two hours before the antibiotic.

Eat Your Magnesium

Many common foods are excellent sources of the mineral…

Nuts
Almonds, 1 oz, 80 mg
Peanut butter, 2 Tbsp, 49 mg
Cashews, 1 oz, 74 mg

Seeds
Pumpkin seeds, 1 oz, 168 mg
Flaxseed, 2 Tbsp, 78 mg
Chia seeds, 1 oz, 111 mg

Whole grains
Brown rice, ½ cup, 42 mg
Dry buckwheat, 1 oz, 65 mg
Shredded wheat, 2 biscuits, 61 mg
Oatmeal, instant, 1 packet, 36 mg
Bread, whole wheat, 1 slice, 23 mg

Beans
Black beans, cooked, ½ cup, 60 mg
Kidney beans, ½ cup, 35 mg
Edamame, ⅓ cup, 50 mg

Fruits and vegetables
Spinach, cooked, 157 mg
Potato with skin, 3.5 oz, 43 mg
Banana, 32 mg
Raisins, ½ cup, 23 mg
Avocado, ½ cup, 22 mg
Broccoli, ½ cup, 12 mg
Apple, 1 medium, 9 mg
Carrot, raw, 1 medium, 7 mg

Meats
Salmon, 3 oz, 26 mg
Chicken breast, 3 oz, 22 mg
Beef, 3 oz, 22 mg
Halibut, 3 oz, 24 mg

Dairy and dairy replacements
Milk, 1 percent, 1 cup, 39 mg
Yogurt, 1 cup, 30 mg
Soy milk, 1 cup, 61 mg

Melatonin: Sorting Fact from Fiction

Cinthya Pena-Orbea, MD, a sleep specialist at the Cleveland Clinic, Ohio.

For anyone who has ever suffered from insomnia, an over-the-counter supplement like melatonin is alluring. But before you stock up, it's helpful to have a realistic understanding of what this hormone can—and can't—do.

Natural Melatonin

Your body already makes its own melatonin. Nestled in the center of the brain, the pineal gland communicates with receptors in the retina—the back of the eye—to know when it's light or dark. When it senses darkness, it releases high levels of melatonin to prepare you for sleep. When it senses light, it shuts melatonin production down.

Around age 40, your body begins to produce less melatonin, which can lead to age-related sleep problems. By age 90, melatonin levels are a mere 20 percent of what they were in your young adult years.

Whatever your age, you can help melatonin do its job by taking a few simple steps…

•**Keep the lights low before bed.** Even dim light can interfere with a person's circadian rhythm and melatonin secretion. Just eight lux—less than a table lamp—has an effect.

•**Avoid blue light from computers, smartphones, and tablets for two to three hours before bed.** If you can't avoid them, try using a blue-light filter or an app, like F. Lux or Night Shift to adjust your screens to night-time mode. Compact fluorescent lightbulbs and LED lights produce more blue light than incandescent lightbulbs.

•**Dim red light is the best choice for nightlights.**

•**Get exposure to daylight during the morning.** Sunlight helps your body produce serotonin, which is the precursor to melatonin.

Melatonin can also be found in various foods, including corn, cucumbers, asparagus, olives, pomegranate, nuts, seeds, barley, and rolled oats. Studies have reported that consumption of kiwis, tart cherry juice, and salmon may improve sleep, too.

Supplemental Melatonin

Melatonin affects when you fall asleep, not how quickly, so taking a melatonin supplement is far from a cure-all for insomnia. In fact, studies show that it may shave a mere seven or eight minutes off your wait to fall asleep and lengthen sleep time by about the same—hardly a cure for standard insomnia. The American College of Physicians guidelines strongly recommend the use of cognitive behavioral therapy for insomnia (CBT-I) instead. (See sidebar.)

But sleep disorders that aren't simple insomnia are different. Because melatonin af-

Cognitive Behavioral Therapy for Insomnia

Cognitive behavioral therapy for insomnia (CBT-I) helps people with insomnia identify and replace thoughts and behaviors that cause or worsen sleep problems with habits that promote sound sleep. *The therapy has multiple components…*

•**Sleep hygiene.** These are practices that foster and maintain sleep, such as keeping the bedroom dark and quiet, participating in regular exercise, and limiting the consumption of caffeine, alcohol, and tobacco.

•**Stimulus control therapy** trains your brain to associate your bed with sleep or sex and nothing else. It means no working, watching television, or worrying while lying in bed.

•**Relaxation training** uses practices such as progressive muscle relaxation and diaphragmatic breathing to create a positive state for sleep.

•**Cognitive therapy** helps you identify and challenge incorrect and unhelpful thoughts about sleep, such as "I know this is going to be a bad night. I won't feel rested tomorrow. Why can't I sleep like everyone else?"

To find a CBT-I provider, visit https://cbti. directory/index.php/search-for-a-provider. The Cleveland Clinic offers a six-week-long online program, *Go to Sleep*. Learn more at https://clevelandclinicwellness.com/pages/ GoToSleep.htm.

—Dr. Cinthya Pena-Orbea

fects your circadian rhythm, it can help with issues such as delayed sleep phase syndrome, which is when you consistently fall asleep very late and wake up late the next day.

It may help shift workers, who often struggle to work at night when melatonin levels naturally rise and to sleep during the day when they fall. Studies suggest, however, that light therapy is more effective than melatonin supplements.

The strongest case for supplemental melatonin comes from studies on jet lag. Multiple studies show that taking melatonin close to bedtime when you arrive in a different time zone can help reduce lag symptoms.

Dosage

There is no general consensus regarding dosage. Melatonin supplements often come in doses of 3 to 5 milligrams (mg), but studies suggest that as little as 0.3 to 0.5 mg per day might be more effective than higher doses in many people. Taking too much of the hormone can cause morning grogginess, headaches, reduced focus, and dizziness, so it's best to start small. (You might have to get a 1 mg tablet and cut it in half to do so.)

Take melatonin about an hour or two before bedtime to give it time to work. Don't take it in the morning, as it can reset your internal clock in an unintended way.

Safety

Short-term use of melatonin supplements appears to be safe, but there isn't enough data to assess long-term safety. Be careful of mixing it with other drugs. Melatonin can have interactions with other drugs such as blood thinners, anticonvulsants, some blood pressure medications, and diabetes medications. Melatonin may stay active for a longer time in older people, and it can cause dizziness and drowsiness that can increase the risk of falls.

In 2017, researchers tested 31 melatonin supplements and found that the amount of melatonin in the product didn't match what was listed on the product label in most cases. They found serotonin in more than a quarter of sampled products.

Prebiotics Could Help With Sleep Disruption

Michael Breus, PhD, is a clinical psychologist and sleep expert in private practice, Manhattan Beach, California, commenting on a study published in *Brain, Behavior and Immunity.*

Rodents with disrupted sleep cycles slept better when fed prebiotics—starchy foods such as artichokes and onions that allow gut bacteria to flourish, according to a recent study. While further research may uncover more about the effects of prebiotiotics on sleep, including them in your diet might help with jet lag or if you work a night shift.

The Science Behind Acupuncture

Ania Grimone, MS, a licensed acupuncturist and Chinese herbalist with the Northwestern Medicine Osher Center for Integrative Medicine in Chicago.

For 3,000 years, acupuncture has been a staple of Chinese health care, where it is regularly used to treat conditions as diverse as insomnia, pain, and the symptoms of menopause.

In the United States, the history of the practice is shorter—the first legal acupuncture center opened in 1972—but acupuncture is now the most widely used alternative medical practice in the nation.

It's supported by an impressive body of research, offered by some of the most respected academic medical institutions, including the Mayo Clinic and Harvard Medical School, and covered by several major insurers. Even the U.S. Army endorses it as a treatment for chronic pain.

Theory of Acupuncture

In acupuncture, thin, sterile needles are gently inserted through the skin at different points in the torso, limbs, and head. These points are positioned along a network of pathways called meridians that are dotted with acupuncture points, also called acupoints.

Traditional Chinese medicine practitioners believe that organs, tissues, muscles, and ligaments are all connected, and that meridians run the length of the body, so the needle placement is often unexpected. For example, chronic headaches may be treated with needles on the hands and ankles as well as the head. Upper back and shoulder pain, for instance, is associated with a blockage in the bladder meridian, which has 67 acupoints starting at the eye, crossing the forehead, running down the back of the head, past the buttocks, and ending at the pinky toes.

When an acupuncturist stimulates acupoints with needles, it signals the brain and body to produce endogenous opioids, powerful pain-relieving chemicals, anti-inflammatory compounds, immune-boosting compounds, hormones, and vasodilators that increase blood circulation. Traditional acupuncturists also believe that stimulating acupoints releases blockages in the body's flow of energy, called *qi* (pronounced chee). For many people, that stimulation translates to pain relief.

Proven Pain Relief

In a report published in the National Institute for Health Research Journals Library, researchers reviewed 29 clinical trials and concluded that adding acupuncture to standard medical care (anti-inflammatory medications and physical therapy) reduced the severity of neck and lower back pain, significantly reduced the number of headaches and migraines, and eased the pain and disability of osteoarthritis. The American College of Physicians recommends acupuncture and other non-pharmacologic therapies as first-line treatments for patients experiencing chronic low-back pain.

It's even used for pain relief in veterinary medicine. Studies show it can ease chronic spinal and osteoarthritic pain, as well as acute pain from neuromusculoskeletal injuries and surgery. Since animals don't have expectations for a treatment to work, veterinary applications offer exciting evidence that acupuncture offers more than a placebo effect.

Alzheimer's Disease

In a 2019 review article published in *Frontiers in Psychiatry*, researchers reported that acupuncture may be beneficial for people with Alzheimer's disease. They cite multiple small studies that have found that acupuncture can improve mood and cognition and increase verbal and motor skills. A clinical trial with 87 patients found that acupuncture improved cognitive function better than the medication *donepezil* (Aricept), with benefits that lasted for 12 weeks.

Hot Flashes

Acupuncture also appears to ease hot flashes from breast cancer treatment and menopause. In a *Journal of Clinical Oncology* study of breast cancer patients experiencing treatment-related hot flashes, those who received weekly acupuncture as part of a three-month self-care regimen including exercise, nutrition, and psychological support had hot flash scores (calculated as the frequency of hot flashes multiplied by the average severity) that were 50 percent lower than those in the acupuncture-free self-care protocol. Importantly, the benefits continued for six months after the acupuncture ended.

In another study, women who underwent five weeks of acupuncture had fewer hot flashes, less frequent and less severe night sweats, and fewer sleep, skin, and hair problems than women in the control group.

Acupuncture may provide these benefits by dilating blood vessels, similar to what hormone replacement therapy does, and triggering the release of endorphins (stress- and pain-relieving chemicals) and hormones related to mood regulation.

Fight Insomnia and Depression

After reviewing 46 clinical trials, researchers reported in the peer-reviewed *Journal of Al-*

ternative and *Complementary Medicine* that acupuncture independently improves sleep quality and duration and amplifies the benefits of other insomnia interventions. A different team in 2020 reported that eight weeks of electroacupuncture (acupuncture with mild electrical stimulation) improved the quality and quantity of people's sleep, and significantly improved depression symptoms.

Depression and Anxiety

Many studies have reported that acupuncture can ease depression. At least one has found that it may be more effective than medication. Similarly, studies show that it can treat both general and preoperative anxiety. The quality of these studies, however, tends to be low—but so are the risks as long as you visit a certified acupuncture practitioner who uses sterile or single-use needles. (To find an acupuncturist, visit NCCAOM.org.)

What to Expect

For many people, the largest barrier to trying acupuncture is a fear of needles, but the most you should feel is a small pinch, if anything at all. Once the needle is in, you may have a mild awareness that something is there, but you won't experience pain.

On average, sessions last about 25 minutes. Many acupuncturists will treat acute issues twice a week and chronic conditions once a week, continuing until the problem is resolved or you've hit a plateau in improvement. In general, newer health problems resolve more quickly than chronic issues.

Acupuncture tends to have very few side effects, although some people may experience minor bleeding or soreness at the insertion sites. It can lower blood pressure and blood sugar levels, depending on which acupoints are stimulated, so be sure to hydrate and eat before your session.

Home Remedy for Knee Pain: Pectin and Grape Juice

Terry Graedon, PhD, medical anthropologist and leading authority on the science behind folk remedies, and cohost of *The People's Pharmacy* radio show and website, writing at PeoplesPharmacy.com.

Although there is no scientific research to back up the claims, many people swear that this folk remedy eases arthritis knee pain.

To try it: Liquid pectin, such as Certo brand used for making jams and jellies, is easiest to use. Mix one tablespoon of liquid pectin in eight ounces of purple grape juice, and drink daily.

Alternative: Some people get more relief taking the mixture two or three times a day. To do that, mix two teaspoons of liquid pectin in three ounces of purple grape juice per dose.

Natural Remedies for Warts

Healthline.com

Aloe vera—remove a leaf from an aloe plant, apply the gel to the wart, and repeat daily. *Apple cider vinegar* can help peel away infected skin—mix two parts of the vinegar with one part water, soak a cotton

Bananas for Poison Ivy

If you've been exposed to poison ivy, first wash the area with soap and water to remove the urushiol resin that causes the extremely uncomfortable blisters and itching. If you start to get itchy, you may get some relief by rubbing the rash with the inside of a banana peel—the riper, the better. Scientists have yet to study this, but there's plenty of anecdotal evidence that it helps.

Joe Graedon, pharmacologist and cofounder of The People's Pharmacy. PeoplesPharmacy.com

ball in the solution, place it on the wart and leave it on for three to four hours. *Banana peel*—try rubbing the inside of the peel on the wart daily. *Dandelion weed*—break apart a dandelion, squeeze out the sticky white sap from the stem, and apply to the wart once or twice a day for two weeks. *Garlic*—crush a clove, mix with water, apply to the wart, cover with a bandage, and repeat daily for three to four weeks. *Pineapple*—rub fresh pineapple on the wart daily. *Potato*—cut a small one in half, rub the cut side on the wart, and repeat twice a day. There is little or no scientific evidence for most of these remedies, but they are easy to try, and some people report success using them.

Drinking Tea Boosts Brain Health

Study by researchers at National University of Singapore, published in *Aging*.

Brain regions of people age 60 and older who had been drinking tea at least four times a week for 25 years were more efficiently interconnected than the brain areas of people who did not drink tea. The type of tea did not matter—the effect was found with green, oolong and black tea. This means that long-term tea drinking may help protect against age-related declines in cognitive function.

Chapter 12

PAIN RELIEF AND AUTOIMMUNE DISEASE

Drug-Free Headache Relief

People who suffer from chronic headaches have seen some exciting therapeutic advances over the past few years, but, for many, the excitement is short-lived. Even the newest medications don't help everyone, and side effects can range from uncomfortable to intolerable.

Lawrence Taw, MD, has met and treated hundreds of these patients with headaches in his role as director of the UCLA Center for East-West Medicine, where he recommends a more holistic approach. Here, he explains how incorporating natural medicine can make a world of difference for some patients.

How do natural healing approaches treat headache pain?

Dr. Taw: Headaches are often triggered or worsened by things like skipping meals, losing sleep, or even changing altitude. The body likes a healthy routine, and it perceives disruptions to our daily rhythms as stress on the system.

In response to this perceived stress, the body protects itself by tightening up. Most patients struggling with headaches have co-existing tension in their neck and shoulder muscles, but there's tension below the surface, too. Constriction of blood vessels and changes to blood flow may also contribute to headache pain.

How can people ease that tension without medications?

Dr. Taw: One way to reduce this tension is to do a mind-body exercise called tai chi, which combines continuous movement with gentle stretching and deep breathing—the body's way of turning off the stress response. While scientists don't know the exact mechanisms at play, we suspect that tai chi is effective because it relaxes the body and muscles.

In a study conducted at the UCLA Center for East-West Medicine, we learned that patients who participated in a 15-week-long tai chi program had less headache pain as well as more energy and better emotional well-being. Because tai chi is so gentle, it's an excellent option for people of any age or ability. You can start with a five-minute

---

Lawrence B. Taw, MD, the director of the UCLA Center for East-West Medicine–Torrance. Dr. Taw is board certified by both the American Board of Internal Medicine and the American Board of Integrative and Holistic Medicine and is also certified in Oriental Medicine, Acupuncture and Herbology by the National Certification Commission for Acupuncture and Oriental Medicine.

session and work your way up to about 30 minutes.

You can find a tai chi class near you by visiting the Tai Chi Foundation at TaiChiFoundation.org to use their class directory. You can also purchase DVDs or find free videos on the Internet so you can practice in your own home.

What is the role of acupuncture in managing headaches?

Dr. Taw: In our clinic, acupuncture consistently shows positive results. It reduces tension, promotes local circulation, and causes the body to release its own endorphins, which are natural painkillers. Researchers using functional MRI studies have demonstrated that acupuncture stimulation of a commonly needled point on the hand has specific effects on the limbic system, the stress and emotional regulatory center of the brain.

A review of 22 clinical trials that was published in the *Cochrane Database of Systematic Reviews* found that acupuncture may be as effective as migraine preventive medications. Headache frequency decreased by half in up to 59 percent of the 5,000 people who were in the study, and, for some people, the effects lasted for more than six months.

What do you suggest for people who don't have access to an acupuncturist or who are not comfortable with the needles used in the practice?

Dr. Taw: At the UCLA Center for East-West Medicine, we teach patients how to apply acupressure to specific points, which can produce similar effects to acupuncture. *For example...*

• **Large intestine 4.** Applying pressure to this point, which lies on the hand between the thumb and index finger may relieve stress, neck tension, and headaches.

• **Gallbladder 20.** Also, when resting your head between both hands with fingers interlaced, you can use both thumbs to apply pressure on the points where the neck muscles attach to the base of skull to help alleviate neck tension and headaches.

• **Triple heater 3.** Applying pressure between the knuckles of the pinky and ring finger may ease neck pain, shoulder pain, and tension headaches.

At the UCLA Center for East-West Medicine, we suggest that patients apply pressure to targeted points for 30 to 60 seconds twice per day.

What supplements can help people with headaches?

Dr. Taw: There are several promising over-the-counter supplements...

• **Magnesium** is a well-studied supplement that relaxes muscles and, as a result, has a wide range of therapeutic applications. It eases constipation, improves asthma symptoms, may help you sleep better, and shows promise in treating tension headaches.

A common starting dose is 200 to 400 milligrams (mg). Magnesium oxide is difficult to absorb, so look for magnesium glycinate or citrate.

If you get loose stools (a common side effect and the reason it's often used as a treatment for constipation), lower your dose. If you have kidney disease, talk to your doctor before taking magnesium.

• **Feverfew,** some studies suggest, may help prevent migraine and other types of headaches, reduce their frequency, and lessen related symptoms such as pain, light sensitivity, nausea, and vomiting.

The recommended dosage is 50 to 150 mg daily. Don't take feverfew if you are sensitive to ragweed, as it can cause an allergic reaction.

• **Riboflavin** (vitamin B2), has been shown to reduce both headache frequency and the need for pain-relieving medications.

The recommended dosage is 400 mg daily. Don't take riboflavin before bed, as it can give you a boost of energy that may interfere with sleep.

• **Coenzyme Q10** can reduce the severity, frequency, and duration of migraine headaches.

The recommended dosage is 100 mg three times daily. It is best to take this during the day, as it may help fatigue.

• **Essential oils.** Menthol, eucalyptus, rosemary, and lavender oils have a calming effect that may ease tension and headaches. But be careful because, for some people, strong smells can trigger a headache

---

The Problem with Pain Medications

Harrison Linder, MD, offers pain management therapies at The Center for Interventional Pain Medicine at Mercy Medical Center in Baltimore.

D o you take painkillers every day for head pain? Your headaches might begin to feel worse.

Any acute pain medication can serve as a trigger of what we call medication overuse headaches (MOH), but it's not seen as often in nonsteroidal anti-inflammatory drugs (NSAIDs), such as aspirin, as it is with migraine and opiate medications.

According to the most recent diagnostic definitions, MOH is a headache occurring 15 or more days per month, along with overuse of acute headache medication for more than three months. The exact mechanism of MOH is unclear, but experts think the overuse of headache medications may deplete serotonin while increasing the production of other neurotransmitters to increase sensitivity to pain.

Typical treatment involves weaning off the overused medication. Some studies have shown that it's better to completely avoid the medication than to use it less frequently. While transitioning off the medication, you can use headache medications from another class and focus on nonpharmacologic treatments, such as cognitive-behavioral therapy, relaxation training, lifestyle modification, and trigger avoidance. There can be an initial worsening of headaches within the first few days of weaning. Typically, withdrawal symptoms are thought to last up to 10 days.

Regardless of whether NSAID use is contributing to chronic headaches, these medications can be associated with gastrointestinal discomfort and ulcers, along with effects on the heart and kidneys, so it's important to use them only as directed. If your headaches continue to occur daily, you may need to see a headache/migraine specialist for further exploration.

Fatty Fish Reduces Headache Frequency

A diet high in fatty fish and low in vegetable seed oils reduces headache frequency by up to 40 percent. Fatty fish such as tuna and salmon triggers production of molecules that seem to reduce pain in headache-relevant tissues...while the linoleic acid in vegetable oils has the opposite effect.

For cooking: Choose low linoleic acid oils such as olive, coconut, and macadamia—or butter.

Daisy Zamora, PhD, assistant professor at University of North Carolina at Chapel Hill and co-lead author of a National Institutes of Health–funded study of 182 migraineurs published in *The BMJ*.

New Treatments for Migraine Pain

Brian M. Grosberg, MD, director of the Hartford HealthCare Headache Center and professor of neurology at University of Connecticut School of Medicine, Farmington. He was named one of Connecticut's Best Doctors in 2019 by *Connecticut Magazine* and is a member of the Migraine Research Foundation's Medical Advisory Board. HartfordHealthCare.org

I f you've ever had a migraine—almost 40 million people in the US suffer them regularly—you know that it is far more than a typical headache. Yes, there is intense, throbbing pain, typically on just one side of the head, that can last between four hours and three days. But a migraine can be accompanied by nausea and vomiting...dizziness... numbness in your arms, legs and/or face... and extreme sensitivity to light, sound, and odors. You also may experience aura—a visual or other disturbance that signals a migraine is on the way.

Migraine runs in families and can be triggered by many things—stress...consumption of alcoholic and caffeinated beverages...caffeine withdrawal...eating aged and unpasteurized cheeses and cured meats...lack of or too much sleep...overexposure to the sun... changes in weather...and use of certain medications such as birth control pills.

Thankfully, new treatments are available now and more are in development.

•**New medications.** Doctors used to believe that migraine was simply caused by overdilation and constriction of blood vessels in the head. But new research shows that migraine involves a cascade of events in the brain, including activation of the trigeminal nerve—a large nerve in the skull that is responsible for sensation in the face and motor functions such as biting and chewing—and the release of calcitonin gene-related peptide (CGRP). It appears that CGRP irritates nerve endings in the brain and inflames and dilates blood vessels. *This discovery has led to the development of new types of migraine-preventive medications...*

•CGRP monoclonal antibodies. One of the drugs in this class, *erenumab* (Aimovig), mimics the shape of CGRP and binds to the CGRP nerve receptors so that the peptide has no place to attach when it arrives at a nerve cell—this prevents pain. The other three drugs in this class—*galcanezumab* (Emgality)...*fremanezumab* (Ajovy)...and *eptinezumab* (Vyepti)—attach to CGRP itself, changing its shape so that it can't fit into the receptor. Aimovig, Ajovy and Emgality can be self-administered monthly or quarterly via an autoinjector. Vyepti is administered intravenously every three months by a health-care provider.

•Gepants. Also known as CGRP inhibitors, gepants work similarly to CGRP monoclonal antibodies, but they contain smaller molecules and so can be taken orally. *Ubroge-*

pant (Ubrelvy) and *rimegepant* (Nurtec) are taken as needed to stop migraine attacks. Recently, Nurtec received approval for use as a preventive treatment, too, meaning that it can be taken regularly during the month to help prevent migraine. *Atogepant* (Qulipta) also has received FDA approval for migraine prevention. *Zavegepant* is awaiting FDA approval.

•Ditans. *Lasmiditan* (Reyvow) is the first approved drug in the "ditan" family, another new class of medication for migraine treatment. Ditans are close relatives of triptans (see below) but are more selective in their effects on the brain—meaning that they work on different types of serotonin receptors than triptans. This allows them to have no effects on the cardiovascular system.

Warning: Ditans are potentially sedating, so lasmitidan has been labeled a controlled substance with a restriction against driving for eight hours after you take it. This side effect limits the drug's widespread use, but it may be helpful for people whose migraine attacks usually occur at night or awaken them from sleep.

•**Standard medications.** Before CGRP inhibitors became available a few years ago, the class of drugs known as triptans was used to treat migraine. The first triptan—*sumatriptan* (Imitrex)—was approved by the Food and Drug Administration (FDA) in 1991. Others have since been released, including *almotriptan* (Axert), *eletriptan* (Relpax), *frovatriptan* (Frova), *naratriptan* (Amerge), *rizatriptan* (Maxalt) and *zolmitriptan* (Zomig). Depending on the triptan, these drugs are available as pills, injectables and nasal sprays. For some people, a single dose of a triptan can bring migraine relief within a few hours. But for 20 percent to 30 percent of people impacted by migraine, a second dose is needed.

•**Gepants vs. triptans.** *There are pros and cons for gepants and triptans...*

•Heart problems. Triptans may constrict blood vessels, which could cause heart attack or chest pain in people who have ischemic heart disease and/or poorly controlled high blood pressure. Gepants appear to be safer because they don't narrow blood vessels.

•Rebound headaches. Gepants aren't as likely as triptans to cause rebound headaches from overuse of the medication.

•Efficacy Gepants often aren't as effective as triptans—only about 20 percent of people impacted by migraine find complete relief within two hours after taking a gepant (versus 64 percent for injectable sumatriptan).

But: Gepants are more likely to be effective when a migraine is already underway. Triptans, on the other hand, work best when taken at the very start of a migraine.

•**Nondrug treatments.** There are a number of brain-modulating devices that have recently received FDA clearance for migraine treatment. They can be used safely by all people impacted by migraine and are particularly helpful for people who don't find relief with medications or don't want to take medications. These devices effectively eliminate head pain in 30 percent to 40 percent of sufferers within two hours of using them. *Examples…*

•Cefaly Dual is a small device that is placed on the center of the forehead to prevent migraine as well as to stop an attack in progress. It delivers electric stimulation to small branches of the trigeminal nerve. It may take daily use for a few months to see a preventive benefit.

•Nerivio is an armband device that you control via a smartphone app to stimulate nerves in the arm and indirectly address migraine pain. It also is being studied for migraine prevention.

•Relivion is a headband that goes around the forehead to electrically stimulate nerve branches in the front and back of the head to treat headache pain.

Oral CGRP for Migraine Approved

U.S. Food and Drug Administration

The U.S. Food and Drug Administration (FDA) has approved *atogepant* (Qulipta)

for migraine. This is the first calcitonin gene-related peptide (CGRP) receptor antagonist that is taken orally. All other CGRP drugs are injected. In a study submitted to the FDA, participants experienced three to four fewer migraine days per month after taking the medication for 12 weeks. Possible side effects include constipation, nausea, and fatigue.

Botox Injections Can Reduce Migraine Days for People with High-Frequency Episodic Migraines

Daniele Martinelli, MD, neurologist at Mondino Hospital-Istituto Neurologico Nazionale IRCCS, Pavia, Lombardy, Italy.

Investigators administered 155 units of Botox (onabotulinumtoxinA) into study participants' heads and necks four times over 48 weeks. Thirty-four percent of the patients had at least a 50 percent reduction in the number of migraine days. The injections were also associated with a significant reduction in the use of pain medications.

Don't Let Arthritis Slow You Down: Reach Your Fitness Goals Without Pain

Brian Feeley, MD, chief of sports medicine and shoulder surgery at the University of California San Francisco.

Exercise is a fundamental tenet of good health, and that doesn't change with the onset of arthritis. With a few modifications, you can maintain your cardiovascular fitness and strength, and even reduce some of the pain and stiffness of arthritis.

Both resistance training and aerobic exercise are associated with less pain and disability from arthritis and better performance, but that's just the start of what exercise can do for you.

Cardiovascular Exercise

Cardiovascular (aerobic) exercise can strengthen the heart, lower blood pressure and LDL (bad) cholesterol, raise good HDL, regulate insulin levels, and lower blood sugar. It can improve body weight, fight insomnia, strengthen the immune system, improve cognitive performance, and boost mood.

For good health, you need about 150 minutes per week of moderate-intensity activity or 75 minutes per week of vigorous exercise.

• **Walking** is a safe way to relieve arthritis pain, strengthen muscles, and reduce stress for almost everyone. The workload can be easily adjusted by choosing flat or hilly ground or changing your speed. If you're outside, look for smooth, dirt trails, which are easier on your joints than sidewalks or the street. A treadmill in your home or at a gym can keep you moving even in inclement weather.

• **Water exercise.** Take your walk to the pool to halve the weight on your joints. Swimming and water aerobics classes deliver cardiovascular results with less strain on joints. Water-based exercise is ideal for people who are heavier or have advanced arthritis.

• **Cycling.** Riding a bicycle boosts cardiovascular fitness while also strengthening the muscles in your lower body. As with walking, you can adjust the intensity by choosing a flat or hilly trail and by changing your speed.

Make sure your seat is at the correct height: When your leg is extended on the down pedal, your knee should be slightly bent. If a traditional bicycle is uncomfortable, a recumbent bike provides more support. If you take an indoor cycling class and feel pain when you stand and pedal, remain seated.

• **Running.** While high-intensity exercise has traditionally been frowned upon for people with arthritis, the science is quite mixed. While running may be uncomfortable for some people, studies show it can be beneficial and safe for joints for others. The best approach is to listen to your body. If you are an avid runner and nothing is bothering you while you run, keep going. If you do start to experience pain, pay attention to when it happens. If you feel pain at mile three, try shortening your distance but increasing your pace. Instead of running every day, run three days a week and alternate with cycling, swimming, weight training, or yoga.

Strength Training

Weight training strengthens the muscles that help support and protect joints. Strong muscles help you more easily perform a wide variety of activities, from standing up from a chair to getting out of a car. It improves bone density and helps boost your metabolism too.

If you are starting a new weight training program or looking to get stronger, aim for three days per week. If you're looking to maintain your current strength and muscle mass, two days per week is sufficient. Don't work the same muscle group two days in a row. Arthritis can make some exercises you're used to doing uncomfortable, but simple modifications can get you the same results without the pain.

• **Knee pain.** If you have knee pain when doing squats or lunges, don't dip down as far. As you bend your knee, there is progressively more load on your joint and it is distributed less broadly, which can cause pain. By reducing the angle of your bent knee, you can decrease that load. You can also lower the weight that you're holding. To maintain the intensity of the exercise, increase the number of repetitions or speed them up.

There is one exercise that you should never do: Leg extensions. These are done in a chair or a machine where you sit with your leg bent over the edge of the seat and straighten it against resistance. This exercise puts excessive load on the kneecap.

• **Back pain.** If you suffer from low-back pain, the first thing you need to do is sit less. The most load that we put on the spine is by sitting. Get up and move around every 15 to 20 minutes to relieve it. To strengthen the back, focus on core stability with exercises like planks, side planks, and squats. Good form is imperative. Doing an exercise incorrectly can potentially cause more damage to your back.

• **Shoulder pain.** Shoulder exercises like military presses are safe—as long as your form is good. But many people, especially as they age, get in trouble when they take up activities like CrossFit and use maximal exertion to fatigue with heavy weight and high repetitions. This can put the shoulder at risk for dislocation. People who do heavy chest presses for years can also increase the risk of shoulder arthritis.

Rhythm of a Workout

There's a pattern to every workout that helps prevent injury and reduce discomfort. Always start with a warm-up. Spend five to 10 minutes moving gently with range-of-motion exercises or easy cardiovascular work, and then transition into your work phase. Start slow and build up to harder work, whether that's heavier weights or a faster walking speed. At the end of the active portion of your workout, slow back down to let your heart rate and breathing return to normal. End the session with gentle stretches of any of the muscle groups that you used.

If you're continuing on an existing exercise program and these modifications ease your pain, you're all set to work out on your own. If you're trying to achieve new goals, however, a professional, such as a physical therapist or trainer, can help ensure that your form is good.

How to Exercise with Back Pain

Carol B. Espel, MS, program and wellness director at the Pritikin Center for Longevity in Miami. In 2012, she was named "Fitness Director of the Year" by the World IDEA Health & Fitness Association.

Back pain: It's become a reality for many people as poor posture, excessive sitting, and slouching have had deleterious effects on the back, core, and hips. While exercise is undoubtedly healthy, it's important to take special care of your back.

Don't make the mistake of thinking you can work through the pain, believing it's due to muscle inactivity. Working through pain leads to poor form and exercise execution and, in the end, leads to serious and chronic injury and more pain. It's important to ease into exercise slowly, and to heal, strengthen, and stretch the back and core muscles first. You can then start to add exercise and activities that are appropriate, effective, and safe.

Brace Yourself

Bracing the core muscles (primarily the abdominal and oblique muscles) is critical to alleviating back pain when standing. An easy way to activate the "brace" is to take a deep breath in and then exhale fully. At the end of the exhalation, to expel any remaining air, forcefully exhale, making a "huh" sound. This will tighten and tone the abdominal wall. Supporting your body posture this way sets you up for pain-free movement, activity, and exercise. The following exercises are gentle and safe for people with back pain.

Cat Cow

Start and end each session with this exercise. Start on all fours. Inhale as you round your back up like a cat, fully contracting your abdominals. Drop your chin into your chest and look at your belly button. Try to stay there for two to four counts. Exhale as you slowly lengthen your spine, lifting your head up and out, gazing slightly upward, and arch your back. Stay for two to four counts. Slowly repeat as many times as you enjoy.

Bird Dog

Start on all fours. Look slightly forward and down. Brace your abdominal muscles and then slowly and fully extend your right leg straight back. Return to the starting position. Next, slowly extend your left arm in front of you, then return to the starting position. Repeat on the other side. Complete one to three sets of six to 12 repetitions on each side.

Modified Curl-up

Lie on your back. Place both hands behind your head, lightly supporting it. Let your elbows drop and open out, as close to the floor as possible. Bend both of your knees and place your feet flat on the floor. Contract your abdominals in and down as you slowly lift your entire torso off the floor. Return to the floor completely. This should be a small movement. Your focus must be up toward the ceiling throughout the exercise. Complete one to three sets of six to 12 repetitions.

Hip Extensions

Lie on your back, with both knees bent and your feet flat on the floor. Place both hands on top of your pelvis. Better yet, place a foam block on top of your lower belly and pelvis. The purpose of the foam block is to make sure both hips are pressing upward equally,

avoiding one side dropping lower than the other. Lift both hips off the floor, squeezing the gluteal muscles, but not arching the rib cage. Return to the starting position. Complete one to three sets of six to 12 repetitions.

The key to long-term success for better back health involves a daily commitment to performing regular back and core strength, flexibility, and mobility exercises. This will help you to enjoy doing the things you like to do with greater ease, freedom of movement, and joy.

Unlearn Pain: Use Your Brain to Fight Chronic Back Pain

Yoni K. Ashar, PhD, postdoctoral associate in the department of psychiatry at Weill Cornell Medical College in New York City. Dr. Ashar is the lead author of the *JAMA Psychiatry* study on PRT for chronic back pain.

Acute low back pain, which is incredibly common, can last from a few days to a few weeks. But for about 20 percent of people, the pain persists. When it lasts more than 12 weeks, it's considered chronic, and some people suffer for years.

New research suggests that part of the problem is that many doctors are treating the wrong body part. The brain—not the back—causes about 85 percent of chronic back pain, Yoni K. Ashar, PhD, wrote in *JAMA Psychiatry* in September 2021.

The good news is that it's entirely possible to teach your brain how to unlearn pain.

How the Brain Causes Pain

Pain is like an alarm that goes off to warn you of danger. Acute pain triggers brain pathways that cause fear, worry, and anxiety. Brain researchers have a saying: "Nerves that fire together wire together." That means that, over time, the brain pathways between pain, fear, and anxiety become like the grooves made by wagon wheels: They are easy to follow, and they go both ways. When you think you are going to have pain, your brain produces it. When you have a twinge of pain or mild pain, your brain produces fear and anxiety. People with chronic primary pain live in a vicious cycle of worry, fear, avoidance, and months or years of pain.

Unlearning the Pain

The study that Dr. Ashar and his colleagues published in *JAMA Psychiatry* was the first clinical trial of pain reprocessing therapy (PRT).

PRT was developed by psychotherapist Alan Gordon, LCSW, to treat primary chronic back pain. It starts with education about the cause of primary pain. Once the patient accepts that pain does not always mean harm, he or she learns that pain is reversible.

The next stage, somatic tracking, teaches patients to pay attention to bodily sensations in a focused manner, such as during guided meditation. Patients are taught to develop a more open, accepting, and fearless approach to pain sensations.

Finally, in the exposure therapy stage, patients resume activities that they had avoided. If the therapy works, they find that they no longer have pain while gradually resuming normal activities.

Gordon and his colleagues were getting remarkable results in their clinical practice, so they wanted to test their results in a controlled clinical trial. They, along with Dr. Ashar, recruited 151 people who were diagnosed with primary chronic back pain by a physician. The average number of years with back pain was about 10. The patients reported back pain of at least four on a scale of one to 10.

Before treatment started, all study participants had brain imaging that showed the areas of the brain responsible for pain. The researchers measured the brain's pain responses before and after the trial during a mild task that caused back stress. People in the trial were randomly assigned to receive two PRT therapy sessions per week for four weeks, to get an inactive back injection of saltwater (a placebo), or to continue whatever they were doing for back pain (usual therapy).

At the end of treatment, 66 percent of people in the PRT group were pain-free or nearly pain-free. Their average pain scores were reduced to one out of 10. Importantly, at a one-year follow-up visit, people in the PRT group continued to score their pain between one and two out of 10.

About 20 percent of people in the placebo group were pain-free or almost pain-free. And ten percent of the people in the treatment-as-usual group were pain-free or almost pain-free.

The results surprised even the research team. That amount of pain relief is very rare in pain studies using medications, injections, physical therapy, and surgery.

Future Trends

PRT and other mind-body treatments don't have to be the only treatment for chronic primary pain, but they should be part of the treatment. Primary chronic back pain is real pain, and there is no single approach that works for everybody.

For years, chronic pain has been treated with medications, injections, physical therapy, or surgery. The role of the mind in chronic pain can't be ignored any longer.

What to Know Before You Buy Your Next Mattress

Michael J. Breus, PhD, clinical psychologist in Los Angeles, a Diplomate of the American Board of Sleep Medicine and author of *Energize! Go from Dragging Ass to Kicking It in 30 Days.* TheSleepDoctor.com

From TV commercials to ads on social media, it seems like every day brings a new mattress company trying to outdo the others with technical advances and layering systems that promise better sleep and less morning stiffness. But don't select a mattress simply because it has the newest bells and whistles. Instead, determine the features that make sense for your needs, and then look for a mattress that satisfies them. *To help with that, we asked sleep expert Michael J. Breus, PhD, for his top picks in the world of mattresses, the features you should consider and which gimmicks to avoid...*

The Anatomy of a Mattress

Mattress materials have evolved over the last 150 years since the creation of the innerspring, a network of bouncy springs or coils. Memory foam, originally created by NASA, started being used for mattresses about 30 years ago to provide relief for pressure points such as shoulders and hips while contouring to your body. Some newer entries to the market have reimagined latex mattresses, which were introduced nearly a century ago. Like memory foam, latex relieves pressure but has more of the bounce of an innerspring mattress and is very durable.

The latest trend is toward hybrids—a combination of these and other materials in layers. A mattress needs to deliver two separate things—support underneath you and comfort close to your body.

Support will keep your spine aligned regardless of sleeping position. This allows for better blood flow so nutrition can be administered throughout the body, enabling muscles to rejuvenate. It also helps avoid nerve impingement. A mattress's support comes from the bottom eight inches of structure and material. Innersprings, for instance, do a great job of providing support.

The comfort part of a mattress is the top five inches. This cushioning is very important to cradle your body's pressure points if you're a side or stomach sleeper. Natural latex, a material made from the sap of rubber trees, is excellent—in addition to its responsiveness and adaptability, latex helps regulate the mattress's temperature to keep you cool. Natural latex is processed in two ways—Dunlop with a firmer feel...and Tala-

lay with a slightly softer feel. Synthetic latex is an option but is less durable.

"Pillow top" mattresses offer an additional layer of comfort with padding sewn on top. The padding may be filled with different materials, including foam, latex, cotton, wool or some combination.

You're also likely to see mattresses described by level of firmness, on a scale of one to 10, with one as the softest. Next in order are medium-soft, medium-firm and firm at 10.

Matching Your Needs

You and your bed partner should start by asking yourselves what you need from the mattress beyond restful sleep...

• **If you sleep warm,** which often happens to women after menopause, look for materials that help regulate temperature. A hybrid mattress does a better job of keeping you cool than one that's all memory foam. Latex is naturally cooling, so it's a good pick for hot sleepers.

• **If you need extra cushioning,** consider a pillow-top mattress. Often the body's subcutaneous fat layer (which also helps you regulate temperature) gets thinner with age, meaning that you have less natural cushioning of your own.

• **If you're older and/or have mobility issues,** look for ones with springs or a hybrid mattress but not one that's only memory foam, which may be hard to get in and out of and to turn while sleeping. If you need to sit on the edge of a mattress before standing, you need one that has edge support, a reinforcement you can grab onto so you don't slide off.

• **If you have low back pain and need better support,** an innerspring mattress with coils at its core offers more firmness. Coil technology has advanced—these aren't your parents' innersprings. Plus, you can look for designs that feature comfortable materials in the top layer such as a mix of foam and latex.

• **If you snore…or your partner snores… or one of you has GERD**—or if you enjoy sitting up in bed to read before sleep—an adjustable base under the mattress can form a slight incline to raise the bed. Look for a mattress specifically designed to work with this kind of base. The Purple Ascent Adjustable Base is a great one and works with mattresses other than its own, such as the Nectar.

• **If you want to have better sex,** an innerspring or hybrid will be better than memory foam, which is less effective in supporting your body during sex.

Making It to Tryouts

There's no substitute for in-person mattress shopping. This often is possible even with offerings from online companies—some have brick-and-mortar stores or sell their mattresses through furniture stores.

Example: Raymour & Flanigan stocks Casper, Nectar, Purple and more.

If you don't know what level of firmness you like, try out the choices. Be sure to wear loafers to the mattress store so you can kick off your shoes during your test. It might feel awkward to roll around on a mattress in public, but it's important to take the time to do it correctly. When you lie down on a bed, it takes four to five minutes for your body to recalibrate from standing and for your muscles to relax. It will take a few more minutes for you to sense what the bed actually feels like to you. At that point, write down how much you like the mattress's comfort, support and firmness on a scale of one to 10. If you have a partner, he/she should do the same. Repeat these steps with all the mattresses you're considering, and then compare notes.

Some companies allow you to try out a bed in your home for a certain period of time. One of the biggest mistakes people make is giving up on a new mattress too soon. It can take three weeks before you'll know if a mattress is a good fit. Some companies even insist that you keep their mattress for at least 30 days.

Reason: The return rate goes down the longer a mattress is in your home. But regardless of timing, if you determine that a mattress is not a comfortable fit for you, do not hesitate to return it.

What About Box Springs?

Before the popularity of the platform bed and its cousin, the futon, innerspring mattresses came with a box spring—a separate base with coils that supported the mattress and gave it more lift. Many mattresses today go directly on what's called a "foundation," or a "base," some of which might be made of attractive wood or covered in upholstery. Many companies still term it a "box spring," but there are no springs.

What About Price?

It is hard to get a great mattress for $600 to $800—these beds-in-a-box are fine for a guest room or limited use. But expect to pay closer to $2,500 (or more) for a great queen-size mattress, topper and base. The ultimate bed comes from the Swedish company Hästens. It's handcrafted to your needs, and most models start in the tens of thousands of dollars and can go into the hundreds of thousands for the top-of-the-line model. This product goes beyond customized—it will be tweaked in your home until the perfect balance of natural materials, including flax and horsetail hair, is achieved. Also available is an adjustable base that operates through your smartphone as well as a remote.

Do You Really Need a New Mattress?

Beyond sagging and wear-and-tear, if you wake up more than three days a week with body-wide stiffness that lasts 20 minutes, then goes away, you likely need a new mattress.

Alternative: A latex topper for your existing bed. It can help with heat regulation and offer extra comfort.

Simple Solutions for Hip Pain

Sanjeev Bhatia, MD, an orthopedic surgeon at Northwestern Medicine Central DuPage Hospital in Winfield, Illinois. He serves on the Northwestern Medicine Hip and Knee Joint Preservation Center Team.

If your normally active life is suddenly upended by hip pain, your response may depend on your age. A middle-aged runner may assume it's a severe injury, while a retiree might suspect arthritis and the need for hip replacement.

But there's good news for people of any age: The most common causes of hip pain are usually managed successfully with no surgery required.

Pain Location Provides Clues

Hip pain can arise from structures that are outside of the actual ball-and-socket joint (extra-articular) or from the cartilage inside the joint (intra-articular). *The location of your pain can provide clues to what is occurring and guide treatment decisions…*

• **Front of the hip.** If you have pain in the front of your hip, it's likely to be an intra-articular condition. If you feel a sharp pain after twisting, squatting, pivoting, or getting in and out of the car, you may have hip impingement. This condition strikes when the bones of the ball and socket don't fit together properly. The mismatch can lead to tears in the labrum, a ring of cartilage on the rim of the hip-joint socket. Hip impingement and labral tears can cause pain, but they can also hinder normal motion, destabilize the hip joint, and, in severe cases, lead to advanced arthritis.

• **Side of the hip.** If you feel pain when lying on your side, sitting with your legs crossed, walking, or climbing stairs, greater trochanteric pain syndrome (GTPS) may be to blame.

This extra-articular condition affects structures that surround the large bony prominence on the side of the hip (the trochanter). GTPS is one of the most common causes of side hip pain in adults and affects women more than men. One study in adults ages 50 to 75 found that 15 percent of women and 6.6 percent of men were affected.

In the past, it was called trochanteric bursitis, because it was generally accepted that it was caused by inflammation of the bursae—fluid-filled sacs that keep tendons and muscles from rubbing directly against the trochanter. Recent ultrasound and MRI studies, however, suggest that the pain is often caused by inflammation of the gluteal abductor tendons in addition to bursitis and tightness in the iliotibial band. The iliotibial band is a stretch of fibrous tissue that runs from the hip to under the knee.

• **Back of the hip.** Hip pain that is more posterior in nature often arises from extra-articular causes such as discomfort in the sacroiliac joint, which connects the hip bone to the sacrum, or conditions such as sciatica that stem from the lumbar spinal nerve roots (lumbar radicular pain).

Muscular causes of posterior hip pain can include tendinopathy of the muscles in the back of the thigh (hamstring). Tendinopathy can be caused by the inflammation of a tendon (tendinitis) or degeneration of a tendon's collagen (tendinosis).

Nonsurgical Treatment

Nonsurgical treatment is almost always the first choice for hip pain, and the success rate is as high as 90 percent for extra-articular conditions and 50 percent for intra-articular causes. Although the intra-articular rate is lower, it still suggests that a nonsurgical approach may be beneficial.

Nonsurgical treatments include physical therapy, over-the-counter medications such as *acetaminophen* (Tylenol) and *ibuprofen* (Advil and Motrin), prescription antirheumatic drugs and biological response modifiers, and injections and infusions of medications such as corticosteroids. Dietary supplements such as glucosamine and chondroitin may help as well. Many people benefit from losing excess weight and participating in low-impact exercise.

Several studies have shown that mental and emotional factors, such as stress and anxiety, can affect the perception of hip pain, especially in the postoperative period. As such, stress reduction techniques may be beneficial.

This type of integrative approach to musculoskeletal pain may become the norm in the future as more research begins to support these efforts.

Minimally Invasive Procedures

If these efforts fail, it doesn't mean hip replacement is needed. Advances in minimally invasive procedures mean that surgeons can address issues such as hip impingement, labral tears, and gluteus medius tears with only tiny incisions in same-day procedures.

Another option, orthobiologic therapy, uses injections of substances like bone marrow or plasma that are already in your body to relieve pain and promote healing. Consider platelet-rich plasma therapy. A small amount of your blood is drawn and run through a centrifuge to concentrate the platelets. When those concentrated platelets are injected into the joint or tissue, they release growth factors and cytokines that boost healing and regenerate injured tissue. Similarly, stem cells may be taken from your bone marrow and injected into the site of injury to regrow tissue.

Preventing the Pain

One of the best things people can do to prevent pain is to help their cartilage remain healthy with a low-impact exercise program that preserves motion and strengthens the hip. That includes things like using elliptical machines, swimming, biking, yoga, and practicing Pilates. Additionally keeping one's core, gluteal, and lumbar back muscles strong helps decrease the incidence of extra-articular hip problems.

Steroid Injections for Hip Pain May Cause Rapid Hip Deterioration

Kanu M. Okike, MD, orthopedic surgeon with Hawaii Permanente Medical Group in Honolulu and lead author of a study published in *The Journal of Bone and Joint Surgery*.

Steroid injections into the hip are a common treatment to alleviate pain.

Recent finding: Risk for rapidly destructive hip disease (RDHD) increases substantially following a high-dose injection or multiple injections. Serious hip damage—including joint-space narrowing and collapse of the femoral head—can occur within months. Risk following a single low-dose injection is low.

New Peptide Helps Medical Marijuana Relieve Pain Without Cognitive Side Effects

Rafael Maldonado, PhD, professor, University Pompeu Fabra, Barcelona, Spain.

A new peptide could allow medical marijuana to relieve pain without cognitive side effects. Researchers created a peptide that disrupts the interaction between the receptor that is the target of tetrahydrocannabinol (THC), the psychoactive component of marijuana, and another that binds serotonin, a neurotransmitter that regulates learning, memory, and other cognitive functions. Mice given the peptide along with a THC injection exhibited better memory than those given THC alone. The pain relief was not diminished.

Overdose Drug Can Help Chronic Pain

University of Zurich, University of Queensland, Memorial Sloan Kettering Cancer Center, University of Michigan.

Low doses of *naltrexone*, a form of the drug used to reverse opioid overdoses, reduced pain intensity and improved quality of life among participants in a new clinical trial. Naltrexone acts on glial cells to calm the overactive nervous system.

How to Stop Achilles Heel Pain

Mitchell Yass, DPT, creator of The Yass Method, which uniquely diagnoses and treats the cause of chronic pain through the interpretation of the body's presentation of symptoms. Dr. Yass is author of several books, *Overpower Pain: The Strength-Training Program that Stops Pain without Drugs or Surgery, The Pain Cure Rx: The Yass Method for Diagnosing and Resolving Chronic Pain* and his latest, *The Yass Method for Pain-Free Movement: A Guide to Easing through Your Day without Aches and Pains.* Mitchell Yass.com

You've probably heard the phrase "Achilles' heel" used to describe a vulnerability that has the power to bring a person down despite his/her overall strong character. That's ironic because when it comes to actual Achilles heel pain, neither the Achilles tendon nor the heel bears any responsibility at all. In most cases, heel pain is caused by weakness in the muscles that support the hips or in the leg muscles.

Painful chain of events: One gluteus medius muscle sits on each side of the pelvis and is responsible for keeping the pelvis level when you are standing on one leg, as you do every time you take a step. When the gluteus medius on one side is weak, the lower back muscles on the other side try to compensate

Credit Card Debt Causes Pain—Literally

People with consistently high unsecured debt, such as credit cards and payday loans, were 76 percent more likely to have pain and stiffness later in life, according to a recent study. Even if they managed to mostly pay off such debt, risk for pain and stiffness was 50 percent. Taking on new unsecured debt during middle age was particularly damaging.

Adrianne Frech, PhD, associate professor of health sciences at University of Missouri in Columbia and leader of a study of 8,000 adults published in *Social Science & Medicine—Population Health.*

to keep the pelvis level. That shortens the back muscles and elevates the hip on the side opposite the weak gluteus medius. This means that the distance the foot must travel to the floor is increased causing a greater load to develop as the foot reaches the floor. This excess load, in turn, makes it more difficult to push off that leg when walking. And then that leg ends up hurting because of the undue strain on the calf, the primary muscle responsible for propelling you forward. Because the Achilles tendon connects the calf to the heel, strain in the calf often leads to pain in and above the heel.

If you have Achilles heel pain on both sides, there's likely a strength imbalance between the hip flexor/quad muscles and the gluteus maximus/hamstrings. Such an imbalance can develop from running, stair-climbing and exercises that tend to overdevelop muscles in the front of the legs while neglecting those in the back. This imbalance causes a forward center of mass that must be picked up by a muscle in the back of the body or you would fall forward. In this case, the excess load ends up being supported by the calves, resulting in pain in both Achilles tendons.

Three Exercises for Relief

The exercises below will strengthen your gluteus medius muscles, gluteus maximus muscles and hamstrings—all the muscles involved in creating optimal posture. The descriptions below are for single-sided weakness, but if your pain is bilateral, perform the exercises on both sides.

Complete three sets of 10 repetitions for each exercise (resting 45 to 60 seconds between sets). Repeat the workout three times a week with one day between workouts. The level of resistance should feel like you are working reasonably hard to complete the set. Stay with this resistance level until it feels fairly easy to complete the set, then increase the resistance. This process can continue until you are strong enough to perform your daily activities without pain.

Important: For single-sided pain, work the leg that is opposite the side where the heel pain occurs. If you work the same side, you'll inadvertently increase the imbalance between the two sides and the pain will continue.

For pain on only one side, the most important exercise is the hip abduction exercise. For pain in both Achilles tendons, perform the three exercises with both legs.

Hip Abduction (*gluteus medius*)

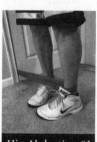
Hip Abduction #1

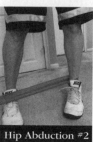
Hip Abduction #2

Knot both ends of a resistance band together, and put the knot behind a closed door at ankle height. Standing perpendicular to the door, place the loop of the band around the ankle farthest from the door (the working gluteus medius). Start with your feet together. Turn the toes of the working leg in so that the foot is pointing about 10 degrees in front. Keeping your nose aligned over the standing leg, lift the moving leg slightly and move it until the outside of the ankle is aligned with the outside of the hip. Put the foot down. Now shift your weight until your nose is over the moved foot. Immediately move the foot and your body to the start position with your nose over the standing leg again.

Hip Extension (*gluteus maximus*)

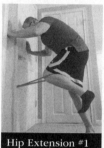
Hip Extension #1

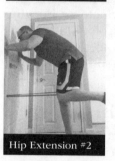
Hip Extension #2

Close the knot of the resistance band in the door at about knee height. In a standing position facing the door, place the loop of the resistance band behind your knee. Start with the hip flexed to about 60 degrees. Bring the knee about 10 degrees behind the hip. Then return to the start position. Make sure your back is rounded and the knee of the leg you are standing on is not locked.

Hamstring Curl (hamstrings)

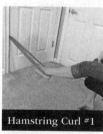
Hamstring Curl #1

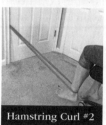
Hamstring Curl #2

Close the knot of the resistance band in the door at about knee height. In a seated position facing the door, place the resistance band around the back of the ankle. Begin with the exercising leg pointing straight out with the knee unlocked. Begin to bend the knee until it reaches 90 degrees, then return to the start position. To isolate the hamstrings better, the toes of the exercising leg should point upward toward the face as the exercise is being performed.

Exercise photos courtesy of Mitchell Yass.

265

Diverticulitis: How to Stop the Pain

Anne Peery MD, a gastroenterologist and associate professor of medicine at the University of North Carolina Chapel Hill School of Medicine. Dr. Peery is a national expert in diverticulitis and recently coauthored a report outlining best treatment practices for the American Gastroenterological Association.

One day, seemingly out of nowhere, you're hit with intense lower abdominal pain. It's difficult to stand up straight.

You have a fever and you may also have nausea, constipation, diarrhea, or symptoms reminiscent of a urinary tract infection, such as an increased urge to urinate or burning while doing so. Gastroenterologists see this constellation of symptoms quite often, and a singular diagnosis usually springs to mind: diverticulitis.

What Is Diverticulitis?

One of the most common gastrointestinal diseases, diverticulitis is an inflammation of tiny sac-like protrusions that form in the wall of the colon. These marble-sized pouches, called *diverticula*, are found in more than half of Americans over age 60, but most of the time, they don't cause trouble. The existence of the pouches is called diverticulosis, and it's generally harmless. Most people don't even know they have them. But for about 5 percent of people with diverticulosis, those pouches will become inflamed or infected. When that happens, the condition progresses to diverticulitis, which demands immediate medical attention. In fact, the painful condition is responsible for nearly 2 million outpatient visits and 208,000 inpatient admissions a year.

Who Develops Diverticulitis?

We are just now starting to truly understand why people get diverticulitis. It has long been blamed on a low-fiber diet, but while a high-quality diet is associated with reduced diverticulitis risk, the truth is that genetics, not diet, are responsible for about 50 percent of one's risk. Siblings of patients with diverticulitis, for instance, are believed to have a threefold higher risk of developing it themselves. Researchers using genetic markers very recently found that genes related to obesity and type 2 diabetes are associated with an increased risk of diverticulitis.

That said, nutrition does have an impact, with a diet high in fruits, vegetables, whole grains, poultry, and fish linked with reduced diverticulitis risk, and vegetarians enjoying some protection over carnivores. A high-fiber diet is important to manage diverticulitis or possibly even avoid it in the first place. When researchers followed 50,000+ health professionals for 24 years, they found that those who consumed the most fiber (an average of 28.5 grams a day) had the lowest risk of developing diverticulitis, and those who consumed the least fiber (12.5 grams a day, on average) had the highest risk. Fiber should come from foods, not supplements.

Vigorous physical activity is also associated with a reduced risk. Diverticulitis is more common among men than women at younger ages, but over age 60, rates are higher for women. Regular use (at least twice a week) of aspirin or nonsteroidal anti-inflammatory drugs such as ibuprofen increases risk, as does obesity, smoking, and the use of hormone replacement therapy for menopause.

Immunocompromised patients—those with cancer or rheumatological conditions, for example—tend to experience diverticulitis at higher rates than the general population, possibly due to chronic steroid use. Interestingly, these patients often present with milder symptoms, delaying diagnosis. They also experience more complications.

Pain Is the Number One Symptom

The pain usually appears suddenly, most often in the left lower quadrant of the abdomen. Patients often describe it as the worst pain they've ever had. Even a mild episode can make it difficult to walk. Other symptoms can include fever, constipation (excess inflammation may prevent stool from moving through the colon), diarrhea, and urinary symptoms because an inflamed colon is sitting atop the bladder.

Most people see their primary care physician or visit an emergency room when the pain begins. Your doctor will draw blood to see if you have an elevated white blood cell count, which indicates possible infection. He or she may also run blood tests to confirm inflammation and will rule out a urinary tract infection. An abdominal CT scan is also strongly recommended with the first episode to identify and diagnose diverticulitis and also help determine severity.

Three Types of Diverticulitis

Most people have *acute uncomplicated diverticulitis*. Somewhere between 94 and 97 percent of these patients can be successfully treated on an outpatient basis with rest and a clear liquid diet for a few days. The pain *usually* improves within about two weeks.

A small (less than 10 percent) proportion of uncomplicated diverticulitis patients continue to experience symptoms for weeks to months. This is called *smoldering diverticulitis* and indicates ongoing inflammation, like a fire that is almost extinguished, but not quite. This type of diverticulitis may require antibiotics or surgery to remove the inflamed part of the colon. Fortunately, about 75 percent of patients will never have another episode. The rest will experience recurrences once a year or even multiple times a year.

About 5 percent of people with acute uncomplicated diverticulitis will go on to develop *complicated diverticulitis*, involving an abscess or hole in the wall of the colon, through which gas and fluid escape. These patients are almost always hospitalized, require antibiotics, and may need to have a temporary drain inserted in their abdomen to promote healing. Surgery to remove part of the colon may be necessary in some cases.

What Happens After a Flare-Up?

Your gastroenterologist will tell you when to progress from a clear liquid diet (during an episode) to low-fiber solid foods (eggs, cooked fruit, pasta, dairy foods) and then, once all symptoms have subsided, to a high-fiber routine (produce, beans, brown rice, bran and whole-grain cereals). It's important to maintain communication with your doctor during the clear liquid diet phase to ensure you don't lose too much weight.

Some people with diverticulitis will experience chronic gastrointestinal (GI) pain and, eventually, be diagnosed with irritable bowel syndrome (IBS). In a Swedish trial, periodic abdominal pain was reported by nearly half of uncomplicated diverticulitis patients at one-year follow-up. This IBS pain is sometimes treated with a low dose of a tricyclic antidepressant such as *amitriptyline* (Elavil), *imipramine* (Tofranil), or *nortriptyline* (Pamelor). These drugs help reduce stomach sensitivity by blocking pain signals sent from the GI tract to the brain.

Six to eight weeks after diverticulitis symptoms resolve, you should have a colonoscopy to rule out malignancy, as colon cancer can resemble diverticulitis on a CT scan. The risk is higher in patients with complicated diverticulitis.

New Crohn's Guidance

Christina Ha, MD, an associate professor of medicine and director of the inflammatory bowel disease fellowship at Cedars-Sinai Medical Center in Los Angeles. Dr. Ha is also chair of the Professional Education Committee of the Crohn's & Colitis Foundation's National Scientific Advisory Committee.

You wouldn't fight a forest fire with a garden hose, right? But for many years, that's how doctors approached Crohn's disease treatment, tamping down painful, debilitating symptoms before opting for advanced therapies that actually douse the spark—a hyperactive immune system.

Reduce Crohn's Symptoms

Diet and lifestyle changes typically aren't enough to treat Crohn's, but it might be possible to lessen symptoms by eating smaller, more frequent meals and avoiding these triggers...

- **Carbonated drinks**
- **Popcorn**
- **Vegetable skins**
- **Nuts**
- **High-fiber foods**

—Dr. Christina Ha

More than 500,000 Americans are believed to have Crohn's, a type of inflammatory bowel disease that counts diarrhea, nausea, cramping, anemia, fatigue, and joint pain among its day-to-day symptoms. The chronic condition can also produce swelling, blockages, and pockets of infection throughout the gastrointestinal (GI) tract as well as excruciating tunnels called fistulas that connect the intestine to other organs or tissues.

For patients with moderate to severe Crohn's, frequent hospitalizations or surgery to remove damaged intestinal tissue are ever-present concerns. But new clinical guidelines from the American Gastroenterological Association (AGA) offer doctors an updated treatment strategy, recommending aggressive therapy sooner with a rapidly expanding group of medications called biologics that calm the immune system.

While these guidelines are new, this proactive approach to treating Crohn's isn't. It formalizes a strategy many gastroenterologists have used for years: prescribing the right drugs for the right patients to protect them from worsening problems that interfere with their lives.

Plan of Attack

Biologics are already used to treat immune-based conditions such as multiple sclerosis, psoriasis, and rheumatoid arthritis. Because the GI tract breaks down proteins,

pills won't work for this type of medication, so they're given by injection or infusion.

But while the route of administration may not be as convenient as taking a pill, biologics target Crohn's better than the two medications that used to be the standard first-line treatment. Corticosteroids and aminosalicylates were part of a "step-up" approach to tamp down intestinal inflammation and prevent Crohn's complications. But those drugs work like a leaky bandage that does nothing to fix the underlying problem, and steroids, in particular, come with a host of harmful side effects, including bone thinning, serious infections, cataracts, and elevated blood sugar levels.

Biologics, however, are antibodies that stop specific proteins in the body from causing inflammation. Biologics work best when they're given earlier, not after other drugs fail. Prescribing them sooner for patients considered at high risk of worsening Crohn's will help stop the disease in its tracks, before bowel damage progresses. It aims a fire hose on the blazing forest.

There are many biologic drugs available. The AGA recommends starting with a type of biologic called an anti-tumor necrosis factor agent, such as *infliximab* (Remicade), *adalimumab* (Humira), or *certolizumab pegol* (Cimzia), or either *ustekinumab* (Stelara), or *vedolizumab* (Entyvio).

Your physician will work with you to choose the medication that best suits your individual needs.

Chronic Fatigue Syndrome: Get the Help You Need

Chris Iliades, MD, retired ear, nose, throat, head, and neck surgeon who now dedicates his time to educating patients through his medical writing.

Since 1934, chronic fatigue has gone by many names, but today it's called myalgic encephalomyelitis/chronic fatigue syndrome (ME/CFS). This disorder affects as many as 2.5 million Americans, mostly women, but despite that number, ME/CFS is not taught in many medical schools, many doctors don't take it seriously, and few are prepared to treat it.

Myalgic encephalomyelitis means muscle pain and inflammation of the spine and brain, even though not all people with this condition have muscle pain or clear evidence of inflammation. What people with ME/CFS do have is life-changing fatigue that is relentless and unrelieved by sleep.

Symptoms and Diagnosis

No tests can diagnose ME/CFS: It is a diagnosis of exclusion. Anemia, depression, white blood cell cancers, celiac disease, Lyme disease, multiple sclerosis, and fibromyalgia must all be ruled out first.

Since there are no tests, diagnosis rests on the symptoms. To be diagnosed, a person needs to have two types of symptoms for more than six months. *They must first have three core symptoms…*

•**Chronic fatigue that is unexplained,** not reduced by rest, and severe enough to affect daily activities.

Worsening symptoms after physical activity or emotional stress, called post-exertional malaise (PEM). People with ME/CFS may describe it as a relapse or a crash.

•**Disturbed or unrefreshing sleep.** Sleep disturbance may include insomnia, but the main symptom is not feeling rested or refreshed after sleep.

For an ME/CFS diagnosis, they must also have either cognitive impairment or orthostatic intolerance. Cognitive impairment is problems thinking clearly, paying attention, or making decisions. People with ME/CFS often call this brain fog. The brain fog gets worse after any physical effort or emotional stress.

•**Orthostatic intolerance** is the worsening of symptoms upon standing.

Other common symptoms include muscle pain, headache, sore throat, constipation, diarrhea, chills, night sweats, shortness of breath, and heart palpitations.

Treatment and Prognosis

There are no approved drugs or treatment guidelines for ME/CFS. Cognitive behavioral therapy and graded-exercise therapy had some early research support, but follow-up studies found they were not effective. Trials of antiviral drugs, antibiotics, steroids, vitamins, supplements, and antidepressants have all failed.

What may help is managing specific symptoms…

•**For orthostatic intolerance,** increasing fluids and salt intake along with wearing support stockings may keep blood pressure from falling.

•**Over-the-counter pain medications may reduce pain.**

•**Working with a mental health-care provider can help anxiety and depression.**

•**Prescription medications are sometimes used to treat muscle spasms,** insomnia, depression, anxiety, or brain fog.

Addressing Sleep

People with ME/CFS often have problems sleeping, but even those who sleep well often feel tired when they wake up. The ME/CFS and Fibromyalgia Self-Help Program, founded by Bruce Campbell, PhD, notes that this is most likely due to insufficient delta sleep—the deepest and most restorative sleep phase. To improve your sleep, follow the principles of sleep hygiene. Create a comfortable environment that is dark, quiet, and cool. If you have a partner who snores, sleep separately. Go to bed and get up at the same time each day. Turn off electronic devices and television at least 30 minutes before bedtime. Try taking a warm bath or shower before bed. If you can't fall asleep, get out of bed and read or listen to soft music until you are sleepy. Use relaxation or breathing exercises to lower stress and ease tense muscles. Avoid caffeine, alcohol, and tobacco. Ask your doctor or pharmacist if any of your medications

What's in a Name? A Brief History

1934. ME/CFS was first recognized when there were sudden outbreaks of the symptoms that we still see today. At first, it was blamed on polio, but it was later recognized as a new disorder called *benign neuro myasthenia*, which means nonfatal, nerve-related muscle weakness.

1970. There was an epidemic of benign neuro myasthenia in London. Ill-informed doctors blamed it on mass hysteria because there were no obvious physical findings and most of the patients were women. They changed the name to *myalgia nervosa* (nervous muscle pains).

1980s. An outbreak occurred in New York and Nevada. At first, it was blamed on the Epstein-Barr virus, which causes mononucleosis. The name was changed to chronic *Epstein-Barr virus syndrome*.

1987. A committee created by the U.S. Centers for Disease Control and Prevention changed the name to chronic fatigue syndrome (CFS). At about the same time in Europe, the name was changed to *myalgic encephalomyelitis* (ME).

2015. The World Health Organization recognized both ME and CFS as real diseases of the nervous system, but even today, the name is controversial. People living with ME/CFS say chronic fatigue is too mild to describe how sick they feel.

2022. ME/CFS may not be the name much longer. The National Academy of Medicine has advised changing it to *systemic exertion intolerance disease* (SEID), a name that actually describes the condition.

cause sleeplessness or daytime drowsiness. Talk to your doctor about trying over-the-counter (OTC) supplements such as valerian, melatonin, passionflower, or chamomile.

If none of those steps help, you may want to see a sleep specialist who can assess you for sleep apnea, a common disorder in which your airway closes off until you wake up, gasp for air, and then go back to sleep. Most people with apnea are unaware that this is happening, but their partners often report excessive snoring. This can happen so frequently that people are chronically exhausted. The good news is that it's treatable with a device called CPAP (continuous positive airway pressure).

Another common disorder, restless legs syndrome, gives you strong unpleasant sensations that make you want to move your legs. It's often worse at night and can interfere with sleep.

Pacing

For PEM, a therapy called pacing is often effective. You figure out what level of physical or mental activity you can tolerate and learn to live inside your "energy envelope." *Here are some suggestions from the Solve ME/CFS Initiative...*

• **Prioritize what you need to do in a day.** Delegate when possible and eliminate nonessential tasks.

• **Complete small segments of activities with rest periods in between.**

• **If you have to do something that takes extra energy, rest before and after.**

• **If you feel dizzy, short of breath, or have other symptoms, immediately stop what you're doing and rest.**

• **Don't push through when you feel unwell or overdo it when you feel good.**

• **Pay attention to emotional triggers.** Worrying and feeling angry can sap you of energy.

For most people, ME/CFS is a lifetime disease, although there may be periods of remission. ME/CFS is not fatal, but it can be very debilitating: About 50 percent of people will be able to return to full- or part-time work, but about one-fourth will be housebound or bedridden at times.

Now that ME/CFS is finally being taken seriously, researchers may start finding answers to the mystery of its cause, and develop more effective treatments, and maybe even a cure.

Integrative Approaches for Rheumatoid Arthritis

Lawrence Taw, MD, director of the UCLA Center for East-West Medicine in Torrance, California. Dr. Taw is board-certified by both the American Board of Internal Medicine and the American Board of Integrative and Holistic Medicine. As director of the Center's Integrative East-West Inflammation Program, he collaborates with UCLA's division of rheumatology to use an integrative medicine approach for patients with various inflammatory joint and connective tissue disorders.

Marked by widespread joint pain, tenderness, swelling, and stiffness, rheumatoid arthritis can leave you fatigued, steal your appetite, provoke low-grade fevers, and even cause heart, lung, blood, nerve, eye, or skin problems.

But it's the pervasive pain that can sap energy and stop normal life in its tracks. The ever-expanding arsenal of drug options for RA often works far better at calming joint-damaging inflammation than quashing pain.

A Whole-Body Approach

Prescription medications—which include disease-modifying antirheumatic drugs, biologics, corticosteroids, and nonsteroidal anti-inflammatory drugs (NSAIDs)—are typically front-and-center in RA care and with good reason: These conventional treatments can slow disease progression and diminish pain. But lingering pain—bad enough on its own—also launches a damaging cascade, tampering with well-being, thwarting sleep, and ultimately tanking your mood. If you need more than just medication to live comfortably with RA, integrative medicine may fill the void.

An umbrella approach that treats the whole person, integrative medicine complements traditional Western medicine in a yin-yang embrace. Western medicine typically works better to stabilize acute RA symptoms or curb flare-ups, while integrative medicine shines at managing day-to-day RA symptoms and helping patients reduce or even eliminate certain medications. It also targets disease aspects that exacerbate pain that medications alone can't fully address. Integrative approaches to RA pain can be broken down into four main buckets: nutritional, physical, psychological, or a combination. Here are easy ways to incorporate them.

Nutritional Approach

In RA, certain foods might make pain worse, with common culprits including dairy, gluten, and processed sugars. An elimination diet can help you identify your personal triggers. Don't remove all possible triggers at once: Eliminate dairy first for two weeks and pay close attention to any possible joint effects. Then try another food group. This trial-and-error approach requires patience and vigilance.

You may also want to add RA-fighting foods to your diet…

- **Omega-3 fatty acids.** Found in fish and dietary supplements, omega-3s were shown in sweeping 2017 research to improve pain. Since most Americans don't eat much fish, fish oil capsules are an easy alternative. If you're vegan or don't appreciate the "fishy burps" some get with supplements, try flaxseed, which is also rich in omega-3s and can be sprinkled on foods.

- **Turmeric.** This golden spice, readily found in teabags and curry powder, helps block proteins that promote inflammation and can soothe pain as effectively as some NSAIDs. For best absorption, use turmeric with black pepper.

- **Ginger.** Little beats a cup of ginger tea in the morning to jump-start stiff and painful RA joints by promoting circulation that actually makes joints feel warmer. Research points to this herb's anti-inflammatory effects.

While fish oil, turmeric, and ginger supplements are widely available, they're more potent than food-based forms and raise the risks of excess bleeding. If you're on an aspirin regimen or prescription blood thinners, avoid these supplements and consume the nutrients only in foods, which requires no special considerations.

Physical Approach

The last thing you may feel like doing when your joints hurt is to move more. But exercise and other consistent physical activity targets RA pain and swelling by warming joints and muscles, relaxing soft tissues, and promoting healing blood flow. Much research also points to pain relief benefits from endorphins, feel-good chemicals that have been dubbed the body's natural opioids.

One of the easiest ways to get moving is in water. Swimming is gentler on joints than most land-based exercise and is often an effective bridge to get RA patients more active on terra firma as well. Since pool water is often heated, joints immediately feel better. Ask your doctor about aquatic physical therapy. Moist heating pads or warm baths can work wonders as well.

Acupuncture can fight pain as well. This traditional form of Chinese medicine is considered one of the oldest natural pain remedies, with research indicating it lowers levels of inflammatory chemicals and eases chronic pain. Using thin needles placed strategically around the body, the technique stimulates pressure points, releasing muscle tension and promoting blood flow that's crucial to healing.

Using the same principles as acupuncture, self-massage applies pressure on key pressure points around the body to stimulate relaxation, circulation, and the body's healing response. This can be done with hand and finger pressure, heat, or a small TENS (transcutaneous electrical nerve stimulation) device that delivers tiny electrical impulses through the skin. Ask your health-care provider for more information.

Magic of Menthol

Menthol, a chemical compound derived from peppermint, is a natural pain reliever. Rub mentholated ointment into achy joints, which also benefit from its circulation-promoting properties. *Diclofenac* gel (brand name Voltaren) is a topical anti-inflammatory that may augment these effects.

—Dr. Lawrence Taw

Psychological Approach

Consistent stress relief efforts can relax unconscious muscle tension that can significantly worsen RA pain. Common techniques include journaling, talk therapy, and deep breathing exercises. Working with the mind-body connection pays off in other ways as well, promoting overall well-being and sounder sleep that improves pain tolerance.

Combination Approach

Practices like tai chi blend elements of both exercise and stress reduction. This gentle martial art involving a series of slow movements has been shown in research to ease various types of pain and promote strength, flexibility, and balance. Tai chi also provides proven immune-enhancing effects and incorporates deep breathing, dampening the body's stress response.

Beware Snake Oil

Pain makes us vulnerable: When it's bad, we just want it gone. Discouragingly, some nefarious businesses and products prey on such desperation. Beware of exploitative and baseless online ads touting quick RA pain relief from intravenous or vitamin therapy. Also, certain botanicals promising less RA pain, such as the herb *Tripterygium wilfordii* (thunder god vine), can cause serious side effects like bone-thinning and male infertility.

Any supplement can potentially interact with RA drugs or other medications you're taking, both prescription and over-the-counter, so tell your doctor about everything you take. Natural doesn't necessarily mean safe.

Air Pollution Appears to Worsen Rheumatoid Arthritis

European Congress of Rheumatology

Exposure to even low levels of air pollution is associated with an elevated risk of arthritis flares and higher levels of C-reactive protein (a marker of inflammation). Researchers are planning additional studies to determine if the relationship is causal.

Eczema Is Linked to Autoimmune Diseases

Study by researchers at Karolinska Institute, Stockholm, Sweden, published in *British Journal of Dermatology*.

People with atopic dermatitis, commonly known as eczema, are nearly twice as likely to have autoimmune disorders, especially those that affect the gastrointestinal tract, skin or the body's connective tissue.

Blood Pressure Meds Linked to Psoriasis

Study titled "Antihypertensive Drug Use and Psoriasis: A Systematic Review, Meta- and Network Meta-analysis," by researchers at Ewha Womans University, Seoul, South Korea, published by the *British Journal of Clinical Pharmacology*.

Psoriasis is a chronic skin condition that is manifested by swelling and skin irritation. It can also affect the eyes and joints. Psoriasis is considered to be an autoimmune disease, where the body's immune system overreacts and attacks vital organs and tissue. When you have psoriasis, your immune system causes noticeable skin inflammation. Although the cause is not known, certain

factors may increase a person's risk of contracting psoriasis.

Psoriasis Might Be a Reaction to Blood Pressure Medications

A recent review of 21 studies involving about 12 million people concludes that one of the risk factors for psoriasis is taking a blood pressure medication known as an antihypertensive. This link between antihypertensives and psoriasis is not new, but there has not been a consensus on whether antihypertensives actually increase risk for psoriasis.

Although some studies have found a link, others have not. Previous studies have also found an increased risk of psoriasis in people with high blood pressure, so it's not clear if high blood pressure or high blood pressure medications increase the risk of psoriasis.

Doctors Should Monitor High Blood Pressure Patients for Psoriasis

The new review of studies was conducted by researchers at Ewha Womans University in Seoul, South Korea, and published in the *British Journal of Clinical Pharmacology*. They found that all high blood pressure drugs were associated with a higher risk of psoriasis. There was a significant increased risk with drugs called ACE inhibitors, calcium channel blockers, beta-blockers, and thiazide diuretics. The pooled risk for these drugs ranged between a 40 percent increased risk and doubling of risk.

The researchers say that this review confirms an association between blood pressure medications and psoriasis risk. Although this association does not prove that blood pressure medications cause psoriasis, it does suggest that patients who take blood pressure medications should be followed closely by their doctors for signs of psoriasis.

Other Risk Factors for Psoriasis

Other risk factors for psoriasis include a family history of the disease and skin injury from trauma, burns or radiation. Infections, stress, alcohol, smoking, and obesity may also be risk factors. Beta-blockers and other drugs that include lithium, chloroquine, steroids, and non-steroidal anti-inflammatory drugs (NSAIDS) may worsen psoriasis.

The reason why high blood pressure or high blood pressure medications are associated with psoriasis has not been determined. Psoriasis is associated with other diseases of inflammation (comorbidities). According to the National Psoriasis Foundation, successful treatment of psoriasis can reduce the risk of comorbidities and treatment of comorbidities can make psoriasis easier to treat. Comorbidities include high blood pressure, heart disease, diabetes, obesity, high cholesterol, and inflammatory bowel disease.

Psoriasis Complications

Zhanna Mikulik, MD, a rheumatologist at The Ohio State University Wexner Medical Center and rheumatology and immunology faculty member at its College of Medicine.

People tend to think of psoriasis as a skin condition, and it's easy to see why. The most visible symptom is red patches covered by silvery plaques that appear anywhere on the body. But those plaques are more than skin deep. They're just one manifestation of an immune system malfunction that causes certain white blood cells to overproduce proteins called *cytokines*, leading to chronic inflammation. You can see the effects of inflammation on the skin, but the damage is happening internally, too.

Common Complications

The low-grade, systemic inflammation that comes with psoriasis can contribute to a host of hidden complications, such as increased insulin resistance, oxidative stress, endothelial cell dysfunction, and atherosclerosis (plaque buildup in the arteries), increasing the risk for other diseases.

●**Heart disease.** Cardiovascular disease (CVD) is one of the most significant conditions that can occur with psoriasis.

It's one result of the dramatic snowball effect of systemic inflammation: First, the inflammation leads to insulin resistance. That's when cells in your liver, muscles, and fat don't use the hormone insulin to effectively tap the glucose, or sugar, in your blood for your energy needs. Your pancreas is then tasked with making more insulin to help the process along, but at some point, it may not be able to keep up, setting the stage for diabetes.

●**Inflammation-induced insulin resistance is thought to lead to endothelial dysfunction**—when the endothelial cells that line your arteries don't work as they should, causing blood vessels to narrow. This creates what's called vascular stiffness and increases the risk for atherosclerosis, dangerous plaque buildup along the arteries. Treating psoriasis and monitoring its effects on your heart can help protect your heart health.

●**Eye conditions.** Many people with psoriatic disease also develop autoimmune eye diseases. Inflammation of the iris, uvea, or retina (uveitis) is the most common disorder, but any part of the eye can be affected, including the cornea (keratitis), the edges of the eyelids (blepharitis), the membrane that lines the eyes and eyelids, called the conjunctiva (conjunctivitis), the whites of the eyes, called the sclera (scleritis), and the tissue between the conjunctiva and the sclera (episcleritis).

●**Psoriatic arthritis.** In about one-third of people with psoriasis, the immune system will attack the joints in what's called psoriatic arthritis (PsA). As with many other types of arthritis, inflammation leads to painful, stiff, and swollen joints. The arthritis can be severe and lead to permanent joint damage.

●**Obesity.** Being overweight can cause inflammation, but there's also a link between obesity and psoriasis. A study in the *British Journal of Dermatology* reported that people who lost weight saw a 50 percent reduction in psoriasis symptoms within about five months.

- **High blood pressure.** Hypertension is more common in patients with psoriatic disease. People with late-onset psoriasis or obesity have the highest risk, researchers reported in *Clinical Rheumatology* in 2019.

- **Other autoimmune diseases.** Having psoriasis makes having another autoimmune disease more likely. There's genetic overlap between psoriasis, Crohn's disease, ankylosing spondylitis, primary sclerosing cholangitis, and ulcerative colitis.

Researchers reported in the journal *Immunology* that two autoimmune disorders, vitiligo, which causes skin-pigmentation loss, and alopecia areata, which causes hair loss, are linked to psoriasis.

Guarding Against Complications

Just as many complications are interrelated, there's overlap among prevention steps. For instance, sticking with your psoriasis treatment, losing weight, eating a healthier diet, and exercising more will all help you avoid obesity, diabetes, high blood pressure, and cardiovascular disease. *Here are more specifics…*

- **Quit smoking.** Smoking stimulates inflammation, and quitting is one of the strongest recommendations in the 2018 American College of Rheumatology/National Psoriasis Foundation guideline for PsA treatment. There is strong evidence that smoking makes the disease worse and even reduces the efficacy of biological medications.

- **Control stress.** Physical activity, deep breathing, meditation, and cognitive behavioral therapy can help you manage both your physical and mental health.

- **Get a good night's sleep.** Deep sleep strengthens the immune system, while too little weakens it and may increase your pain perception.

- **Practice good sleep hygiene.** Shut off screens at least an hour before bed, go to bed at the same time every night, and keep your bedroom dark and cool. Pain can make it hard to get good rest, so tell your doctor if your symptoms aren't under control. Adjusting your medications may help you get the deep sleep you need.

- **Aim for daily exercise.** Regular physical activity can lessen joint pain and improve your mobility, energy level, endurance, and sleep quality. Go for low-impact activities like walking, bicycling, swimming, and water exercises to avoid stressing your joints.

Exercise will also help with weight loss. Gentle stretching for at least five minutes before and after activity can help you warm up, expand your range of motion, and avoid injury.

- **Eat a quality diet.** New research published in the *Journal of Investigative Dermatology* found that too much sugar and saturated fat can upset the gut microbiome and worsen inflammation, psoriasis, and PsA.

The Mediterranean diet is a great anti-inflammation approach to good health, incorporating fish, grains, fruits, vegetables, and extra virgin olive oil, which research shows has anti-inflammatory properties.

- **Get regular health checks.** In addition to working with a rheumatologist to control psoriasis, get regular blood pressure checks and blood tests that measure cholesterol and glucose levels. High levels of all of these can increase the risk for heart disease and diabetes.

Prevent Total-Knee Replacement with Realignment Surgery

Codie Primeau, PhD candidate, Collaborative Training Program in Musculoskeletal Health Research, Western University, London, Ontario. His study was published in *Canadian Medical Association Journal*.

High tibial osteotomy straightens limbs in patients with bowed legs and knee arthritis. It shifts knee loads to improve pain and function. In a study of 643 knees in 556 patients, 95 percent did not have knee replacement within five years…79 percent did not have knee replacement within 10 years. The surgery is especially suitable for younger, more active patients with less severe joint damage.

A Possible Cause for a Mysterious Condition

Study titled, "Assessment of Cytokines, MicroRNA and Patient Related Outcome Measures in Conversion Disorder/Functional Neurological Disorder (CD/FND): The CANDO Clinical Feasibility Study," by researchers at the University of York and Hull York Medical School, UK, published in *Brain, Behavior, & Immunity-Health*.

Conversion disorder/functional neurologic disorder (CD/FND) is a mysterious condition that brings about such symptoms as weakness, paralysis, or even blindness. The most distressing thing about this disorder is that no cause can be found. People with CD/FND have symptoms that can drastically affect their quality of life. Treatments such as psychotherapy, physical therapy and hypnosis have had limited success.

A study from researchers at University of York and Hull York Medical School in the UK has found evidence that the cause is stress-related inflammation. The study was small, only 15 people, but the researchers believe that their findings can lead to larger studies into the cause of CD/FND and possibly to new treatments. Their study is published in the journal *Brain, Behavior, & Immunity-Health*.

Stress Triggers Inflammation

Patients recruited for the study were diagnosed with CD/FND. Their past and present stress levels were explored. Over 80 percent of the patients had significant or repeated childhood traumas, called adverse childhood experience, and an above-average score on current stressful life events. Stress is known to trigger inflammation. The researchers found elevated levels of several stress markers, called *cytokines*. Cytokines are small proteins that trigger the immune system to cause inflammation.

CD/FND is known to affect close to 800,000 people in the UK alone.

More Research Needed to Find a Viable Treatment

The researchers were able to recruit patients who could remain actively involved in the study despite the disabilities caused by their symptoms. They found evidence of childhood and current life stress, and they linked the stress to elevated cytokine levels. This type of initial study is called a pilot study or feasibility study. One of the main goals is to find out if future studies are projected to yield results…and the researchers concluded that future studies are feasible. The researchers also hope to delve into the areas of treatment, since the usual pathways for psychosomatic disorders have not been successful with CD/FND.

Redheads Feel Less Pain

Study by researchers at Massachusetts General Hospital, Boston, published in *Science Advances*.

Red hair is caused by a variant form of certain pigment-producing skin cells.

Recent mouse study: The variant also alters the body's balance between opioid receptors that inhibit pain and receptors that perceive pain.

Result: A higher pain threshold. Confirming this finding could lead to new drugs to manage pain.

Chapter 13

PHYSICAL INJURY AND BONE HEALTH

Tennis Elbow: Anyone Can Get It

You don't have to play tennis to get tennis elbow. In fact, most people who develop this painful condition are not racket-sports enthusiasts. Instead, they are hairdressers, gardeners, knitters, or anyone who puts repetitive strain on the muscles and tendons of the forearms. Some people develop tennis elbow after an injury. Others develop it without any apparent cause.

The condition, formally known as lateral epicondylitis, can be so painful that people abandon favorite sports or hobbies or can no longer do their jobs.

The good news: It's treatable, usually without surgery.

To understand what causes the pain in the first place, it helps to know a little anatomy. The muscles in your forearm are responsible for the extension of your wrists and fingers. Your forearm tendons, or extensors, attach these muscles to your upper arm bone at a bony point in your elbow called the lateral epicondyle. Over time, heavy use of your wrists and forearms can cause the tendon to pull away from the bone and develop small tears.

Getting a Diagnosis

The main symptom of tennis elbow is a distinctly painful spot on the outer elbow. The pain usually starts gradually and gets worse over time. It tends to be most noticeable when you use your wrists and forearms, especially with twisting motions. For some people, even shaking hands is painful.

If you go to your doctor with elbow pain in the spot typically associated with tennis elbow, he or she likely will press on the spot to confirm the location of the discomfort and ask how long you have had the pain and when you tend to notice it most. In many cases, you also will get an MRI scan to confirm the diagnosis.

If you have a clear-cut case of tennis elbow, you might not need any other tests. But if the diagnosis is not clear, you might get a more extensive workup. For example, you might get an X-ray to rule out arthritis in your elbow.

What to Try First

Once you know you have tennis elbow, the first thing to try is resting the affected arm

Steve K. Lee, MD, Chief of the Hand and Upper Extremity Service at Hospital for Special Surgery in New York City.

for about a month. Stop or cut back on activities that aggravate your condition. That's not too hard if your pain is caused by recreational tennis or backyard gardening, but if the aggravating activities are part of your job, taking a break can be tougher. If needed, a doctor may write to your employer saying that you temporarily need different duties or a few weeks off.

During this time, try wearing a brace on your wrist. While wearing a wrist brace when your elbow hurts might seem counterintuitive, the idea is to support and rest the affected tendon at the point where it originates. Look for a brace that gently holds the wrist in a "cocked up" position. These are widely sold in drug stores and online.

You can take ibuprofen, naproxen, or other other-the-counter analgesics to control pain for a few days. But, because taking those medications for a long time can have side effects, such as ulcers and stomach bleeding, you might want to try an anti-inflammatory gel that you can apply directly to the painful area. Effective products containing the active ingredient *diclofenac* are available over the counter. Studies suggest they produce fewer side effects than pills do.

Some doctors also advise applying ice when your elbows hurt, especially when you first notice the pain. Apply ice or cold packs for 10 to 15 minutes several times a day. Put a cloth under the ice to protect your skin.

What to Try Next

If you still have symptoms after a month of rest, bracing, and pain management, your next stop should be a physical therapy clinic. A therapist can work with you on gentle exercises to stretch and strengthen the muscles in your forearm.

When Tennis IS the Cause

Sometimes tennis elbow is caused by playing tennis or other racket sports, but an aching elbow doesn't mean it's game over. Instead, you should work with a coach or trainer to see where you might make improvements in your equipment or technique that could ease the strain on your elbows. Common modifications include restringing your racket to reduce string tension, adjusting the grip size on your racket, or using a different backhand technique.

If your pain persists, you may want to try a shot of cortisone, a potent anti-inflammatory agent that is injected directly into the painful area. Tennis elbow is not caused by inflammation, but the shots seem to help some people. If one shot does not provide adequate relief, your doctor may recommend a second shot after six to eight weeks.

Some doctors offer an additional therapy known as platelet-rich plasma (PRP). Platelets, which are blood cells that aid clotting and contain substances that might aid healing, are obtained from your own blood and injected into the affected area. Studies of the therapy have produced mixed results. Another experimental approach is using ultrasound or shock waves to promote healing.

Whatever approach you take, you should know that most patients get better within several months.

Turning to Surgery

If you don't get better after six to nine months, you may be among the 10 to 20 percent of patients who are candidates for surgery. In the most common procedure, your surgeon will make one cut over your injured tendon and remove the damaged tissue. The tendon is then repaired. Less commonly, surgery is done with an arthroscope, a thin tube with a tiny camera and light that is inserted through a few small cuts. The surgeon uses a video monitor to see and remove the unhealthy part of the tendon. Neither kind of surgery requires an overnight hospital stay.

After surgery, you may need to wear a splint on your arm for a couple of weeks and then a wrist brace for a couple more. After that healing period, you will start gentle exercises to restore motion, followed by several weeks of strengthening exercises.

About 80 percent of people who have tennis elbow surgery get relief from their pain and can return to their usual activities as long as they take care to prevent new damage by using proper form during sports and hobbies and avoiding overdoing it at work, for instance.

Others may have to make bigger lifestyle changes or try repeated treatments to keep their elbows in good working form.

Elbows Can Be Replaced

Elizabeth Nolan, MD, clinical assistant professor of orthopaedic surgery at The University of Oklahoma, Oklahoma City.

Osteoporotic patients who fracture their elbows or people who develop arthritis after injuries are undergoing replacements. Part of the upper arm bone and part of one or both bones of the lower arm are replaced with metal implants.

Recovery time: Six weeks with no weight on the arm…then 12 weeks of physical therapy. Patients should not lift more than five to seven pounds with that arm for the rest of their lives.

Hand Therapy: Simple Exercises Can Preserve Function

Timothy G. Havenhill, MD, a hand specialist and orthopedic surgeon at Northwestern Medicine McHenry Hospital, Crystal Lake, Illinois.

Physical therapy can be beneficial for both arthritis and carpal tunnel syndrome. For arthritis, physical therapy emphasizes range of motion, joint functionality, strength, flexibility, and dexterity.

Arthritis Exercises

Try these simple exercises at home. For each one, do 10 repetitions on each hand.

• **Fist formation.** Fully extend your fingers, and then draw them in to form a fist with your thumb outside of your fingers. Don't squeeze. Hold the fist for three breaths; then slowly extend your fingers again.

• **Finger bends.** Fully extend your fingers, and then curl one finger at a time as far as you can into your palm. Hold each finger stretch three breaths and repeat 10 times.

• **Form an O.** Fully extend your fingers, and then slowly curve your fingers and thumb into an "O" shape. Release.

• **Hitchhiker bend.** Place your hand on a table with your thumb pointing up as if you are about to shake someone's hand. Curl your fingers into your palm to make a hitchhiker's sign. Release.

• **Finger lift.** Place your hand on a table, palm up. Raise each finger, one at a time, as high as it will go.

• **Wrist flex.** Extend your right arm and hand with your palm facing down. Use your left hand to press down on the back of the right hand until your palm is facing you. Hold for three breaths; then return to your original position. Repeat with your left arm.

• **Grip strengthener.** Squeeze a soft ball or rolled-up sock as hard as you can for three breaths. Release.

Carpal Tunnel Exercises

For carpal tunnel syndrome, physical therapists use what are called nerve-glide exercises. The carpal tunnel is a narrow passageway in the wrist. Carpal tunnel syndrome occurs when that passageway compresses the median nerve that runs through it. The nerve-glide exercise can help reduce pressure on the nerve to reduce symptoms, while tendon-glide exercises may improve range of motion.

• **Nerve-glide exercise.** Apply heat to your wrist and hand for 15 minutes. Make a fist with your thumb outside your fingers.

Hold this and each subsequent position for three seconds.

- Extend your fingers while keeping your thumb close to the side of your hand.
- Keep your fingers straight and bend your hand back toward your forearm.
- Keep your fingers and wrist in position and extend your thumb.
- Keep your fingers, wrist, and thumb extended and turn your palm up.
- Keep your fingers, wrist, and thumb extended and use your other hand to stretch the thumb.
- Ice your hand and arm for 20 minutes.
- **Tendon-glide exercise 1.** Apply heat to your wrist and hand for 15 minutes. Hold your hand in front of you with your wrist straight. Your fingertips should be pointed to the ceiling. Straighten all of your fingers. Hold this and each subsequent position for three seconds.
  - Bend the tips of your fingers into a "hook" position, with your knuckles up, and hold for three seconds.
  - Make a fist with your thumb over your fingers and hold for three seconds.
- **Tendon-glide exercise 2.** Apply heat to your wrist and hand for 15 minutes. Hold your hand in front of you with your wrist straight. Your fingertips should be pointed to the ceiling. Straighten all of your fingers. Hold this and each subsequent position for three seconds.
  - Bend your fingers at the bottom knuckle. On your right hand, the shape looks like the number seven. Hold for three seconds. Bend your fingers at the middle joint and touch your palm.
  - When you've done the series, ice your hand and arm for 20 minutes.

More Exercises

- **Wrist extension.** Hold your hand as if you're telling someone to stop, and straighten your arm. Use the opposite hand to gently pull your palm toward you until you feel a stretch in your forearm. Hold for 15 seconds, release, and repeat five times.

Don't Delay

Exercises like these, as well as nighttime splinting, can effectively stop the progression of carpal tunnel syndrome symptoms, but only if they are caught soon enough. In most cases, once strength and sensation are lost, they can't be brought back, even with surgery. The most important thing you can do is seek an evaluation with a hand specialist or orthopedic surgeon. An occupational therapist can help develop strategies to work around hand impairments.

- **Wrist flexion.** Keep your arm straightened, and bend your wrist so your palm and fingers are pointing down. Use your opposite hand to pull your hand toward your body until you feel a gentle stretch on the top of your forearm. Hold for 15 seconds, release, and repeat five times.

Don't Treat a Sprain with Ice...Counter-Wisdom for Injury

Paul A. Offit, MD, attending physician in the division of infectious diseases at Children's Hospital of Philadelphia and the Maurice R. Hilleman Professor of Vaccinology at Perelman School of Medicine at University of Pennsylvania. He is author of *Overkill: When Modern Medicine Goes Too Far*. Paul-Offit.com

Many things we do to heal ourselves and stay healthy are based not on modern science but on outdated theories and unproven practices.

Belief: Treat a sprain with R.I.C.E. (Rest, Ice, Compression, Elevation).

Truth: Treating a sprain with R.I.C.E. can delay healing.

When an ankle is sprained, the damaged ligaments surrounding it release substances that promote inflammation, which triggers the body to boost blood flow to the injured area. Increased blood flow steers clotting factors and immune cells to the injury, where they help stop internal bleeding and remove damaged cells. Inflammation also promotes production of the protein collagen, which is needed for recovery. In other words, inflammation fuels healing.

But inflammation also causes pain. That's why the R.I.C.E. protocol, created by sports medicine physician Gabe Mirkin in 1978, gained traction, and many medical groups, including the American Academy of Orthopaedic Surgeons and National Athletic Trainers' Association, have endorsed it for treating sprains and other minor injuries. Rest, ice, compression (wrapping) and elevation all feel good in the moment, but ice and compression decrease blood flow to the injured area—the opposite of what is needed for healing.

Result: A prolonged period of healing and, possibly, improperly healed ligaments.

Important finding: There is "limited evidence supporting the efficacy" of the R.I.C.E approach, concluded a 2020 study in *World Journal of Orthopedics.* And in 2015, Dr. Mirkin himself renounced his own popular advice.

What to do instead: Try to tough out the pain without ice and compression. After the initial swelling has decreased, applying warmth to the area—a heating pad or a warm, damp cloth—for an hour may provide some relief. Elevation also may help.

Also: After a few days of rest and once the swelling has gone down, try gentle ankle movements to increase blood flow to the area.

Example: Draw an imaginary alphabet with your foot.

Protect Yourself from Falls

Carrie Ali, editor, *Bottom Line Health.* BottomLine Inc.com

Close to one-third of people ages 65 or older fall every year, and about 10 percent of them suffer serious injuries.

Even those who escape injury often develop a fear of falling that can have a devastating effect on activity levels and quality of life. *Fortunately, a few simple steps can help reduce your risk…*

•**Exercise.** Both group- and home-based exercise programs can reduce the rate of falls by up to 23 percent. Tai chi and exercises that improve leg strength and balance are particularly effective. Exercise can also reduce the risk of injury: Weight-bearing activities such as jogging, weightlifting, or using resistance bands stimulate the growth of new bone tissue, making bones stronger.

•**Monitor your vision.** Visit your eye doctor every year or two and update your glasses as needed. Bifocals and progressive lenses can distort distance vision and lead to falls on stairs. Consider alternating between two sets of glasses instead. If your glasses tint in reaction to sunlight, wait for them to adjust before going from outdoors to indoors.

•**Stand slowly.** If you experience sudden dizziness when standing up, stand slowly, and if you start to feel dizzy, sit or lie down and allow any dizziness to pass.

•**Consider footwear.** Something as simple as the shoes you choose can make a big difference. Flip-flops, high heels, slippers, and socks can increase your risk of slipping and falling. Even when you're in the house, opt for sturdy shoes with non-slip soles to reduce risk.

•**Manage medication.** Medications such as antidepressants, antipsychotics, benzodiazepines, antiepileptics, opioids, and antihypertensive agents have been linked to a higher risk of falls. Talk to your physician about swapping high-risk drugs for safer options.

These quick tweaks can keep you on your feet and mobile for many years to come.

Best Exercise to Prevent a Potentially Devastating Fall

Rudolph Tanzi, MD, Joseph P. and Rose F. Kennedy Professor of Neurology, Harvard Medical School, and Tara Stiles, founder of Strala Yoga, and author of *Clean Mind, Clean Body: A 28-Day Plan for Physical, Mental and Spiritual Self-Care.*

While exercise, in general, is an excellent way to improve stability and balance, a form of tai chi specifically designed to reduce the risk of falls is particularly effective, researchers reported in *JAMA Network Open* and *JAMA Internal Medicine.* Tai Ji Quan: Moving for Better Balance (TJQMBB) emphasizes exercises that include coordinated eye-head-hand movement, head-shoulder-trunk alignment and rotation, unilateral weight bearing, and weight shifting. TJQMBB specifically targets modifiable fall risk factors including gait abnormalities, impaired balance, and reduced lower- extremity strength.

Researchers randomized 670 people who were 70 years of age or older and who had impaired mobility or a history of falls to one of three groups. In all three groups, participants exercised for one hour twice per week for 24 weeks. Each exercise session consisted of a warm-up, an active exercise, and a cool-down. Group 1 participants completed TJQMBB exercises. Group 2 participants completed aerobic conditioning as well as strength, balance, and flexibility activities. They used hand and ankle weights, resistance tubing, and balance foams. Group 3 participants performed seated breathing, stretching, and relaxation activities.

Throughout the study and the six-month follow-up, participants recorded any falls and whether they required medical care. Falls that resulted in sprains, strains, contusions, or abrasions requiring no medical care were considered mildly injurious,

"Toe Test" Assesses Risk of Falling

Researchers have devised an easy way to predict if an elderly person is at risk of falling.

Enhanced paper grip test: The healthcare practitioner slides a small card beneath the patient's foot and then tries to pull it out while asking the patient to grip the card with his/her big toe. Inability to hold the card in place signals that the patient lacks strength and balance needed to avoid a dangerous fall.

Study by researchers at Staffordshire University, Stoke-on-Trent, UK, published in *Gait & Posture.*

while those that resulted in admission to an emergency department or hospital were deemed to be seriously injurious.

The researchers reported that, after one year, participants in the TJQMBB and multimodal exercise groups had significantly fewer falls than those in the stretching group.

But when they looked at falls that resulted in serious injuries, the results were more striking: Participants in the TJQMBB group reported 11 seriously injurious falls compared with 29 in the multimodal exercise group and 50 in the control group.

Other studies have found equally compelling results with nonspecific tai chi interventions. A review published in *BMJ Open* in 2017 analyzed 18 trials with 3,824 participants and concluded that traditional tai chi, especially Yang style, significantly reduced the risk of falls in older adults. The U.S. Centers for Disease Control and Prevention also recommends tai chi as an effective fall-reduction strategy. For exercise examples and instructions, go to YouTube.com and search "TJQMBB 8 forms."

Alternative Ways to Ease Long-Term Concussion Disorders

Rebecca Acabchuk, PhD, is a senior scientist at RoundGlass, a global holistic wellness company, and an associate research professor affiliate at University of Connecticut in Storrs. She is lead author of a meta-analysis of 22 studies published in *Applied Psychology: Health and Well-Being.*

Chronic concussion symptoms are eased by yoga, meditation, and mindfulness.

These practices reduce fatigue and depression while boosting quality of life for patients dealing with long-term symptoms from brain injury, such as headaches, disturbed sleep and impaired academic/job performance. They are low-risk modalities that promote healing and can be used as part of a recovery plan.

Osteoporosis Linked to Hearing Loss in Women

Study titled "Osteoporosis, Bisphosphonate Use, and the Risk of Moderate or Worse Hearing Loss in Women," by researchers at Brigham and Women's Hospital and Harvard University, published in *Journal of the American Geriatrics Society.*

Among the many pitfalls of aging are hearing loss and low bone density. Could one possibly cause the other? Previous studies have found that hearing loss is more common in women who have low bone density (LBD) or osteoporosis. However, the studies have been inconsistent, and few studies have followed hearing loss in women over time (called a longitudinal study).

Hearing loss that comes with age, called age-related hearing loss, is not reversible. Yet animal studies suggest that drugs called bisphosphonates may reduce hearing loss caused by noise damage. Bisphosphonates are used to treat osteoporosis.

Head Injury Links to Brain Damage

A Single Head Injury Increases the Risk of Dementia in Later Life

Researchers recently discovered that a person with a single head injury had a 1.25 times higher risk of developing dementia than someone with no head injuries. A history of two or more injuries more than doubled the risk. Overall, 9.5 percent of all dementia cases in the study population could be attributed to a head injury.

Andrea L.C. Schneider, MD, PhD, assistant professor of neurology, University of Pennsylvania School of Medicine, Philadelphia, Pennsylvania.

More Than One-Third of Kids With Concussions Experience Mental Health Problems

Recent finding: 37 percent of children who had concussions developed problems with anxiety, depression, withdrawal, or PTSD, and 20 percent developed problems with aggression, hyperactivity, or attention—and some problems persisted for years. While a history of mental health issues raises risk for more after a concussion, 26 percent of the children with such issues had no history of them.

Vicki Anderson, PhD, pediatric neuropsychologist at Murdoch Children's Research Institute, Parkville, Australia, and leader of a study of 90,000 concussion cases, published in *British Journal of Sports Medicine.*

Can Bisphosphonates Curb Hearing Loss?

Researchers from Brigham and Women's Hospital and Harvard University wanted to see if a longitudinal study would confirm the risk of hearing loss in women with osteoporosis and if taking bisphosphonates reduces the risk. To find out, they used data from the long-running Nurses' Health Studies. Since 1976 (NHS) and 1989 (NHSII), nurses have been sending in data to Harvard University every two years on a wide range of health issues.

Nearly 144,000 women from NHS and NHSII were included in the study. Their ages ranged from 31 to 61. These women had reported hearing loss or worsening of hearing, a diagnosis of osteoporosis or LBD, any hip or spine (vertebral) fractures, and medications (including bisphosphonates). Hip and vertebral fractures are the most common fractures in women with osteoporosis. The results of the study were published in the *Journal of the American Geriatrics Society.* These were the key findings…

• **Compared to women without osteoporosis or LBD,** women with osteoporosis or LBD had a 14 to 30 percent higher risk of hearing loss.

• **The risk of hearing loss was the same in women who used bisphosphonates** as in women who did not use bisphosphonates.

• **Having a hip fracture did not increase the risk of hearing loss,** but having a vertebral fracture increased the risk by 31 to 39 percent.

Theory for an Osteoporosis– Hearing Loss Link

The researchers were unable to determine exactly how osteoporosis or LBD might cause hearing loss or why vertebral fractures, but not hip fractures, increased the risk in women. They suspect that the difference between hip and vertebral fractures may be due to the difference in the type of bone structures. One theory of how osteoporosis or LBD may cause hearing loss is that if density changes in bones that surround and protect the hearing nerves in the inner ear, this could have an effect on nerve function and eventually initiate hearing loss.

Although bisphosphonates may not reduce the risk of hearing loss, there is some hope for other remedies. Previous research by the team shows that a heathy diet, exercise, a healthy weight, and not smoking reduces the risk of hearing loss.

Age-Proof Your Bones

Ann Louise Gittleman, PhD, CNS, a holistic nutritionist based in Post Falls, Idaho, and The New York Times best-selling author who has written more than 35 books, including Radical Longevity: The Powerful Plan to Sharpen Your Brain, Strengthen Your Body, and Reverse the Symptoms of Aging. AnnLouise.com

Calcium gets all the attention, but your body requires other key minerals to properly deposit that calcium where it's needed. *Here are the key players*…*

• **Magnesium,** found in leafy green vegetables, nuts, seeds, and legumes, helps create strong, more flexible bones.

Recommended: 400 mg to 800 mg of magnesium per day.

• **Boron** plays a key role in maintaining calcium and magnesium levels. Prunes are an excellent source.

Recommended: 3 mg/day—about 10 prunes.

• **Selenium.** Selenium is an antioxidant protector that helps support bone health. Found in Brazil nuts, fish and beans.

Recommended: 100 mcg/day to 200 mcg/day—about two or three Brazil nuts, depending on size.

• **Vitamin D,** found in eggs, fatty fish, beef liver and mushrooms, supports calcium absorption.

Recommended: 2,000 IU/day to 5,000 IU/day. You also can get the recommended amount by exposing your arms and legs to 15 to 20 minutes of midday sunshine.

• **Vitamin K** activates the critical protein *osteocalcin,* which integrates calcium into bones. Food sources include green leafy vegetables such as collards, kale, and spinach.

Recommended: 90 mcg per day—up to one cup.

*Be sure to ask your doctor before starting to take any new supplements. Vitamin K, in particular, can interfere with medications such as coumadin.

Evenity Effective for Osteoporosis

Arthritis Advisor

A study presented at the American Society for Bone and Mineral Research Annual Meeting showed that in patients who took *romosozumab* (Evenity) once per month for 12 months, bone density increased an average of 14 percent in the lumbar spine and 6.6 percent in the hip. Romosozumab is an anabolic agent that stimulates bone formation and decreases bone resorption. It is FDA-approved for postmenopausal women at high risk for bone fractures.

How Massage Heals and Strengthens Muscles

Studied titled "Skeletal Muscle Regeneration with Robotic Actuation-Mediated Clearance of Neutrophils," by researchers at Harvard's Wyss Institute for Biologically Inspired Engineering, Boston, published in *Science Translational Medicine*.

The hands-on practice of massage has been helping to heal sore and injured muscles throughout human history. And several modern studies support the use of massage to soothe body aches and pains. But how does it work? A new study from researchers at Harvard's Wyss Institute for Biologically Inspired Engineering may have found the answer.

Skeletal Muscles and Mechanotherapy

Researchers know that immune cells, the cells of your body's defense system, play a role in the skeletal muscles' response to injury. Skeletal muscles are the muscles you use to move your bones. To search the link between muscle repair and the immune system, the research team studied the effects of compression and stimulation on damaged muscles in mice. This type of muscle massage is called *mechanotherapy*.

In their study, which is published in the journal *Science Translational Medicine*, the team caused muscle damage in the hind legs of mice by injecting the leg muscles with a substance called myotoxin. To treat the damaged muscles with mechanotherapy, the team developed a robotic device that would compress the muscle at a pressure and rate that could be measured and regulated. At the same time, the team used ultrasound imaging to measure muscle regeneration and repair.

No More Inflammatory Substances, No More Pain

Two groups of mice received the myotoxin injections, but only one group received mechanotherapy. The researchers discovered that muscle repair was faster and stronger in the mice receiving 14 days of mechanotherapy. The reason is that mechanotherapy compressed inflammatory cells called *neutrophils* out of the muscles, which improved the muscles' ability to heal and regenerate muscle cells.

Neutrophils are the body's way of removing germs and damaged tissues. They release inflammatory substances called *cytokines* and *chemokines*. The research team showed that neutrophils help in the early stages of muscle damage, but the inflammatory substances interfere with muscle repair and regeneration.

Neutrophils and inflammatory substances were lower in the treated muscles than in the muscles that were left to heal on their own. To confirm the removal of neutrophils during mechanotherapy, the team injected tiny fluorescent molecules. The researchers could witness these molecules vacating the muscle fibers during mechanotherapy. They also grew muscle tissue in the lab and observed the effects of neutrophils on a molecular level.

Soon after a muscle injury, the neutrophils stimulated the growth of cells called *muscle progenitor cells*, but the inflammatory substances released by the neutrophils slowed down the growth of the progenitor cells into fully active muscle cells. When the team analyzed muscle fibers in the treated and untreated mice, they found that the mice who received mechanotherapy were able to grow larger and stronger muscle fibers than the untreated mice.

The team would like to continue their research in larger animals and eventually in humans. This could lead to mechanotherapy devices that would treat injured muscles, improve muscle performance, and may even treat age-related muscle loss, bringing the ancient art of massage into the twenty-first century.

For more information on how massage can relieve pain: Visit the National Center for Complementary and Integrative Health website at NCCIH.NIH.gov/health/massage-therapy-what-you-need-to-know.

Avoid Injury When Pushing and Pulling Objects

Harvard Health Letter. Health.Harvard.edu

Use your core and leg muscles, and don't arch your back.

For pushing: Stand close to the object, knees slightly bent with one leg slightly behind the other and elbows braced against your sides. Tighten your abdominal muscles and push the object forward.

For pulling: Face the object, knees slightly bent and feet close to the object, hip-width apart and elbows braced against your sides. Grab onto the object, tighten your abdominal muscles and take a step backward, pulling the object with you.

Exercising Barefoot Helps Balance and Mobility

The neural feedback to the brain provided by thousands of nerve endings in our feet encourages subtle muscle adjustments to optimize strength and balance. Wearing shoes smothers those communications.

To start: Walk barefoot in your house for 10 minutes a day…stand barefoot on both feet and turn your head from side to side… balance barefoot on one foot for five seconds and work up to a minute on each side.

Stacey Vachon, a certified personal trainer and owner of Core V3 Fitness Studio in Vail, Colorado. COREV3.com

Best: If you have a choice, pushing is safer than pulling—people can push about twice as much weight as they can pull.

Compression Socks Preserve Strength After Training

Study by researchers at Tohoku University, Sendai, Japan, published in *European Journal of Applied Physiology.*

Wearing below-the-knee compression garments during exercise helped avoid loss of strength for 24 hours, meaning that the wearer could go back to maximal-intensity strength training sooner. Because of the mechanical support and tissue compression provided by the socks, they also can decrease risk for musculoskeletal injury.

Chapter 14

PREGNANCY AND REPRODUCTIVE ISSUES

New Hope for Pregnancy in Early Menopause

Human procreation does not adhere to equality of the sexes. Unlike men who can produce millions of sperm into their senior years, women only have a certain number of eggs available for reproduction. Once a woman runs out of eggs, ovulation stops and so does the possibility of a spontaneous pregnancy. For some women, ovulation stops before age 46, a condition called early menopause.

When Menopause Happens Too Soon

Early menopause occurs in about five percent of women. Premature menopause is menopause before age 40. This type of menopause is rare, occurring in only about one percent of women. The cause of early menopause is often unknown. Some factors that increase the risk of early menopause are smoking, cancer treatment, a family history of early menopause and autoimmune disease such as rheumatoid arthritis or inflammatory bowel disease.

IVF Not a Sure Thing

The only hope for these women is in vitro fertilization (IVF) with donor eggs. During IVF, mature eggs are taken from productive ovaries. The eggs are fertilized with sperm in a lab. The fertilized eggs are placed into the uterus of the woman seeking to become pregnant. The success rate varies and is dependent on a number of factors, such as a woman's age—women under 35 have a success rate average of 50 percent; and for women 42 and over, the rate drops to 3.9 percent, according to recent data from the Centers for Disease Control and Prevention. However, a small pilot study reported in The North American Menopause Society journal *Menopause* may offer hope for these women.

Chemical Messengers and Healing Platelets

In the study, researchers injected a combination of follicle-stimulating hormone and

Study titled "Resumed Ovarian Function and Pregnancy in Early Menopausal Women by Whole Dimension Subcortical Ovarian Administration of Platelet-Rich Plasma and Gonadotropins," by researchers at National Taiwan University Hospital, Taipei, Taiwan, et al., published in *Menopause*, the journal of The North American Menopause Society.

platelet-rich plasma directly into the ovaries of 12 women with early menopause. Their average age was about 44. Follicle-stimulating hormone is a chemical messenger that stimulates ovulation, called a *gonadotropin*. Platelet-rich plasma is blood drawn from a person and processed in a lab to concentrate cell fragments...called platelets. When reinjected, this blood product may help heal or repair injuries.

After the injections, blood tests and the return of menstrual periods indicated that ovulation had returned in 11 of the 12 women. This remarkable finding suggests that women with early menopause may still have some eggs to release if the ovaries are stimulated and repaired, a type of discipline known as *regenerative medicine*. In fact, 13 mature eggs were harvested from six of the women for in vitro fertilization. Ten of the eggs were successfully fertilized. One egg that was transplanted resulted in a pregnancy confirmed by ultrasound imaging.

Regenerative medicine may prolong fertility for women with early menopause. Larger studies are needed to confirm this small study, but the future looks a little brighter for women with early menopause who still want to become pregnant.

Women's Reproductive Lifespan Has Increased

Women's periods are starting 0.8 years earlier, on average, and menopause is starting 1.5 years later—expanding women's reproductive lifespan from 35 to 37.1 years.

Study of 7,773 women over 59 years led by researchers at Texas Tech University Health Sciences Center, Lubbock, published in *JAMA*.

Exercising During Pregnancy Beats Diabetes

Study by researchers at University of Virginia School of Medicine, Charlottesville, published in *Journal of Applied Physiology*.

Exercising during pregnancy might stave off diabetes in children later in life.

Recent study: Female mice that were fed a high-fat diet and exercised during pregnancy were less likely to pass on obesity-linked diseases—including diabetes and other metabolic diseases—to their offspring. More research is needed to show if the same is true for humans.

Secondhand Smoke Danger

Study of 194 nonsmoking pregnant women and their newborns by researchers at Virginia Commonwealth University, Richmond, published in *Environmental Health Perspectives*.

Exposure even to low levels of secondhand smoke during pregnancy increases risk for genetic changes that can predispose infants to diseases and other poor health outcomes later in life. Conditions potentially triggered by these genetic changes include diabetes, cancer and problems involving the cardiovascular system, brain, and nervous system.

Iodine Deficiency in Women: A Growing Problem

Study titled "Iodine Excretion and Intake in Women of Reproductive Age in South Australia Eating Plant-Based and Omnivore Diets: A Pilot Study," by researchers at the University of South Australia, published in *International Journal of Environmental Research and Public Health*.

Iodized table salt may be low on your shopping list these days with all the various gourmet and sea salts available to please the palate. Yet iodine is a mineral essential for thyroid and reproductive health. Since our bodies do not create iodine, it needs to be supplied by the diet. Pregnant women in particular need to watch iodine intake. If iodine levels drop too low, it may affect the baby's intellectual development. A 2017 study found that almost two billon people are iodine deficient worldwide. Diet changes such as switching to vegetarian meals only, plant-based milks and less salt…or salt without iodine…contribute to this deficiency.

Vegan Diets Can Cause an Iodine Deficiency

People who eat a strictly vegan diet or use iodine-free salt are at higher risk for iodine deficiency. Iodine deficiency leads to low thyroid function, and that can be dangerous during pregnancy. Even mild to moderate iodine deficiency has been linked to slower thinking, poor memory, and poor language development in children.

Study details: Researchers at the University of South Australia compared iodine levels (measured through urine samples) and dietary iodine intake in women of childbearing age who ate a plant-only diet versus a diet with meat. This was a small "pilot" study to see if larger studies are needed. The findings are published in the *International Journal of Environmental Research and Public Health*.

There were 31 women in the plant-based diet group and 26 women in the meat-eating group. The World Health Organization (WHO) recommends a level of at least 100 micrograms (mcg) per liter (µg/L) urinary concentration of iodine. Women in the plant-based group took in significantly less iodine in their diets than the meat-eating women. The plant-based urine samples showed an average iodine concentration of 44 µg/L compared to 64 µg/L in the meat-eating group, both well below the recommended level. Women in both groups who used pink or Himalayan salt in place of iodized salt had the lowest iodine levels, about 23 µg/L.

RDA of Iodine for Adults and Pregnant Women

According to the National Institutes of Health, the recommended dietary allowance (RDA) for iodine is 150 mcg per day for adults, 220 mcg for pregnant women, and 290 mcg for lactating women. WHO, UNICEF, and the International Council for the Control of Iodine Deficiency Disorders recommend a slightly higher iodine intake for pregnant women of 250 mcg per day.

Takeaway: Iodine in the diet comes mainly from iodized salt, seaweed, fortified bread, seafood, eggs, and dairy products. The researchers conclude that more studies are needed to raise awareness of the importance of iodine in the diet, especially for women in their reproductive years. They also recommend that new salts and plant milks be fortified with iodine. Be sure to speak with your doctor before changing your diet or increasing your salt or supplement intake.

Good Fish/Bad Fish… How to Tell What's Safe

The US Food and Drug Administration and the Environmental Protection Agency have jointly created a chart that ranks the safety of more than 60 fish and shellfish based on their mercury levels. The chart, which is divided into Best Choices, Good Choices, and Choices to Avoid, was developed as a guide for women who are or might become pregnant or are breastfeeding and for children ages one to 11. It gives recommended serving sizes as well as suggested frequency of consumption.

More information: A PDF of the chart is available at https://bit.ly/3H3T6Ui.

US Food and Drug Administration and Environmental Protection Agency. FDA.gov

Everyday BPA Dangers: Don't Put Yourself or Your Baby at Risk

Chris Iliades, MD, retired ear, nose, throat, head, and neck surgeon who now dedicates his time to educating patients through his medical writing.

B isphenol A (BPA) is an industrial chemical that's used in plastic bottles, inside metal cans, and in the lining of bottle caps.

When it became widely known that BPA was leaching into the foods and drinks inside those containers, many people ditched the cans and bottles, and the U.S. Food and Drug Administration banned the use of BPA in baby products.

A Much Bigger Problem

New research, however, shows that another common product exposes people to up to 1,000 times more BPA than what you might get from food or drink packaged in BPA polycarbonate: thermal paper. That's the thin paper that many receipts, boarding passes, and theater tickets are printed on. A 2016 study found that BPA levels in urine were almost three times higher in cashiers who handled thermal paper receipts than people in a control group.

Not all receipts are printed on thermal paper. The Environmental Working Group found that while McDonald's, CVS, KFC, Whole Foods, Walmart, Safeway, and some U.S. Postal Service locations use thermal paper, Target, Starbucks, and Bank of America automated teller machines do not. You can easily check if paper is thermally treated by

rubbing it with a coin. Thermal paper will discolor when rubbed.

Why It Matters

Many animal studies have warned that BPA can interfere with hormone signals. Hormones are chemical messengers that help control body functions. Studies suggest a link with cancer, diabetes, high blood pressure, infertility, and behavioral problems in children.

The FDA's current stance on BPA was based on a four-year review of more than 300 research studies that was completed in 2014. Since then, new research has emerged. A 2019 study presented to the European Respiratory Society found that pregnant women with high levels of BPA in their urine had children that were at higher risk for poor lung capacity and wheezing. There were more than 2,500 women in the study, and close to 80 percent of them had detectable levels of BPA in their urine. Those with the highest levels gave birth to children with a 23 percent higher risk of asthma.

A 2020 study published in the journal *JAMA Network Open* followed close to 4,000 adults with BPA in their urine over a period of 10 years. People with the highest levels of BPA were 50 percent more likely to die of any cause over 10 years compared to people with the lowest levels of BPA. Although this study does not prove that BPA contributed to those deaths, the researchers conclude that further studies are called for.

Reduce Your Exposure

Lowering your exposure to BPA can be simple with these steps…

• **Avoid plastic when possible.** Glass and metal food storage containers and water bottles are now widely available.

Have You Been Exposed to BPA?

Almost every American adult has been exposed to BPA. Even if you avoid it in food packaging and thermal paper, it has been used in water pipes and has been deposited in enough dump sites to leave trace amounts in air, dirt, and water samples. As a result, BPA has been found in 90 to 93 percent of U.S. urine samples. A 2019 study from Washington State University found levels to be more than 40 times higher than what the FDA deems very low and safe. It has also been measured in blood and breast milk.

• **When you do need plastic,** check for the recycle code and don't use anything with a 3 or 7. Those types of plastic are likely to contain BPA.

• **Don't put any food containers that may have BPA in the dishwasher or microwave.** Heating increases the risk of BPA leaking out.

• **Throw away old plastic containers.** Age breaks down the plastic, releasing BPA.

• **Use plastic containers marked BPA-free with caution.** Studies show that these replacements can also interfere with the body's hormones.

• **Avoid canned foods and metal bottle caps when possible.**

• **Use fresh, frozen, or dried food instead of canned.**

• **If you can't avoid foods in BPA-lined cans,** rinse the food in water before eating.

• **Never heat food in a can.**

• **If you don't need a receipt, don't take it.** If you need a record, ask for an email or text receipt instead.

• **If you save your receipts,** wash your hands when you get home and save your receipts inside a bag or envelope.

• **Do not let children handle thermal paper.**

Speed Bumps Can Be Dangerous for Pregnant Women

Data modeled on crash tests found that, when driven over quickly, speed bumps can cause abdominal pain and other complications in a pregnant woman as well as injure the fetus's brain and cause an abnormal fetal heart rate.

Best: When a pregnant woman is in a vehicle, it should be driven over a speed bump at no more than 28 mph and preferably as little as 15 mph to avoid injury to the fetus.

Study led by researchers at University of British Columbia, Okanagan, Canada, published in *Journal of Biomechanics*.

• **Don't put thermal paper into your recycling.** BPA residue from receipts will contaminate recycled paper.

C-Section Babies Benefit from Mother's Poop

Study titled "Maternal Fecal Microbiota Transplantation in Cesarean-Born Infants Rapidly Restores Normal Gut Microbial Development: A Proof-of-Concept Study," by researchers at the Human Microbiome Research Program, University of Helsinki, Finland, published in *Cell*.

---

t's a cringe-worthy scenario: A brand-new mom transfers healthy microbes to her newborn by adding some of her feces to breast milk. Fortunately, there's a purification process to smooth out the ick factor.

Background: When a baby is born through a vaginal birth, he/she is exposed to microbes present in the mother's vaginal and rectal area. This transfer is key for a baby to develop a healthy colony of microbes (the microbiome) in his/her own intestines. A healthy microbiome is essential for a strong immune system.

Previous studies have shown that babies born by Caesarian section (C-section) do not get this transfer, and their microbiome develops differently. This may put them at higher risk for immune-system diseases, such as asthma, allergies, celiac disease and rheumatoid arthritis later in life. Some researchers have tried swabbing a baby's skin with vaginal fluid right after birth, but results have not been consistent.

Now: A new study from researchers at the University of Helsinki Human Microbiome Research Program in Finland offers a new option that shows promise. Since the most important microbes come from a mother's gut bacteria, the researchers wanted to see if taking a stool sample from a mother before C-section, purifying the stool sample and then adding it to breast milk would be a safe and effective way for C-section babies to develop a healthier microbiome. The study is published in *Cell*.

Study details: Seven mothers volunteered to give a stool sample three weeks before a scheduled C-section. The stool samples were purified and saved. Right after birth, the stool samples were added to the mother's breast milk and fed to the babies as a bottle feeding. Stool samples were taken from the babies' first stool before the feeding and at one-, two- and three-week intervals, with a final sample taken at three months.

There were no adverse effects on the babies. The three-month stool samples were compared with samples from babies born vaginally and babies born by C-section who were not in the study. The stool-fed babies had microbiomes similar to the vaginally born babies...significantly different from the other C-section babies.

Conclusion: This was an early (proof-of-concept) study. It shows that microbial transplantation through stool samples for C-section babies is safe and appears to be effective. If future studies, which will be larger and more controlled, support these findings, the researchers think that this poop-to-breast-milk transfer could become a beneficial and routine part of the C-section procedure. However, researchers warn that you shouldn't try this at home. Stool samples have to be tested and treated for safety.

Why Women Who Breastfeed Have Lower Risk for Heart Disease and Diabetes

Study titled "The Association of Lactation Duration with Visceral and Pericardial Fat Volumes in Parous Women: The CARDIA Study," by researchers at Texas Tech University Health Sciences Center, et al., published in *The Journal of Clinical Endocrinology & Metabolism*.

Breastfeeding has long been hailed as super healthy for the nursing baby. It's also a beneficial practice for the mom, too, lowering her risk for breast and ovarian cancer, among other female-specific conditions. Many studies also have shown that women who breastfeed have a reduced risk for heart disease and diabetes, but the reasons why have never been fully understood. Researchers at Texas Tech University Health Sciences Center had a theory that they tested in a recent study.

Less Harmful Visceral and Pericardial Fats

The theory is that women who breastfeed often have less fat inside the belly, called *visceral fat* and less fat around the heart, called *pericardial fat*, since stored fat is used to provide substance to breast milk. These types of fat are known to increase the risk of heart disease and type 2 diabetes. Visceral and pericardial fat secretes inflammatory proteins called cytokines. Cytokines reduce the response to insulin, which increases the risk for type 2 diabetes. Cytokines also increase the build-up of plaques in the arteries, called atherosclerosis, which leads to coronary heart disease. As implied in the name, pericardial fat puts pressure on the heart, which contributes to cardiovascular conditions.

To test their theory, the researchers used data from an ongoing health study called the CARDIA study. This study, sponsored by the National Institutes of Health, has been active for over 30 years. It has collected health data from over 5,000 women. The research team was able to collect data from over 900 women in the study who had their pericardial and visceral fat measured by CT scan imaging in 2010 through 2011. They compared fat volumes between women who breastfed and women who never breastfed. They also compared fat volume based on how long women breastfed. The results of the study are published in *The Journal of Clinical Endocrinology & Metabolism*.

The Longer Breastfeeding, the Less Fat

The average age of the women when they started the study was 24. *These were the key results...*

- **Women who never breast fed** had a combined fat volume of 122.
- **Women who breastfed for one to five months** had a volume of 113.7.
- **Women who breastfed for six to 11 months** had a volume of 105, and women who breastfed for over one year had a volume of 110.1.
- **The longer women breastfed,** the less fat they had.
- **Women who breastfed also gained less weight.**

The researchers conclude that this study supports their theory. It may explain why women who breastfeed their babies have less heart disease and about a 50 percent lower risk of type 2 diabetes. The researchers plan to do more research on how breastfeeding influences cytokines.

COVID Vaccine Not in Breast Milk

Study titled "Evaluation of Messenger RNA From COVID-19 BTN162b2 and mRNA-1273 Vaccines in Human Milk," by researchers at the University of California, San Francisco, published in *JAMA Pediatrics.*

Whatever fears (or hopes) a lactating woman has had concerning the COVID-19 vaccines entering breast milk, they are, according to a recent study, unfounded. The CDC and the World Health Organization have recommended COVID-19 vaccination for women who are breastfeeding or who plan to breastfeed. The vaccine provides the necessary protection against the virus for the women only. Some research has suggested that antibodies from the vaccine may pass to babies in breast milk and provide them with some

protection against the virus. But a recent study shows that's not the case.

Breastfeeding Women Not Initially Tested

Two of the vaccines currently in use are new types of vaccines called messenger RNA (mRNA) vaccines. These vaccines use a new genetic messenger (mRNA) to deliver the vaccine. They were approved under an emergency use authorization and not tested in women who were breastfeeding. General studies did not determine if the mRNA could get into breast milk, or if mRNA in breast milk would affect a breastfeeding baby.

Because these mRNA vaccines are new and untested during breastfeeding, some women have been vaccinated but stopped breastfeeding. Others have refused the vaccination and continued to breastfeed. Now a recent study from researchers at the University of California, San Francisco, has found evidence to support the recommendation for women to get vaccinated and to continue or start breastfeeding.

The study was done between December 2020 and February 2021. Breast-milk samples were taken from seven mothers who received the Pfizer or Moderna mRNA vaccines. The breast-milk samples were taken before vaccinations and at several points up to 48 hours after vaccination. None of the breast-milk samples showed any trace of the mRNA vaccine. The study is published in the American Medical Association journal *JAMA Pediatrics.*

CDC and WHO: Lactating Women Should Get Vaccinated

The authors of the study say that this research provides early evidence of vaccine safety during breastfeeding. Although the study was limited by its small size, and investigations of larger populations of breastfeeding mothers are anticipated, this early data supports the current recommendations of the CDC and World Health Organization.

For more information: For more details on CDC recommendations concerning the coronavirus vaccine and breastfeeding, visit CDC.gov/coronavirus/2019-ncov/vaccines/recommendations/pregnancy.html.

Marijuana Lasts a Long Time in Breast Milk

Research letter titled "Persistence of Δ-9-Tetrahydrocannabinol in Human Breast Milk," led by researchers at Children's Hospital Colorado, published in *JAMA Pediatrics*.

It's a long-known fact that marijuana intake affects the health of a fetus. Since 1982, studies have followed children born to mothers who smoked the drug during pregnancy. These studies show that the active ingredient in marijuana crosses into the placenta and into a developing baby's blood supply. The children of these mothers have a higher risk of mental problems such as impulsivity, poor attention span, and poor problem-solving skills. The active substance thought to be responsible is THC, the ingredient in marijuana that gets you high.

Although organizations including the American Academy of Pediatrics (AAP), American College of Obstetricians and Gynecologists (ACOG) and the Academy of Breastfeeding Medicine (ABM) all say women should not use marijuana during pregnancy or breastfeeding, the number of women using marijuana has actually increased.

How Long Does THC Last in Breast Milk?

Women are also told to abstain from marijuana during breastfeeding or to "pump and dump" their breast milk until the THC has cleared out of their system. However, there has never been an adequate time span outline for marijuana users to determine how long the THC remains. Now, a study from researchers at the Children's Hospital Colorado is the first to measure how long THC actually stays in breast milk. Their findings were published in the American Medical Association's journal *JAMA Pediatrics*.

Study details: Between 2016 and 2019, 25 pregnant women who tested positive for THC when they were admitted for delivery agreed to participate in the study. All the women said they would abstain from marijuana use during the study while breastfeeding and provide breast milk samples.

Only seven women were able to abstain during the six weeks. The women who used marijuana said that they took it to relieve pain or stress, or to help them sleep.

Marijuana Lasts Long with a Stronger Punch

At the end of the study, all seven women who had abstained still had detectable levels of THC in their breast milk. Although the study does not address the effects of THC on breastfeeding babies, the researchers are concerned that because of legalization, marijuana use is on the rise. And in some cases, today's marijuana has up to six times more THC than before legalization.

The researchers say their study supports the recommendations of AAP, ACOG and ABM. Women are urged to abstain from marijuana during pregnancy and the duration of breastfeeding, especially since its active ingredient can linger for six weeks or more in breast milk.

For more information: To find out more about how marijuana affects the health of a fetus during pregnancy, visit the Centers for Disease Control and Prevention's information page at CDC.gov/marijuana/health-effects/pregnancy.html.

Chapter 15

RESPIRATORY HEALTH AND ALLERGIES

A Lump in the Lung? What to Do...

Hearing that you have a growth in your lung can be terrifying, but for most people, it's an unfounded fear. Less than 5 percent of these nodules turn out to be lung cancer.

A pulmonary nodule is a round, solid growth that forms inside your lung. It is always smaller than 3 centimeters. (A growth that is larger than that is called a pulmonary mass, which is more dangerous.)

Easy to Miss

Because they're too small to cause symptoms, nodules are usually found when a doctor orders a chest imaging study for lung symptoms caused by something else.

Only the largest nodules show up on an x-ray, so most are found on CT scans, where they appear as a dense white spot that radiologists sometimes call coin lesions. While the cause of most nodules is unknown, some can be attributed to benign tumors or cysts, diseases that cause lung inflammation, scar tissue from an old infection, or a lung abnormality from birth.

Evaluating Risk

A very small number of pulmonary nodules are cancerous. To determine if yours should be biopsied (the only way to diagnose a malignant nodule), your doctor will assess the position, and size of the nodule, your personal risk for lung cancer, and the nodule's growth over time.

• **Position.** Nodules that are located in the upper lung or have strands of tissue called *spiculations* radiating from them are riskier.

• **Size.** The smaller the nodule, the lower the risk. Those smaller than 0.6 centimeters have a less than one percent chance of being cancerous.

• **Personal risk factors.** Older age, a history of smoking, a family history of lung cancer, having a long-term lung disease or another cancer, and exposure to chest radiation therapy or toxic substances like dusts, metals, fumes, or asbestos increase the risk of cancer.

• **Growth.** A nodule that increases in size over time is usually biopsied. If your nodule was present on a previous CT scan or chest x-ray, the size can be compared to the recent imaging study. If you don't have a nodule on

---

Chris Iliades, MD, a retired ear, nose, throat, head, and neck surgeon. After retiring from clinical practice, he became a full-time medical writer and regular contributor to *Bottom Line Heath*.

Don't Ignore These Symptoms

Although there are no symptoms of lung nodules, there are symptoms of lung cancer. *Always let your doctor know about...*

- ●**A cough that does not improve,** gets worse, or produces blood-tinged sputum
- ● **Shortness of breath**
- ● **Chest pain,** especially with a deep breath or cough
- ● **Unwanted weight loss**
- ● **Frequent upper respiratory infections**
- ● **Persistent hoarseness**

—Dr. Chris Iliades

an old imaging study, your doctor may take a wait-and-see approach and schedule a chest imaging study in a few months.

If your doctor thinks you are at high risk for lung cancer, you may need an imaging study called a PET scan, which gives more detailed images than a CT scan.

If your nodule is high risk or a PET scan finds changes that suggest cancer, your doctor will perform a biopsy.

A biopsy may be taken through a tube placed down your throat and windpipe into your lung, called a bronchoscopy. If a nodule is very suspicious or difficult to reach, open surgery may be done to remove it (excisional biopsy).

Though lung cancer is always dangerous, these nodules are usually found at an early stage of lung cancer. Surgery may be able to remove the whole cancer, increasing the possibility of a cure.

Smoking Marijuana Damages Lungs

Robert Hancox, MD, is a research professor of respiratory epidemiology at University of Otago, Dunedin, New Zealand, and lead author of a study of 1,000 people published in *American Journal of Respiratory and Critical Care Medicine.*

Recent finding: The more marijuana someone smokes—and the longer he/she

smokes it—the more likely he will develop a particular type of lung damage. The lungs will have to expand more to supply the body with enough oxygen (lung hyperinflation) and will perform less efficiently.

Warning: Quitting stops the damage from getting worse, but it is cumulative—and may be permanent.

Pulmonary Rehab Can Help You Breathe Better

MeiLan Han, MD, national spokesperson for the American Lung Association and serves on its scientific advisory committee. Dr. Han is the director of the Michigan Airways Program and a professor of internal medicine in the Division of Pulmonary and Critical Care Medicine at the University of Michigan in Ann Arbor.

Your desires may be quite simple: to get through the grocery store without needing to stop and rest, to walk the fairways comfortably during your weekly golf game, or to carry packages without running out of breath. But if you have a chronic lung condition, your prescribed medications might not be enough to help you do what you want.

That's where pulmonary rehabilitation comes in. This underused but valuable tool can dramatically improve how you feel and function.

Comprehensive Approach

Combining exercise training, education, and strategic breathing techniques, pulmonary rehab aims to build strength in people with chronic obstructive pulmonary disease (COPD) and other lung diseases. It's normally provided in a small group setting two to three times a week for three to 12 weeks or even longer. A respiratory therapist or exercise physiologist will lead the session, but behind the scenes, your rehab team may include doctors, nurses, physical and respiratory therapists, and dietitians. *Together, they'll develop a program that includes multiple elements...*

Finding a Program

Doctors don't always mention pulmonary rehab. If you want to know what's available to you, be proactive and talk to your health-care provider about what you're able to do now and what you'd like to be able to do more comfortably. He or she will then administer a series of tests to see if you qualify for a rehab program.

If you do, the doctor may recommend a program, or you may need to do some research on your own. *Here are two excellent resources…*

• **The American Lung Association's Better Breather's Network** (Lung.org/help-support/better-breathers-network)

• **The American Thoracic Society's** directory of pulmonary rehabilitation programs (LiveBetter.org).

If you live in a rural area, outpatient centers offering pulmonary rehab are limited and you may have to travel to find a hospital with a program that has space available. Medicare covers pulmonary rehab for COPD if you meet certain requirements and may also cover other lung diseases depending on your location. With private insurance, your out-of-pocket costs will vary.

—Dr. MeiLan Han

Exercise Training

You might not think that you can exercise when just walking across the room makes you breathless, but by starting slowly and building gradually, you'll be able to increase both your strength and stamina. You'll improve endurance and muscle strength by using weights and cardiovascular equipment.

Nutrition Counseling

People with lung disease use much more energy for the work of breathing than those without disease, so proper nutrition is incredibly important, as is maintaining a healthy body weight. *The rehab team will teach you practical tips, too…*

• **Eat smaller meals more often** and avoid large meals to enable your diaphragm to move freely and let your lungs fill and empty more easily.

• **Drink six to eight glasses** of non-caffeinated, non-alcoholic fluids each day to help thin mucous and clear it from the lungs. If drinking during meals makes you too full, drink at other times of the day.

• **Balance your diet.** When your body metabolizes carbohydrates, it produces the most carbon dioxide for the amount of oxygen used, while the metabolism of fat produces the least. A pulmonary rehab nutritionist can help you find the best balance.

• **Avoid foods that cause gas or bloating,** such as cruciferous vegetables. They make breathing more difficult.

Energy-Saving Techniques

Certain movements can make it harder to breathe by sapping precious energy. For example, lifting, bending, and reaching force you to tighten your abdominal muscles, which can make it harder to get your breath. Investing in some simple tools, such as a handheld shower head, a shoehorn, and sock donner, can make a big difference, as can putting a chair in the bathroom so you can sit down while shaving or brushing your teeth.

Breathing Strategies

Certain breathing maneuvers, such as one called pursed-lip breathing, can create much-needed "back pressure" to keep small airways open when you exhale, tackling a common problem in COPD and asthma. To try it, relax your shoulders and neck, then inhale through your nose for two seconds. Exhale through pursed lips (like you're blowing out a candle) for four seconds. In a pulmonary rehabilitation program, you'll learn other techniques like this to increase your oxygen levels, help you take fewer breaths, and keep your airways open longer.

More Education

You'll learn more about your specific breathing-related condition, along with ways to skirt infections and situations that could worsen your symptoms. You'll also get guidance on how and when to properly take your medications and the ins and outs of oxygen use, should you require it. Many pulmonary rehab programs offer social and support groups, and they can provide referrals to other professionals who can help teach you strategies to manage these feelings.

Promising Results

Most of the research on pulmonary rehab has focused on people with COPD, and the results are impressive. COPD patients who start a pulmonary rehab program within 90 days of hospital discharge for a flare-up are significantly less likely to die within a year than those who put off rehab or don't participate at all. Pulmonary rehab may even lower the chances of landing in the hospital in the first place.

Breathe Easy! Exercises to Increase Your Oxygen Intake

Meera Patricia Kerr, a yoga expert, singer, and songwriter. She is coauthor, with Sandra A. McLanahan, MD, of *Take a Deep Breath: A Simple Exercise Guide to Increasing Your Oxygen Intake* and author of *Big Yoga: A Simple Guide for Bigger Bodies.*

Most of us take the act of breathing for granted. It's an automatic bodily function that we barely notice, although we do it up to 30,000 times per day.

While breathing may appear to be simply the act of inhaling and exhaling, it's actually a complex physiological process involving various muscles, blood vessels and organs such as the lungs, heart, and brain. And in truth, many of us never learned how to breathe correctly when we were younger.

Common mistake: If you fill up your lungs and then your stomach with each breath, that's actually known as "reverse breathing" or "shallow breathing." Proper breathing starts deep in the abdomen and then moves up to the lungs.

When breathing is normal, there is little to think about. But when we are not able to get enough oxygen into our bodies, it can hinder our ability to function and it can be frightening.

Examples: Conditions such as asthma, chronic obstructive pulmonary disease (COPD), being overweight (especially if you carry a lot of weight in your middle section) and COVID-19 infection can impair breathing, causing shortness of breath, a recurring cough and constant pain in the chest.

Important: Even if your lungs are damaged by disease, proper breathing can re-awaken portions of the lungs that haven't been used and may improve COPD, asthma and possibly COVID-19 symptoms.

How to Breathe Correctly

Practicing this simple exercise, known as the diaphragmatic breath, for 20 to 30 minutes each day can strengthen your ability to breathe deeply and fully, deliver more oxygen to cells throughout your body and improve alertness and exercise endurance throughout the day. Improved breathing also helps keep stress and anxiety at bay. If you prefer, break it into two 15-minute sessions rather than all at once.

Sit in a comfortable chair that enables proper posture, with feet flat on the floor or on a pillow and your back supported.

1. Inhale for a count of four through the nose. It's better to breathe in through the nose than the mouth because the nostrils moisturize and warm air, purifying the breath as it goes into the body. Inhale from the bottom up as if filling a balloon with air—first expand the lower belly (below the belly button), then the rib cage, then the upper chest, which will fully expand your lungs.

Important: When your lungs are fully expanded, your collarbone may rise up, but keep your shoulders relaxed and below your ears to prevent tension in your neck.

2. Exhale through pursed lips for a count of four from the top down. Initially, the length of your exhalation should be equal to the length of your inhalation. Gradually increase the exhales to last up to twice as long as the inhales. Start by expelling air while pulling in the upper chest, then the rib cage and lastly the belly. At the end of the exhalation, your belly should be pulled in toward the spine. Breathing out in this order is a more effective way to expel all of the stale air and carbon dioxide from your body.

Keeping your lips pursed slows down the breath, giving you more control over the exhalation so you can breathe out more deeply. A secondary benefit is that it relaxes you, particularly beneficial for people with COPD and other lung diseases who become anxious and fearful when short of breath, making it even more difficult to breathe deeply.

Advanced: Work up to inhaling and exhaling for longer counts.

Goal: Inhale for a count of five, hold for a count of 20, and exhale for a count of 10.

Relaxation and Deep Breathing

If you prefer, you can perform diaphragmatic breathing while lying on your back. This "torso opener" exercise opens up the chest, which allows you to breathe even more deeply than when you are sitting in a chair. It even can improve digestion—when seated, having a big belly or hunching over with rounded shoulders can impede digestion.

1. Lie on a yoga mat or towel with your head on a pillow and your arms to your sides. Put a blanket or bolster under your knees or let your legs lie flat.

2. Place an eye mask over your eyes.

3. Practice diaphragmatic breathing and relax in this position for 10 to 15 minutes.

4. Come out of the position slowly to regain your bearings as you stand up.

Strengthening Exercises

It is important to strengthen muscles that support breathing and improve circulation. When muscles are strong and breathing is deep, more oxygen is pushed out to the body's cells. *Perform three to five repetitions of each of the following seated exercises daily...*

Thoracic Toner

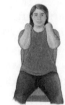

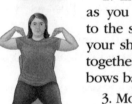

1. Inhale as you touch your fingertips to the tops of your shoulders with your elbows close together in front of your chest.

2. Exhale with pursed lips as you move the elbows out to the side of your body. Feel your shoulder blades squeeze together as you bring the elbows back.

3. Move your elbows back to the first position, and repeat.

Elbow Bends

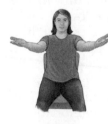

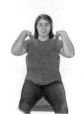

1. Inhale and extend your arms out to the front with your palms facing up. Keep your arms at about the same height as your shoulders.

2. Exhale with pursed lips, bend your elbows and bring your fingertips to the tops of the shoulders. Don't hike your shoulders up.

3. Return to the starting position, and repeat.

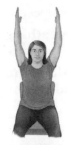
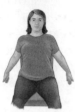

Shoulder Squeeze

1. Inhale and bring your arms straight up overhead. They should be aligned with your ears and your palms should face inward. Don't tense up the shoulders.

2. Exhale through pursed lips, and swing your arms down behind your body keeping your palms facing inward. Squeeze the area between the shoulder blades.

3. Return to the starting position and repeat.

Side Stretch

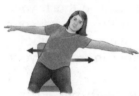

1. Inhale and stretch your arms out to the side. Don't hike your shoulders up. Keep your arms relaxed and your palms facing down.

2. Exhale through pursed lips as you stretch to the left.

3. Inhale and return to the upright position.

4. Exhale through pursed lips, and lean to the right.

5. Return to the starting position, and repeat.

Side Twist

1. Inhale and extend your arms to the sides with palms facing in and down.

2. Exhale with pursed lips, and twist your upper body to the right slowly, progressively rotating from the waist up, bringing your head around last. Turn as far as is comfortable.

3. Inhale and return to the neutral position.

4. Exhale with pursed lips as you twist to the left.

5. Return to the starting position, and repeat.

Illustrations by Alayna Paquette.

Calming Chronic Cough

Rachel Taliercio, DO, a pulmonologist and the director of the Chronic Cough Clinic in the Respiratory Institute at the Cleveland Clinic.

From allergies to influenza, colds to coronavirus, a long list of irritants can spur a cough, the body's natural way of expelling everything from pollen to microorganisms.

It's not uncommon to have a nagging cough for a few days or even weeks, but once you pass the eight-week mark, your cough is considered chronic. For some people, the discomfort, sleep disruption, worry, and even stress incontinence can go on for many months, years, or even decades.

To learn more about managing this bothersome condition, we interviewed Rachel Taliercio, doctor of osteopathic medicine (DO), a pulmonologist and codirector of the Chronic Cough Clinic at the Cleveland Clinic.

Chronic cough is one of the most common reasons for people to visit the doctor. What causes a cough to linger for a long time?

Among nonsmokers, a chronic cough is most often caused by one or more of three conditions…

• **Cough variant-asthma.** While most people with asthma experience breathlessness, wheezing, and chest tightness, some have only a cough. Treatment with inhaled corticosteroids, with or without long-acting bronchodilators, or pills called leukotriene modifiers can provide relief from coughing and treat the inflammation caused by asthma.

• **Upper airway cough syndrome** consists of chronic sinus irritation or infection, post-nasal drip, and allergies or non-allergens that irritate the upper airway. Treatment may include intranasal steroids, antihistamines, decongestants, or antibiotics.

• **Gastroesophageal reflux disease (GERD).** When people have GERD, acidic and nonacidic stomach contents leak into the esophagus, the tube that runs from the throat to the stomach. It can then irritate the nerve that serves both the esophagus and the trachea, the tube that runs from the throat to the lungs. While GERD often causes heartburn symptoms, it can also be silent, causing nothing more than a cough.

What causes chronic cough in people who don't have any of these conditions?

A cough that is unexplained despite looking for and treating the most common causes is called a chronic refractory cough. When we meet such patients at the Cleveland Clinic, we take a thorough history, which can provide valuable clues. The story of the cough is incredibly important. What triggers it? What came before it? What is the character of the cough? What makes it better? Worse?

We also often repeat testing for asthma, upper-airway cough syndrome, and GERD. We have found that initially negative results can turn out to be positive, allowing our interdisciplinary team to treat those conditions.

If that doesn't explain or address the cough and we have ruled out all known triggers and causes, we think about cough hypersensitivity syndrome if the patient's history suggests this condition. Often, a chronic cough starts as part of an illness such as bronchitis, but when the illness resolves, the cough does not.

We think that this may be caused by a neural irritation or injury in the throat or larynx (the voice box). Changes in the peripheral and central nervous system may lead to hypersensitization of the cough reflex.

What treatments are available for patients with cough hypersensitivity syndrome?

The first approach for nerve-related coughing is called neuromodulation therapy. We use low doses of medications that are normally used for nerve pain to try to calm the nerves in the throat. These drugs, such as tricyclic antidepressants and *gabapentin*, are used off-label when treating chronic cough.

In a 2014 study, we found that neuromodulators helped 68 percent of patients. For

Cough-Tracking Apps Are Useful Monitors for Many Health Problems

If your chronic cough is caused by allergies, asthma, acid reflux, COPD or another health issue, an increase in coughing might mean that it's time to see your doctor or adjust your medication or that a particular location is an allergy trigger. Apps such as Hyfe (free for iOS and Android) and Insubiq Cough Tracker (free for iPhone) track coughing more accurately than patients can on their own.

Adithya Cattamanchi, MD, pulmonologist and professor of medicine, University of California San Francisco. UCSF.edu

about a third of them, however, the effects of the medication wore off over time. We call this tachyphylaxis. Ideally, if we find a medication that controls the cough, we continue it for six months, but in 27 percent of patients in our study, the cough returned when the medication dosage was lowered or stopped.

If neuromodulation therapy does not provide relief and we suspect that the person is experiencing laryngeal spasm as a component of the chronic cough, we can perform injection therapy with onabotulinumtoxinA (Botox) or a procedure known as a superior laryngeal nerve block. The nerve block uses a combination of numbing medication and a steroid injection.

Are there any approaches that do not require medication?

Behavioral cough suppression therapy is very promising. Speech language pathologists (SLP) can help patients regain control of the cough spasms without any need for medication. An SLP may start with strategies to interrupt or prevent the cough. For example, a patient can learn how to alter the sensation of an oncoming cough by using breathing techniques, distraction, forceful swallowing, and even voice therapy. The SLP will also educate the patient on how to reduce laryngeal irritation. That includes eliminating irritants (mouth breathing, smoking, and drinking excessive alcohol and caffeine) and increasing hydration. Chewing gum or sucking on hard candies can help some patients by encouraging more swallowing. Some patients can soothe the larynx by learning how to speak in slightly different ways.

What advice do you have for patients who are still looking for the cause of their chronic cough?

You know your body best. When you are reading articles like this and feel like you know what is causing your cough, share that information with your physician. Don't be afraid to get a second opinion if you're not finding answers.

Avoid Bronchitis Overtreatment

Jeffrey A. Linder, MD, the Michael A. Gertz Professor of Medicine and chief of general internal medicine and geriatrics at the Northwestern Medicine Feinberg School of Medicine, Chicago.

A cough that lasts for weeks can get in the way of work and social activities, disturb your sleep and, in the era of COVID-19, earn you some hostile glances at the grocery store. But if the malady causing your cough is a typical case of acute bronchitis, basically, a chest cold, then there's good news: It will go away, usually within three weeks. And you won't need an expensive medical workup or an antibiotic prescription to get better.

The problem is that too many people with acute bronchitis, a common illness, get over tested and overtreated. That's costly for patients and the health-care system. More importantly, it exposes millions of people every year to treatment that does them no good and can cause them harm. It also contributes to a major public health problem: the rise of bacteria that are resistant to antibiotics.

Here's what you need to know when you might have acute bronchitis, and how to feel better safely.

What Is Acute Bronchitis?

Bronchitis is an inflammation of the bronchial tubes, the passages that let air in and out of your lungs. When these airways are inflamed, your chest may feel full or tight and you may cough up mucus. After a while, your cough may become dry. Other symptoms can include shortness of breath, a low-grade fever, and wheezing.

Some people develop chronic bronchitis, long-term inflammation of the bronchial tubes, because of smoking or exposure to other airway irritants. Their symptoms can linger for months and return year after year.

Acute bronchitis is different. It's usually caused by the same common viruses that cause colds and the flu. Less often, it's caused by bacteria. The coughing of acute bronchitis may last longer than the initial cold and flu symptoms but typically subsides within three weeks without treatment.

How Is It Diagnosed?

If you visit your health-care provider with a cough that's been bothering you for a few days or weeks, you should expect to answer a few questions and undergo a quick exam. These days, you should also expect a test for COVID-19. Your provider will also want to rule out some other possible causes, especially pneumonia, an infection of the air sacs of the lungs that can be more serious than bronchitis. A racing heart, rapid breathing, a temperature of at least 100.5 F, and the sound of fluid or other abnormalities in your lungs are possible signs of pneumonia. But if you don't have any of those signs or another condition that would explain your symptoms (such as asthma or chronic obstructive pulmonary disease), acute bronchitis may be diagnosed.

Additional tests, including chest x-rays and tests of your blood, respiratory secretions, and sputum (the mucus you cough up), haven't been shown to be helpful in people with healthy immune systems who appear to have acute bronchitis.

Treatment Disconnect

There's a disconnect in the United States between how acute bronchitis is treated and how expert groups recommend it should be treated. Surveys consistently show that two-thirds or more of patients are prescribed an antibiotic. Antibiotics work only against bacterial infections. Most acute bronchitis cases are caused by viruses, not bacteria. That means that most people get medications that have no chance of improving their symptoms but a good chance of causing side effects such as yeast infections, diarrhea, and long-lasting disruptions in gut microbes. Some people suffer allergic reactions. Even people with bronchitis caused by bacteria are unlikely to benefit from antibiotics in any significant way, studies suggest. In addition, antibiotic overuse promotes the growth of drug-resistant bacteria.

Antibiotic Overuse

The reasons so many people get antibiotics are complex. One is that patients demand them, and doctors want to please patients. Another is that both doctors and patients overestimate the likelihood that bronchitis will progress to pneumonia, which is often caused by bacteria. But studies suggest that giving antibiotics to everyone with acute bronchitis would prevent pneumonia in no more than one in 1,000 cases. One way patients can help is by letting providers know that they want antibiotics only when they really need them.

—Dr. Jeffrey Linder

Better Treatment Choices

The best treatments for acute bronchitis are the simplest: rest, plenty of fluids, and time. People who have a fever or body aches can feel better with some ibuprofen or acetaminophen. If you have wheezing or shortness of breath, you may benefit from an inhaled beta-agonist, a medicine used for asthma. Home remedies, such as honey, warm drinks, humidifiers, and steamy showers, are safe and often helpful.

And while studies have not found clear benefits from cough medicines, over-the-counter medications that contain the ingredient guaifenesin are safe for adults and children over age four. These medicines thin mucus and might reduce coughing.

When to See the Doctor

If you cough for more than four weeks, cough up blood, develop a high fever, experience chest pain, or start to feel worse overall, contact your provider. You might then benefit from additional tests or treatments.

Tongue-Strengthening Device for Mild Sleep Apnea Approved

US Food and Drug Administration, Silver Spring, Maryland.

People with chronic sleep apnea experience interrupted sleep because their tongues fail to keep their airways open. Now the FDA has approved a neuromuscular stimulation mouthpiece, called the eXciteOSA, that strengthens the tongue during waking hours to keep it from collapsing at night. In trials, snoring was cut by an average of 48 percent for 41 of 48 patients. The device is not for people with severe apnea.

When Good Smells Turn Bad...

Murray Grossan, MD, an ear, nose, and throat physician with Tower Ear, Nose, and Throat, Los Angeles. GrossanInstitute.com

An alteration in the sense of smell is called *parosmia*. A patient who regularly bakes may suddenly find that bread smells rotten. An athlete may suddenly find familiar smells, such as sweat in the locker room, unbearable. This distortion of smell can be more bothersome to patients than a loss of smell.

The most common causes of parosmia are head trauma, an injury that causes damage to the nasal anatomy, epileptic seizures, infections involving the nasal passages, sneezing too hard, diving into water incorrectly, and recovering from COVID-19. (The loss of smell some people experience with the novel coronavirus is called *anosmia*.)

Another cause of parosmia is empty-nose syndrome. Inside the nose, there are bony structures covered by soft tissue (called turbinates) that warm and moisten the air flow. Sometimes, during nasal surgery, a surgeon will remove parts of these turbinates, causing atypical air currents that can alter smell.

Parosmia has not been studied well enough to identify reliable treatments, but the following exercise may help some people...

- **Relax the muscles in your face.**
- **Focus on relaxing your jaw.**
- **Relax your shoulders.** Looking in a mirror can help you ensure that you're fully relaxing the muscles.
- **Take a few measured breaths** with a longer exhalation than inhalation.
- **Hold something to your nose that has a pleasant association.** The baker mentioned above may smell fresh-baked bread while remembering a happy family event that she baked for.
- **Regular exercise and good sleep may also reduce symptoms.**

Raspy Voice? Problem Swallowing? Check Your Vocal Cords

Michael J. Stephen, MD, pulmonologist, associate professor at Thomas Jefferson University in Philadelphia, director of its Adult Cystic Fibrosis Center and author of *Breath Taking: The Power, Fragility, and Future of Our Extraordinary Lungs*.

Unless you make your living from your voice, chances are you rarely think about your vocal cords. But that's a mistake.

Even though we associate these two thin strips of fibrous tissue with our ability to speak and sing, they're also involved in a number of other crucial functions.

Examples: When you breathe, your vocal cords must remain open, but they have to close shut when you speak, sing or swallow and even when you need to generate the pushing force that's required for heavy lifting or moving your bowels. *Here's what you need to know to preserve a strong and steady voice and keep your breathing and swallowing capacity in top form...*

How the Vocal Cords Get Overlooked

When people have breathing problems, such as shortness of breath, their doctors may not pay close attention to the voice box, or larynx, the organ that houses the vocal cords.

Example: In a landmark study involving 148 athletes suffering from shortness of breath, most were initially thought to have asthma. When the athletes got a second opinion from a pulmonologist, 70 percent were found to have vocal cord dysfunction (VCD).

VCD causes shortness of breath in a similar way to asthma, obstructing the flow of air at the level of your windpipe, or trachea. During inhalation, instead of the vocal cords opening and staying in a relaxed position until the full breath is taken, people with VCD will let in some air, but then the vocal cords will collapse together prematurely. Asthma and VCD get confused because both create a typical wheeze, the high-pitched musical sound of obstructed air. Also like asthma, with VCD this happens only intermittently, typically when under stress or during physical exercise.

But there's an important distinction: The classic asthma symptom is wheezing when exhaling. If the wheezing occurs while inhaling, that's a telltale sign of a vocal cord problem rather than asthma.

Getting the Right Diagnosis

If you've had a raspy voice, wheeze when you inhale or experience unexplained shortness of breath for more than a week, consider seeing an otolaryngologist (ear, nose and throat specialist). Even better is a laryngologist, an otolaryngologist who specializes in voice, airway and swallowing disorders.

With just a cursory look with a scope, your vocal cords might seem fine because they can quickly return to normal. During a thorough evaluation, it's often necessary to re-create the situation that causes your problem, such as mimicking the fast inhalation that an athlete may take or even having a patient imagine a stressful situation. This could take 30 to 40 minutes. To find a laryngologist near you, consult the American Academy of Otolaryngology—Head and Neck Surgery (ENTHealth.org).

If the evaluation doesn't uncover any underlying problem with your vocal cords but you're still having any of the symptoms described earlier, ask for a referral to a speech pathologist. Your ENT likely will want you to be evaluated by a lung doctor as well, but working with a speech pathologist and doing specific vocal exercises twice a day for three to four months can help if suspicion for VCD is high enough.

Leading Causes of Vocal Cord Problems

VCD most often occurs as you grow older or following a neurologic disorder, such as

Overhead Heating Increases Exposure to Airborne Contaminants

When room air is well mixed, airborne contaminants, such as viruses, are diluted and removed by the heating, ventilation, and air conditioning system. But when heat comes from overhead vents, it creates thermal layers that block the flow of clean air into the middle level of the room—where people are breathing. As a result, exposure to respiratory aerosols can be five to six times higher than it would be in a room with well-mixed air. Portable air cleaners can counteract the effect.

Woody Delp, PhD, mechanical engineer, Indoor Environment and Sustainable Energy Systems Groups, Lawrence Berkeley National Lab, University of California.

a stroke, which can damage the brain's ability to effectively communicate with the voice box. *But VCD also can develop as a result of an underlying cause that may not seem obvious, such as...*

• **Upper-respiratory infections.** These infections, along with postnasal drip and allergies, can involve the vocal cords and cause hoarseness and cough.

• **Laryngopharyngeal reflux (LPR).** Unlike gastroesophageal reflux disease (GERD), LPR—in which stomach acid washes up into the larynx—may not cause heartburn but rather changes in your voice (e.g., hoarseness or raspiness), difficulty swallowing and/or breathing, and a chronic cough.

• **Voice misuse and overuse.** Shouting or singing forces a huge amount of air past the vocal cords, which can injure them. Plus, our vocal cords become more fragile as we age.

Healing your vocal cords from misuse takes a lot more rest than you might think. When hoarseness from overusing your voice occurs, you should avoid talking for a full day or two. For the next seven to 10 days, speak as little as possible, always using a slow and even voice. Then start the exer-

Exercises for Your Vocal Cords

Build up to three to four minutes for each exercise below, and for consistency, aim for a daily regimen. If the exercises seem to be doing more harm than good, stop and consult your physician.

● **"5-2-7" breathing.** This exercise is popular among singers and musicians.

What to do: Breathe in through your nose for a count of five…hold the breath for a count of two…and exhale, with your nose or mouth wide open, for a count of seven.

● **"3-1-3" diaphragmatic breathing.** The diaphragm is the primary muscle used for breathing, and we should use it rather than breathing from the upper chest. Babies breathe this way naturally, but we tend to stop as we get older.

What to do: Sit or lie down, and put one hand on your belly and the other on your chest. Breathe in through your nose for a count of three—you should feel an easy expansion of your belly. Hold the breath for one second, and then, as you tighten your belly muscles, take three seconds to breathe out through pursed lips (as if you're blowing on hot soup)—you should feel your hand sink down as you do this. The hand on your chest should barely move during the exercise.

● **Straw exercises.** A straw can act as an extension of the vocal cords, allowing you to exercise them more fully. When performing straw exercises, breathe in normally and use the straw only for breathing out, with pursed lips. If needed, pinch your nostrils closed to prevent any exhale through your nose. If breathing out through a straw is too difficult, simply blowing out through pursed lips also works.

What to do: Breathe in through your nose for a count of four, and exhale through the straw for a count of eight. Next, make these sounds going up and down your voice register as you exhale through the straw. *Take a break between each of these sounds…*

● **Ooh-ooh-ooh**

● **Coo-coo-coo** (this can be high- and then low-pitched)

● **Shh-shh-shh** (you'll feel this in your neck muscles)

● **Beep-beep-beep**

Four repetitions of each sound at different high-to-low registers completes one cycle. Aim for four complete cycles.

If you close your eyes and focus on your breathing while using the straw, you'll feel vibrations in your throat—try to control this as you slow down and speed up the sounds you're making. This is especially helpful if you have a voice that "cracks" while you talk.

—Dr. Michael J. Stephen

cises in the box above. Drinking herbal teas with honey or lemon also can help heal the larynx and vocal cords.

● **Dehydration.** Your vocal cords are more prone to dehydration than other body tissues because of their poor blood supply. Drinking water, herbal tea and chicken soup is helpful because it provides hydration. Drinking eight to 10 glasses of liquid a day, including sipping while you're doing a lot of talking, will bathe the back of your throat and keep your vocal cords moist. If your voice cracks, that's an indication that your vocal cords are dried out.

● **Poor air quality.** We all do our best to avoid outdoor air pollution, but it's also crucial to limit indoor air pollution. To protect your vocal cords, limit time in front of an open fireplace, and try to stay a safe distance from obvious smoke. If your fireplace screen has glass doors, use them to minimize the amount of particulate matter in the air. Keeping the humidity inside at a consistent level of 30 percent to 50 percent gives your lungs the appropriate hydration.

A humidifier is needed in winter, while a dehumidifier may be necessary on a muggy summer day. Put these in bedrooms to help ensure healthy breathing at night. Air purifiers can be helpful if there are issues with pollen or animal dander in the house. If outside pollen counts are not high and pollution levels are low (check your weather app), opening the windows for fresh air is very healthy.

Beat Inflammation to Boost Immunity, Banish Allergies

Heather Moday, MD, a board-certified allergist and immunologist, and an integrative and functional medicine physician at The Moday Center, Philadelphia. She is author of *The Immunotype Breakthrough*.

To stay healthy, we need to boost our immune systems, right? Not so fast, says Heather Moday, MD, an allergist, immunologist, and integrative and functional medicine physician. The immune system is incredibly complex, and an overactive immune system can be just as bad as one that's underactive. (Rheumatoid arthritis, multiple sclerosis, and allergies are just a few examples of what an overactive immune system can do to your body.)

Immune-System Basics

There's no one-size-fits-all approach to optimizing immunity because we don't all react to threats like viruses and bacteria the same way. Supporting the immune system, then, takes a combination of broad-stroke measures and individualized attention. The first step is to optimize five key elements of your lifestyle.

•**Improve your sleep.** Sleep is a busy time for your immune system. T cells in your lymph nodes are presented with new triggers that the innate immune system picked up during the day. Melatonin, a hormone that is released when it is dark, triggers the release of proinflammatory proteins and tells your immune cells to kill invaders. If you don't get adequate sleep, these immune processes can't work at full capacity.

Even a small amount of light can suppress melatonin production, particularly blue light from phones, computers, and tablets. Turn off all electronic devices 30 minutes to an hour before bedtime and keep your bedroom dark. If you need a nightlight, use red light.

•**Stress.** Relaxing your mind doesn't just improve sleep: Stress reduction can reduce the risk of illness overall. Try creating a daily mindfulness practice or talk to a therapist about cognitive behavioral therapy. Exercise is a stress reducer, as is going outside, so a walk, hike, or run on a nice day is especially beneficial. At least once per month, spend a whole day without social media, news, email, or television.

•**Nutrition and Gut Health.** Eat more plants—beans, whole grains, vegetables, and fruit (organic when possible). In addition, work on reducing your consumption of processed foods, sugar, and alcohol.

To improve gut health, Dr. Moday tells her patients to start with an elimination diet to identify any food intolerances. Try avoiding wheat, soy, dairy, eggs, and corn for 30 days. (Some people add sugar, caffeine, and alcohol to the list.) At the end of the month, add in one food at a time and see if you experience any symptoms within 48 hours. If not, add that food back into your diet and try the next one.

Add fermented foods, such as yogurt, sauerkraut, and kefir, to your diet to restore balance to the gut. You can also take probiotic supplements.

•**Toxins.** Choose organic food, use filtered water, avoid plastic food and drink packaging, and opt for less-toxic personal care and cleaning products. The Environmental Working Group (EWG.org) is an excellent resource to find safer brands. Many are available at regular stores.

Once you address these broad strokes, it's time to target what Dr. Moday calls your immunotype. See the next page to see if you recognize your own health patterns, and then follow the plan for your immunotype.

Smoldering Immunotype

The following supplements help calm excessive inflammation...

Cells and Immunotypes

When your body faces a threat, T cells, key players in your immune system, transform into highly targeted fighters called Th1, Th2, Th17, or regulatory T cells. Under ideal circumstances, each of these fighters does a specific job and then steps aside. But sometimes, the body gets stuck in a loop where a single subtype becomes excessively dominant in the face of any threat—or even no threat at all. *Each subtype can lead to different problems…*

● **Smoldering immunotype (Th1 dominance).** Th1 cells are created in response to bacteria and viruses. They create large amounts of inflammatory cytokines (chemical messengers).

In the short-term, inflammation is beneficial: It helps protect the body and expel invading pathogens. But if Th1 becomes overly dominant, that inflammation doesn't subside, and the body maintains a constant state of low-level inflammation, which has been linked to a wide variety of illnesses, including diabetes, high blood sugar, high blood pressure, coronary artery disease, obesity, gum disease, rosacea, Crohn's disease, or ulcerative colitis.

● **Hyperactive immunotype (Th2 dominance).** Th2 cells are activated when responding to parasites or bacteria that replicate in cavities or on the skin. They tend to stimulate B cells (a cousin to T cells) to make an antibody called IgE. If you have allergies, asthma, chronic cough, ear infections, sinusitis, a physical reaction to strong scents or odors, eczema, itchy rashes, or hives, you may have this immunotype.

● **Misguided immunotype (Th17 dominance).** Th17 cells fight certain types of bacteria and fungal infections. They secrete *highly inflammatory* cytokines, which can lead to autoimmune tissue destruction. People with Th17 dominance have often been diagnosed with autoimmune diseases, such as rheumatoid arthritis or multiple sclerosis. They may have intermittent joint pain, thyroid disease, chronic muscle weakness, or pain. Stress and certain foods may worsen symptoms.

● **Weak immunotype (regulatory dominance).** Regulatory T cells tell the body to tolerate its own tissues, calm inflammation, and balance immune reactions. If they become dominant, the other cell types can be suppressed, and you may have frequent colds or upper respiratory infections that linger for weeks, pneumonia, urinary tract infections, shingles before age 60, cold sores, and chronic fatigue.

—Dr. Heather Moday

● **Curcumin.** Take 1,000 milligrams (mg) in a bioavailable form (e.g., with black pepper) twice daily.

● **Resveratrol** has antioxidant and anti-inflammatory effects. Start with 500 mg per day.

● **Specialized proresolving mediators (SPM)** don't prevent inflammation from occurring, but they block the continued recruitment of new neutrophils to the area. Take 2,000 mg daily.

● **Berberine** downregulates inflammation, reduces oxidating stress, and has antimicrobial properties. Take 500 mg three times per day.

Hyperactive Immunotype

Use these supplements to dampen Th2 activity…

● **Quercetin** interferes with Th2 cytokines and acts as an antihistamine. Take 500 mg twice per day.

● **Astragalus root** lowers IgE antibodies and eosinophils. Take 500 to 1,000 mg daily.

● **Stinging nettle** has antihistamine properties. Take 400 mg daily.

Misguided Immunotype

The following supplements can dampen excessive inflammation, block Th17 cell activity, and increase regulatory T cells.

- **Vitamin D** increases regulatory T cells. If your serum vitamin D levels are below 50 ng/ml, supplement with 2,000 to 4,000 international units (IU) per day.

- **Vitamin A** ramps up regulatory T cells. Take 5,000 to 10,000 IU daily.

- **Skullcap** blocks inflammatory cytokines and Th17 cells. Take 500 mg twice daily.

Weak Immunotype

Try these supplements to shore up weaknesses in the immune system.

- **Melatonin** improves sleep and the immune system. Take 1 to 3 mg a few hours before sleep.

- **Ashwagandha** is useful when you have chronic stress and keep getting sick. Take 300 to 500 mg twice daily.

- **Korean red ginseng** increases T and B cells. Take 1,000 mg daily.

- **Colostrum powder** protects against microbial infection and repairs leaky gut. Take 3,000 mg day.

"Snot" a Cold

Harvard Men's Health Watch. Health.Harvard.edu

A runny nose in winter isn't necessarily a sign of illness. It is the normal, healthy way your nasal passages react to cold temperatures. Breathing cold, dry air causes your nasal passages to secrete water and mucus, thanks to the warm, blood-filled membranes behind your nasal cavities whose job it is to heat up the air you breathe. It is effectively like a mini steam bath in your nose—the resulting condensation runs down your nostrils. Gross and inconvenient, yes…but also perfectly healthy.

Is Your Sinus Headache Actually a Migraine?

Chris Iliades, MD, a retired ear, nose, throat, head, and neck surgeon who is now a full-time medical writer addressing a broad range of topics. He is a regular Bottom Line Health *contributor.*

Does this sound like you? You get frequent headaches over your forehead or around your eyes. Along with the throbbing pain, you have nasal congestion or a runny nose.

The headache may make you feel sick. You take a few over-the-counter (OTC) pills to relieve your sinus pain and pressure and maybe a nasal spray to get through the day. Most people would consider this a classic sinus headache—and most people would be wrong.

True sinus headaches, which are caused by an infection called rhinosinusitis, are uncommon and occur infrequently. Many large studies consistently confirm that about 90 percent of people who diagnose themselves with a sinus headache actually have a condition called migraine with sinus symptoms. This type of migraine causes headache, one-sided facial pain, and nasal congestion.

It can fool doctors, too. Many people with this headache are repeatedly treated with antibiotics, even though their headaches keep coming back. Some even end up with nasal or sinus surgery.

Is It a Sinus Headache?

A real sinus headache, one caused by a sinus infection, causes thick and discolored nasal discharge on one or both sides of your nose. If you have a headache without this symptom, it is probably not a sinus headache. The pain of a sinus headache can be felt between or behind your eyes, over your teeth, or over your forehead. You may also have a loss of smell, a blocked nose, and a low-grade fever.

Sinus infection headaches can follow a head cold and clear up on their own, or the infection can settle in the sinus area and be-

Pre-Headache Clues

About 40 to 60 percent of people with migraines experience what's called prodromal symptoms a day or two before a headache begins. These can include constipation, depression, diarrhea, drowsiness, food cravings, or hyperactivity and irritability.

Another 20 percent of people with migraines experience auras about an hour before the headache begins. These can be visual (such as flashes of light or blind spots), sensory (numbness or tingling), or related to speech or motion.

—Dr. Chris Iliades

come chronic rhinosinusitis. To diagnose rhinosinusitis, a doctor may order an imaging study of the sinuses, like an X-ray, CT scan, or MRI. An ear, nose, and throat doctor may examine the sinus openings by placing a thin scope into the nose (nasal endoscopy).

Is It a Migraine?

You might think your headache can't be a migraine because it isn't serious enough to cause nausea and vomiting, or to send you into a dark room to lie down. Although many people get these types of migraines, a migraine with sinus symptoms can just be a headache you wake up with on one side of your head. *In addition to the absence of thick or discolored nasal discharge, there are some other migraine clues to look for...*

• **You've been treated with antibiotics,** but the headaches keep coming back.

• **The headaches make you feel nauseated.**

• **You have a family history of migraines.**

• **Your headaches are more common if you are overtired,** skip meals, drink alcohol, or get stressed out.

• **Your headaches are triggered by changes in the weather.**

Next Steps

It is important to get the right diagnosis so you can get relief. Although an OTC sinus medicine may help both types of headaches, it is not the best treatment for either one. A true sinus headache may need to be treated with antibiotics. An untreated sinus infection can lead to dangerous complications.

Migraine headaches, however, should not be treated with antibiotics. They don't help, and they can increase antibiotic resistance. Instead, there are prescription medications that can stop a migraine before it gets worse, as well as preventive migraine medications that can reduce the frequency of the headaches. Don't try to be your own doctor if you have frequent headaches.

Chronic Sinusitis Changes the Brain

Chris Iliades, MD, a retired ear, nose, throat, head, and neck surgeon who is now a full-time medical writer addressing a broad range of topics. He is a regular *Bottom Line Health* contributor.

A few years ago, Harvard researchers reported that chronic sinusitis can cause more discomfort and loss of everyday functioning than both back pain and heart failure.

And now there's more: A new study from researchers at the University of Washington School of Medicine has found that, in addition to nasal congestion and headache, chronic sinusitis can cause depression and difficulty thinking and concentrating, too. MRI scans show brain changes that suggest that inflammation from chronic sinusitis interferes with the activity of brain cells responsible for mood and thinking.

As if these complications aren't enough, sinus infections are the most common cause of *orbital abscess*, a severe infection around the eye that can cause loss of vision and a life-threatening brain infection called cavernous sinus thrombosis. A chronic sinus infection can also spread to the bone in your forehead and cause meningitis or a brain abscess.

Sinusitis starts when inflammation, most commonly due to a cold virus, disables the cilia, tiny finger-like projections within your sinus that regulates mucus. Mucus builds up and thickens, creating a perfect breeding ground for bacteria to gather, reproduce, and cause an infection.

The beginning sinus infection is called acute sinusitis. It may go away or may need to be treated with antibiotics. But up to 25 percent of acute sinusitis infections do not respond to treatment or come back after treatment. An infection that lasts for three months or longer is called chronic sinusitis.

Sinusitis Symptoms

How do you know when a simple cold has turned into acute sinusitis? If you have a cold that doesn't go away after 10 days or keeps coming back, it could be sinusitis. Also watch for headache or facial pain, especially around your eye or over your teeth or forehead, thick and discolored (yellow or green) nasal mucus, loss of smell or taste, bad breath, thick postnasal discharge, and fever.

Symptoms of chronic sinusitis are similar to acute sinusitis, but you're less likely to have a fever, and more likely to have fatigue and brain fog.

Preventing Sinusitis

Preventing acute sinusitis is the key to preventing chronic sinusitis...

• **Start by avoiding colds and the flu.** During cold and flu season, wash your hands frequently, and practice social distancing when in crowded places. Get your flu shot.

• **If you have frequent nasal congestion,** get a good nasal exam to make sure you don't have a condition that blocks sinus drainage, like a deviated nasal septum or a nasal polyp. In these cases, an ear, nose, and throat surgeon may be able to do a simple surgical procedure to open your nasal airway and allow better sinus drainage.

• **If you have allergies,** work with your doctor to get them under control. Allergies are a big risk factor for sinusitis.

• **Keep the air in your house moist.** Dry air dries up the mucus you need to clear nasal bacteria. You can use a vaporizer or humidifier.

• **Avoid taking over-the-counter antihistamines.** These medications dry up mucus and decrease sinus drainage.

• **Avoid over-the-counter nasal decongestant sprays.** These sprays open your nasal passages but cause rebound swelling once they wear off. The rebound can be worse than the original congestion and block sinus drainage. Long-lasting sprays like *oxymetazoline* (Afrin) are the worst offenders.

• **Drink plenty of fluids and take an over-the-counter mucus thinner called *guaifenesin* (Mucinex).** Fluids and guaifenesin keep your sinus mucus moist and thin.

• **Sleep with your upper body elevated on a few pillows or a pillow wedge.** Keeping your head elevated helps mucus drain during the night.

Nasal Irrigation

Doing nasal irrigation with a bulb syringe or a neti pot is an excellent way to keep your nasal passages moist and clean and prevent sinusitis, but, according to a warning from the U.S. Food and Drug Administration, using tap water for irrigation might actually

Sinus 911

Sinusitis can cause dangerous complications if the infection spreads to your forehead, eyes, or brain. *Get immediate attention if...*

• **You have redness,** swelling, and pain around your eye (orbital cellulitis)

• **You have a severe headache,** stiff neck, and confusion (brain abscess or meningitis)

• **You have tender swelling over your forehead** (frontal bone infection).

—Dr. Chris Iliades

cause a sinus infection. Tap water may have small amounts of bacteria and other germs. Drinking tap water is safe because stomach acid kills the germs. Forcing it into your sinuses is not safe.

When you use a nasal rinse device as directed, it may come with a sterile irrigation solution or recommend one. If you make your own, use distilled and sterile water from the pharmacy. If you have to use tap water, boil it for three to five minutes and let it cool before irrigation.

Surprising Allergy Triggers

Jeffrey G. Demain, MD, a clinical professor at the University of Washington, Seattle and founder of the Allergy, Asthma and Immunology Center of Alaska.

For many people, allergy symptoms are getting worse with each passing year. *Here are some surprising triggers for this spring misery—and what to do about it...*

Fresh Fruits and Vegetables

Many people suffer from what is known as pollen food allergy syndrome (PFAS). Also known as oral allergy syndrome, PFAS is caused by allergens found in both pollen and raw fruits, vegetables, and some tree nuts. Your immune system can mistake the food for pollen and cause an itchy or tingling mouth, a scratchy throat, and swelling of the lips, mouth, and tongue. In some cases, you may develop hives where the food touched your skin. It is rare, but PFAS can trigger anaphylaxis, a severe and potentially fatal allergic reaction.

If you typically suffer spring allergies, you are likely allergic to birch-tree pollen. Up to 70 percent of people with a birch-pollen allergy also experience an allergic reaction to apples, cherries, kiwi, peaches, pears, and plums, carrots, celery, almonds, peanuts, and hazelnuts. You may have a reaction to these foods only during the spring, when pollen is the highest.

Other fruits, vegetables, and nuts may cross react with different tree and plant pollens that peak at other times of the year. For more information, visit AAAAI.org and search "oral allergy syndrome."

You may be able to eat fruits and vegetables that cause PFAS if you cook them. Heating affects the allergy-causing proteins. Unfortunately, cooking will not alter the proteins in tree nuts.

Most symptoms of PFAS resolve quickly on their own once you stop eating the offending food. However, if you have a reaction to a food, it is a good idea to consult your doctor to determine the cause. PFAS can be confused with a food allergy, so it is important to know what the allergy is and how to treat it. If you have a reaction when eating nuts, in particular, see a doctor as soon as possible. Nuts are more likely to cause anaphylaxis and require medical attention.

Thunderstorms

While a spring rain may help alleviate allergy symptoms by washing pollen away, thunderstorms can exacerbate symptoms and lead to what is known as "thunderstorm asthma." When a heavy storm hits on a day with a high pollen count, grains of pollen get sucked into the storm clouds, where they absorb water and then pop, releasing even smaller grains. These particles are spread from the downdrafts of the thunderstorm and are easily inhaled.

Researchers in Georgia found that visits to the hospital for asthma were 3 percent higher after thunderstorms.

If you suffer from an allergy to pollen, and particularly if you also have asthma, stay indoors and keep windows closed when pollen counts are high and thunderstorms are predicted.

Climate Change

If you're allergic to pollen, which is an allergy trigger for one in five Americans, you may have noticed your symptoms are starting earlier than usual, getting more intense, and lasting longer. That's because allergy season

Allergy-Busting Steps

• **Treat before the symptoms begin.** Start your allergy medications two weeks before allergy season typically begins.

Using a nasal steroid, such as *fluticasone* (Flovent), once a day starting at the beginning of pollen season can reduce your symptoms by about 35 percent. Taking an antihistamine, such as *loratadine* (Claritin) or *cetirizine* (Zyrtec), can lessen symptoms by 25 percent. Using both remedies provides a 45 to 50 percent relief in symptoms.

Eye drops that can help prevent itchy, watery eyes before they start include *olopatadine hydrochloride* (Pataday, Pazeo). Once these symptoms appear, antihistamine eyedrops, including *ketotifen fumarate* (Zaditor), may be effective at alleviating them.

• **Keep your home allergy-free.** Close windows and doors and use an air purifier with a high-efficiency particulate air (HEPA) filter to remove pollens from indoor air. Take your shoes off at the front door to prevent tracking pollen into your house. Take a shower before bed to remove pollens from your skin and hair.

And don't forget pets: Animals can bring pollen in homes on their fur. Try to bathe them once or twice a month.

• **Perform outdoor exercise in the afternoon.** Tree pollen, primarily from birch trees, is the largest spring allergy trigger. Tree pollen cycles begin in the morning, so the best time of day to be outside for a walk, bike ride or some fresh air is the afternoon.

—Dr. Jeffrey Demain

Because spring allergies are starting earlier and are more severe, you need to start your typical allergy-fighting regimen sooner and take extra precautions to successfully treat the symptoms (see sidebar). To determine when allergy season will begin in your area, consult the National Allergy Bureau at AAAAI.org and click on "Check pollen counts" at the top of the home page.

Chia Seeds Can Be a Choking Danger

Rebecca Rawl, MD, gastroenterologist, Carolinas Medical Center, Charlotte, North Carolina, reported in WebMD.

Chia seeds are packed with fiber, protein, and omega-3 fatty acids. But they absorb up to 27 times their weight when exposed to moisture. Seeds swallowed dry can expand in your esophagus into a gel-like obstruction that may require surgery to remove.

Safer: Eat chia seeds only after they have been soaked in liquid and allowed to expand.

Good News If You're Allergic to Sesame

FoodSafetyNews.com

Thanks to a new federal law that adds sesame to the list of major allergens—along with peanuts, milk, eggs, fish, shellfish, tree nuts, wheat and soybeans—it soon will be listed on food labels. Currently, companies often lump sesame in with "spices" or "natural flavors" on labels rather than mentioning it specifically—a problem for the 1.1 million Americans with sesame allergies. The law takes effect in 2023. In the meantime, if you're allergic, check food labels for the sesame-containing ingredients tahini, sesamol and gomasio…or buy from General Mills and

lasts up to 27 days longer than it did only 10 years ago as it gets warm earlier in spring and cold later in winter. A longer frost-free season gives trees and plants more time to grow, flower, and pollinate. Higher temperatures also produce higher amounts of pollen. In fact, a study conducted by the American College of Allergy, Asthma & Immunology found that pollen counts are expected to more than double by the year 2040.

Hershey, which already identify sesame on their labels.

Help! Cold Weather Gives Me the Hives

Thomas B. Casale, MD, professor of medicine, department of internal medicine, University of South Florida, Tampa.

If chilly weather makes you break out in hives, you may have cold urticaria, an extreme reaction to cold. People with this condition have mast cells in the skin that release histamine and other chemicals when exposed to cold. In rare cases, cold urticaria is genetic or associated with a disease such as hepatitis or cancer. Symptoms can occur at a wide range of temperatures, and humidity and wind chill factors are important variables. Sipping an icy drink or eating ice cream can cause the lips or throat to swell in some people with the condition. In severe cases, cold urticaria can trigger anaphylaxis, a serious allergic reaction that can lead to shock, trouble breathing or swallowing, and even death. For example, swimming in cold water can lead to death from anaphylaxis.

To protect yourself, when it's cold outside, bundle up and leave as little skin exposed as possible. Also avoid contact with cold objects, cold food and drinks, and swimming in water below 77°F. Alert your health-care providers as well, as cold IV fluids or surgical procedures can cause an episode.

If these steps don't help, take an over-the-counter (OTC) antihistamine such as *loratadine* (Claritin) when temperatures dip. A doctor might prescribe *cimetidine* (Tagamet), an acid reducer that is also used as an antihistamine, the anti-inflammatory drug *omalizumab* (Xolair), or *epinephrine* (EpiPen), an injection used to treat severe allergic reactions.

Urticaria can be a lifelong condition, but studies show that symptoms go away after about five years for about half of those with this condition.

Where's the Cleanest Indoor Air?

Study by researchers at Georgia Institute of Technology, Atlanta, published in *Indoor Air*.

The cleanest indoor air is inside an airplane. In a comparison of levels of tiny aerosol particles in the air of stores, restaurants, offices and public transportation, levels were lowest in the cabins of airliners at cruising altitude.

Reason: The jets' cabins had high ventilation rates, and clean air was resupplied 10 to 30 times per hour.

Asthma and the Flu

University of Queensland

A subtype of asthma can make you more susceptible to the flu. Paucigranulocytic asthma, a nonallergic form of the condition, suppresses the immune system, allowing the influenza virus to replicate unchecked and to mutate more easily. These findings could have implications for community-wide spread.

Another Reason Not to Vape

Studies by researchers at University of Rochester Medical Center, New York, published in *Tobacco Induced Diseases* and *PLOS One*.

It causes brain fog. Two new studies involving nearly one million students and adults point to an association between vaping and difficulty concentrating. Both smokers and vapers are more likely to report mental fog, and kids who start vaping before age 14 are more likely than their peers to struggle with concentrating, recall and making decisions.

Chapter 16

VERY PERSONAL

Overcome the Stigma of Obesity: Beyond Diet and Exercise

For decades, women with obesity have been told, "Eat less and move more." While those are undeniably helpful behavioral changes, they're rarely sufficient to help people with obesity lose significant amounts of weight. That's because, contrary to popular belief, obesity isn't about a lack of willpower, and it doesn't always neatly follow a Calories Consumed < Calories Burned equation.

Startling numbers: 42 percent of the US population lives with obesity. And 30 percent more is overweight. That means more than 70 percent of Americans are carrying excess weight, a risk factor for more than 200 chronic diseases including hypertension, type 2 diabetes, heart disease, sleep apnea, several cancers and, more recently, increased severity of COVID-19.

In 2013, the American Medical Association officially recognized obesity as a disease. This was an important leap forward, helping to open the public's and the medical community's eyes to the fact that obesity is not a choice but rather the result of com-plex factors, including genetics…socioeconomic status (which impacts access to healthy food)…medications a person may be taking for other conditions…sleep…and more.

A New Medicine That Works

There has been a renewed call by specialists to reshape how we view weight management. A healthy lifestyle that includes whole, nutrient-dense foods, exercise, stress management and restful sleep is at the foundation, but for many people, this isn't sufficient to achieve a healthy weight. They need a more aggressive approach—and that can mean medication.

The Food and Drug Administration recently approved the anti-obesity medication

Robert F. Kushner, MD, medical director of Center for Lifestyle Medicine at Northwestern Medicine in Chicago. He is past president of The Obesity Society and the American Board of Physician Nutrition Specialists, a founder of the American Board of Obesity Medicine (which certifies physicians in the care of patients with obesity) and author of several books including *Six Factors to Fit: Weight Loss That Works for You!* Dr. Kushner was the corresponding author for the 2021 *New England Journal of Medicine* "Semaglutide Treatment Effect in People with Obesity (STEP) 1" study group. *Disclosure:* Dr. Kushner is on the advisory board for Novo Nordisk (manufacturer of *semaglutide*) and receives honoraria.

(AOM) *semaglutide* (Wegovy)—the first such treatment to receive approval since 2014. Originally used to treat type 2 diabetes under the brand name Ozempic, this drug works in the brain to reduce hunger and cravings. Like other AOMs, semaglutide is for patients with a body mass index (BMI) of 30 or higher...or for those with a BMI of 27 or greater who have at least one weight-related condition, such as high blood pressure, high cholesterol, or type 2 diabetes.

Recent study: In a 2021 *New England Journal of Medicine* study, 1,961 adults were injected weekly with 2.4 mg of semaglutide or received a placebo for 68 weeks. All the participants also received individual counseling on diet and physical activity every four weeks. On average, those in the semaglutide group lost 15 percent of their body weight (for example, someone who started at 230 pounds lost 34.5 pounds.) One-third of people on semaglutide lost 20 percent or more of their body weight—a loss approaching that typically experienced after a sleeve gastrectomy, in which the majority of the stomach is surgically removed. Less than 5 percent of those in the placebo group lost 15 percent of their weight via diet and exercise alone compared with 50 percent for the semaglutide group. These results are far superior to those seen with other weight-management medications, which tend to lead to a loss of 6 percent to 11 percent of one's body weight. This means semaglutide is about 1.5 to two times more effective than other AOMs such as Contrave (*naltrexone/bupropion*) and Qsymia (*phentermine/topiramate ER*).

The fact that so many of the study participants taking semaglutide lost 15 percent of their weight is noteworthy because that benchmark is where we often see obesity-related conditions such as high blood pressure and type 2 diabetes begin to reverse or even go into remission. And despite what weight-loss companies and gyms claim, it is very difficult to achieve this degree of weight loss with diet and exercise alone.

Treating Obesity As a Disease

People who struggle with their weight have historically resisted using AOMs and surgeries for a variety of reasons...

•**Stigma.** There's ample stigma surrounding obesity in general and medication for obesity specifically. People trying to lose weight feel as if they should be able to "do it on their own" by working out and cutting calories. These tactics are important, but they're often no match for a genetic tendency toward obesity and they can't undo the impact of living in an area with limited access to fresh food or gyms. There's no shame in needing chemotherapy to treat cancer, but many individuals with obesity feel shame over needing medication.

A person with obesity doesn't just take medicine and instantly lose weight. It needs to be combined with regular physical activity and a healthful, calorie-controlled diet. Most AOMs help dampen appetite...reduce cravings and thoughts about food...and make you feel more content between meals. With those reinforcements, people are better able to adhere to a healthy lifestyle.

•**Lack of coverage.** Medicare explicitly rules out coverage for AOMs. But Medicare Advantage plans provide Part A and Part B coverage along with extra benefits and may offer expanded coverage for weight-loss treatment plans. Medicaid may cover them, depending on the state in which you reside. Coverage from private insurers varies from no coverage at all to limited coverage, meaning there still is a substantial copay. Insurers may not cover these drugs the way that they cover other medications because they do not view obesity as a chronic disease (as opposed to an aesthetic and thus elective issue)...and/or perhaps they realize that with millions of potential candidates, the cost could be astronomical. Certain drugs may be affordable for some people—Contrave and Qsymia (see page 317) may cost about $100 a month after insurance if you work with a mail-order pharmacy. Semaglutide costs about $1,000 a month, rendering it out of reach for most patients.

Should You Try an AOM?

If your insurer covers semaglutide or you can afford the $12,000 out of pocket annually, ask your primary care provider if you are a candidate. Many doctors don't mention AOMs, primarily because they haven't been trained to do so.

Semaglutide comes in two versions. The 2.4-mg version, used in the *NEJM* study, is branded Wegovy and is approved for chronic weight management. The lower, 1-mg dose Ozempic, is approved for type 2 diabetes.

Important: If you have diabetes, the lower dose of semaglutide likely will be covered by insurance.

Semaglutide is self-administered via a weekly injection in the belly, just under the skin. You will start at a lower dose and gradually build up to the full dose over four months. You should notice a reduction in appetite more or less immediately. Side effects include nausea and/or diarrhea, but these tend to dissipate with continued use. The medication should not be used by patients with a personal or family history of medullary thyroid cancer or in patients with the rare condition multiple endocrine neoplasia syndrome type 2 (MEN-2). Your health-care provider will be able to tell you if you are a candidate for its use.

There are several other AOMs on the market. *Two of them, both taken orally and costing about $100 a month, are...*

• **Contrave.** This combination of the drug *naltrexone* used to treat alcohol dependence and prevent relapse of opioid addiction and the antidepressant *bupropion* leads to an average weight loss of 8 percent of one's weight. Side effects can include headaches, constipation, insomnia and dry mouth. People with uncontrolled hypertension, a history of seizures or a history of opioid use or dependence should not use Contrave. Smokers may experience an added benefit, though—bupropion assists with smoking cessation by reducing cravings in the reward center of the brain.

• **Qsymia.** This is a combination of the stimulant *phentermine* and *topiramate ER,* commonly used to treat migraines and epilepsy. Patients can expect to lose 7 percent to 11 percent of their body weight. Side effects include dizziness, insomnia, constipation, dry mouth, tingling of the fingers and altered taste. People with hyperthyroidism, uncontrolled hypertension, coronary artery disease or glaucoma should avoid Qsymia, as should those who are sensitive to stimulants.

AOMs need to be taken long term. Be sure you have reasonable expectations about how effective the medicine will be. Work with a counselor or registered dietitian to understand these medications and craft a nutrition and exercise plan.

If cost is a barrier: Semaglutide and other AOMs are costly. Ask your doctor for a referral to an obesity medicine specialist, who can determine if you are a good candidate for any of them. Some are available in generic form, which increases affordability.

If you are employed, contact your human resources department to encourage your employer to include AOMs as part of its group health insurance plan. You also can join the Obesity Action Coalition (ObesityAction.org), a national advocacy group composed of like-minded people that provides educational resources and advocates for more access to treatments.

New Advances in Hair-Loss Treatment

Sara Wasserbauer, MD, ABHRS, FISHRS, a hair restoration expert in private practice with offices throughout the San Francisco Bay area.

About half of women and even more men experience age-related thinning of the hair, but recent advances can slow the loss and, in some cases, even help hair regrow.

The most common type of hair loss is called *androgenetic alopecia,* a.k.a. female-pattern baldness (all-over thinning) or male-pattern baldness (a receding, M-shaped hairline plus thinning at the top of the head). It's caused by age, hormones, and genetics. Chronic underlying illnesses such as untreated thyroid disorders or anemia can accelerate hair loss, but when the illness is treated, that hair loss usually reverses.

Medical Therapies

When it comes to slowing or reversing hair loss, therapies fall into two main categories: medical and surgical. *Here are the most common medical treatments…*

• *Minoxidil* (**Rogaine**). Applied twice daily to thinning areas, topical minoxidil keeps hair in the growing phase, which means that treated hairs don't shed as frequently as they normally would. It also stimulates regrowth.

For patients who experience scalp irritation, there is an oral formulation. Oral minoxidil was originally used as a high blood pressure medication, but when used in very low doses (around 1 milligram [mg]/day or less, versus the standard 10 to 30 mg/day dose for blood pressure), it stimulates hair regrowth and reduces shedding. It can improve existing high blood pressure, too. Patients with heart failure should avoid oral minoxidil.

• **Dandruff shampoo.** When lathered into hair and left on for five minutes a day, two to three times a week, dandruff shampoo may calm hair-damaging inflammation while killing a common yeast, *Malassezia*, that causes hair loss, itching, and dandruff. Ask your doctor for a prescription for an antifungal shampoo containing 2 percent *ketoconazole*, which a 2019 *Biomedical Dermatology* study found to be as effective as 2 percent minoxidil in women with female-pattern hair loss. (Ketoconazole is the active ingredient in the OTC dandruff shampoo Nizoral AD, but it contains only 1 percent ketoconazole.) Other options include

COVID-19 and Hair Loss

COVID-19 can cause hair loss, typically about three months after infection. The shedding may be the result of a high fever, weight loss, emotional distress, or anything that overstresses the mind or body. In a 2021 *Lancet* study, 22 percent of more than 1,700 hospitalized COVID patients were still experiencing hair loss several months after discharge. In most cases, the hair loss naturally reverses, but the experience can be disturbing, nonetheless.

Head & Shoulders, Selsun Blue, and Neutrogena T/Gel, which contain different active ingredients with similar effects.

• *Finasteride* (**Propecia**) and *dutasteride* (**Avodart**). These daily oral medications are a mainstay of treatment for male-pattern hair loss. They block *dihydrotestosterone*, a naturally occurring steroid that promotes hair thinning. Like minoxidil, they can help maintain and possibly regrow existing hair, but they won't work with complete baldness. Combining Propecia or Avodart with Rogaine can enhance effects. Postmenopausal women may be candidates for use, but women of childbearing age shouldn't even touch these drugs, let alone use them, as they can cause fetal abnormalities during pregnancy.

• **Scalp micropigmentation (SMP).** This camouflage technique uses medical-grade ink to create hundreds of tiny dots on the scalp, mimicking the look of individual hairs. SMP differs from tattooing in that the pigment is different and isn't deposited as deeply.

In someone with complete baldness, this can be done in a way that resembles a buzz cut, almost like a permanent five-o'clock shadow on the skull. For all-over or patchy thinning, it creates the illusion of fullness. Results are instant and last five to 10 years. No recovery is needed. Because UV light breaks down the pigment, wearing a hat when outdoors can reduce the need for touch-ups. Depending on the area treated, expect to spend one to three hours with your SMP specialist, with a total cost of $3,000 to $6,000.

Surgical Therapies

If medical management isn't effective, there are two surgical procedures: follicular unit extraction (FUE) and follicular unit transplantation (FUT or "strip method"). In both, hair is surgically removed from the back and sides of a patient's head (the "horseshoe" region) and strategically transplanted to areas of baldness or thinning. The patient is under local anesthesia. This hair in this area is genetically different from the hair on the top of the head in that it rarely thins with age, so once it's moved to the top, it can grow there for decades.

In FUE, the donor site is shaved before individual follicles (each follicle usually contains one to four hairs) are removed and transplanted. You can expect small scars where follicles are removed, which usually end up concealed by existing hair. Recovery takes three to five days.

With FUT, which doesn't require shaving, a long, thin strip of scalp is removed before individual follicles are harvested and transplanted. The donor area is stitched back up, leaving a barely visible scar (unless you buzz your hair shorter than a #2 on a pair of standard clippers or razor shave your head), and stitches are removed after seven to 10 days. FUE may be better suited to patients with moderate hair loss and FUT for more significant loss.

Both FUE and FUT are day-long procedures that typically cost between $10,000 and $20,000, depending on where you live and the amount of hair transplanted. Results are permanent and, with a skilled surgeon, appear very natural. There is no more "hair plugs" look.

Hemorrhoid Fundamentals

Nimalan A. Jeganathan, MD, a colorectal surgeon and assistant professor of surgery at Penn State Health in Hershey, Pennslyvania.

It's the most common medical problem that no one likes to talk about. But, with millions of people experiencing discomfort from hemorrhoids every year, it's also a problem that doctors are very familiar with. Fortunately, there are straightforward ways of getting relief.

Though people often use the term hemorrhoids to describe a medical condition, hemorrhoids are actually just another part of the human anatomy: Everyone has these veins inside the anal canal that help support the sphincter muscles and maintain continence. When they become enlarged, and the tissues that support them weaken, people develop the condition of the same name.

What's Going On

There are two types of hemorrhoids: internal and external.

Internal hemorrhoids originate in the anal canal. You may find out you have them only from a colonoscopy report. If you strain on the toilet, one may create a small amount of bleeding that you'll see on the toilet paper or in the water. (Keep in mind that a single drop of blood can turn the whole toilet bowl red, so it's important not to panic.)

If a hemorrhoid gets larger and starts to bleed more, however, you should not ignore it. An internal hemorrhoid can grow and develop a stalk that gets longer until it actually protrudes from the anus. This prolapsed hemorrhoid can cause discomfort or pain, irritation, and possibly itching as well.

Exterior hemorrhoids form outside the rectum. (You can see them with a mirror.) These veins can be irritated and/or painful if the area is inflamed and swollen. Typically, there isn't much bleeding, but an external hemorrhoid can swell suddenly to the size of a walnut in a condition called thrombosis. That can lead to increased pain, inflammation, and swelling, and needs to be evaluated by your doctor.

Besides being a natural consequence of aging, hemorrhoids can develop from everyday habits that increase pressure in the anal canal. Constipation because of a low-fiber diet, heavy lifting, straining to pass stool or simply sitting for long periods on the toilet, not getting enough exercise, and being overweight all contribute to their formation.

When to Seek Treatment

Hemorrhoids are treated only when symptoms like bleeding or pain become bothersome, not just because a hemorrhoid is enlarged. If you have bleeding during bowel movements or discomfort that doesn't improve after a week of home care, talk to your doctor. Don't let any feeling of embarrassment stand in your way—hemorrhoids are a condition that colorectal specialists see every day.

For 90 percent of patients, hemorrhoid treatment is focused on adding fiber to the diet and other lifestyle remedies to prevent progression, encourage regular bowel movements, and avoid straining.

Some people swear by topical treatments, like *phenylephrine* (Preparation H) or witch hazel. While these may provide temporary relief, they are usually not a good long-term solution. *To address the underlying problem, follow some simple guidelines…*

- **Increase fiber.** Getting more fiber in your diet with fruits, vegetables, and whole grains helps soften stool, increase its bulk, and reduce constipation, which in turn prevents the straining that leads to hemorrhoids.

As a bonus, fiber also has other tremendous health benefits, including weight loss and reduced risk of diabetes, stroke, heart attack, and high blood pressure. The recommended daily fiber intake is between 25 grams for women and 38 grams for men. Consuming enough from your diet can be difficult and usually requires taking over-the-counter fiber supplements.

- **Drink plenty of fluids.** Aim for the often-suggested eight glasses of water to help keep stool soft and help fiber supplements do their job.

- **Rethink bathroom habits.** Stop scrolling on your phone and doing other types of reading on the toilet. This extra sitting time leads to extra straining and more intra-anal pressure. It's also important to go to the bathroom as soon as you feel the need to go.

If you delay, stool can actually harden and become difficult to pass.

- **Lose weight if needed.** Extra pounds put a strain on anal veins. In addition to changes in diet, try to move more. Sitting all day isn't good for health or hemorrhoids, and regular exercise also helps you stay regular.

- **DIY.** If you have a protruding internal hemorrhoid, you can push it back into the anus yourself. This isn't dangerous to do and may help alleviate some swelling.

Next Steps

When lifestyle changes aren't enough to alleviate hemorrhoids, the next step is in-office procedures, such as rubber-band ligation, which involves tying the hemorrhoid off, and sclerotherapy, which involves injecting a liquid agent into the vein. Both usually involve several office visits. The procedures carry a small risk of a local infection, usually in the first few days, and your doctor will alert you to red flags to watch for, such as severe pain, fever, and the inability to urinate.

Sometimes surgery is needed. A hemorrhoidectomy can reach the very base of the hemorrhoid and remove it along with any affected surrounding tissue. Improvements in surgical techniques have gone a long way toward reducing the pain associated with the procedure, but there is a lengthy recovery: It may take up to four weeks for all pain and bleeding to resolve.

The first few days can be especially difficult, though anesthetics injected in the area during surgery should help in the immediate aftermath. Nonsteroidal anti-inflammatory drugs are the first-line medication for managing pain. Doctors try to avoid prescribing opioids, not only because of the risk of addiction, but because constipation is a major side effect—and that's the last thing you want when recovering from anal surgery. Soaking in a tub and applying warm compresses help some people, while others find relief with a cold pack.

The Other Reflux

Steven Sandberg-Lewis, ND, a professor at the National University of Natural Medicine and co-founder of Hive Mind Medicine, Portland, Oregon. Dr. Sandberg-Lewis' is the author of the textbook *Functional Gastroenterology* (2nd edition, 2017) and offers both in-person and telehealth care.

Every day, the fiery sensation that comes with gastroesophageal reflux disease (GERD) sends one in five uncomfortable Americans to the pharmacy in search of relief. For some, an over-the-counter or prescription drug puts out that fire, but for a surprisingly large subset of sufferers, these drugs offer no relief. In some cases, that's because another disorder is lurking silently in the background: bile reflux.

GERD vs. Bile Reflux

In GERD, acidic fluid from the stomach flows up through a weakened esophageal sphincter into the throat. But in bile reflux, bile travels from the small intestine, through a weakened pyloric valve, into the stomach. For people who have bile reflux without GERD, symptoms can include abdominal pain, nausea, vomiting, heartburn, and unintended weight loss.

• **In a person with GERD,** however, the bile continues its journey into the esophagus along with the stomach acid. While medications such as antacids, proton-pump inhibitors (PPI), and H-2-receptor blockers can neutralize the acid, they do nothing to stop the burn of bile.

• **If you have GERD that doesn't respond to treatment,** especially if you've had your gallbladder removed or suffer from diabetic enteropathy, a digestive issue that may be associated with prediabetes or diabetes, it's time to consider the possibility of bile reflux. Not only can it make GERD treatment difficult, but studies also suggest that bile can be more damaging to the lower esophagus, increasing the risk of Barrett's esophagus, a long-term complication of GERD and possibly precancerous changes and cancer of the esophagus.

Treating Bile Reflux

There are no standard treatments for bile reflux, but many patients find relief with a multi-pronged approach...

• **Reduce pressure.** When pressure below the diaphragm is high, it tends to move things upward. There are several ways to lower that pressure, such as doing simple breathing exercises and not holding your breath when exerting yourself or having a bowel movement.

Some people also benefit from treating underlying small intestine bacterial overgrowth (SIBO), a condition in which normally friendly bacteria overgrow in the intestine. As those bacteria convert carbohydrates into gas, it can increase abdominal pressure. Diarrhea or constipation, abdominal pain, distension, or bloating, and an uncomfortable feeling of fullness all suggest the possibility of SIBO.

People with this condition often have good results by following a low-fermentation diet, which is designed to deprive the bacteria of their preferred food source, fermentable carbohydrates, such as grains, beans, starchy vegetables, seeds, legumes, fruits and fruit sweeteners, agave, roots, and herbs. Visit Siboinfo.com for details on the SIBO diet.

• **Improve the composition of the bile.** Some research suggests that *ursodiol* (URSO, Actigall), a prescription bile salt, and *tauro-ursodeoxycholic acid* (TUDCA), an over-the-

Promote Downward Flow

If you still feel full four to five hours after a meal, you may have delayed gastric emptying. In these cases, prokinetic medications, such as *cisapride* (Propulsid) and *metoclopramide* (Reglan), can cause the contents of the stomach to empty faster. For some patients, this one strategy can eliminate their reflux.

— Dr. Steven Sandberg-Lewis

counter (OTC) bile acid, can make bile less irritating to the esophagus. For people with bile sludge, a mixture of mucus and particulate matter that forms in bile, OTC lecithin and N-acetyl cysteine can help the bile flow. The dosages of these supplements are highly individualized, so it's important to work with a specialist who is familiar with bile reflux before taking them.

• **Strengthen the pyloric and esophageal sphincters.** Huperzine A, an OTC extract, can boost levels of acetylcholine, a neurotransmitter that promotes good muscle tone in those valves. Further, mindfulness and relaxation techniques can strengthen the vagus nerve, which plays an important role in controlling muscles in the digestive tract. Strategies like alternate nostril breathing and therapeutic gargling may also strengthen the vagus nerve.

• **Protect and bolster the mucous membrane.** Several medications can help the mucous membranes of the stomach and esophagus better withstand irritants. These include agents that form a soothing film, called demulcents, such as deglycyrrhizinated licorice, aloe vera, and a prescription called *sucralfate* (Orafate, ProThelial, Carafate).

Safe and Easy Way to Treat Anal Fissures

UniversityHealthNews.com

Anal fissures are small tears in the inner lining of the rectum. They can cause blood in the stool and pain during bowel movements, but they're generally not dangerous and are easy to treat by getting a lot more fiber, either as a supplement or by eating more fruits and vegetables. Also increase how much water you drink.

Helpful: An over-the-counter stool softener and soaking in a warm tub for 10 to 20 minutes, especially after a bowel movement. If the above steps don't help sufficiently or for recurrent fissures, talk to your doctor.

IBD Alerts

Inflammatory Bowel Disease and Microplastics

People with inflammatory bowel disease (IBD) have more microplastics in their feces. A research team obtained fecal samples from 50 healthy people and 52 people with IBD. The feces from IBD patients contained about 1.5 times more microplastic particles per gram than those from healthy subjects. The most common types of plastic were polyethylene terephthalate (used in bottles and food containers) and polyamide (found in food packaging and textiles).

Zehua Yan, PhD, is a professor at Nanjing University, Nanjing, China.

Engineered Bacteria Can Diagnose Inflammatory Bowel Disease

Researchers have created a strain of Escherichia coli that senses pH and glows when it encounters acidosis, a condition that often occurs during flareups of inflammatory bowel diseases like colitis, ileitis, and Crohn's disease. The team suggests that the bacterium could be added to food and programmed to turn toilet water blue to warn patients when a flareup is just beginning.

Jeffrey Tabor, PhD, associate professor of bioengineering and biosciences, Rice University, Houston, Texas.

Lipoma Lowdown

Erum N. Ilyas, MD, MBE, FAAD, a board-certified dermatologist at Schweiger Dermatology, King of Prussia, Pennsylvania.

Most of us would be alarmed to find a lump on our bodies, especially near the breast and armpit areas. These discoveries most definitely have to be checked by a physician. But often the lumps are lipomas, very common tumors that can pop up anywhere. Made of adipose or fatty tissue, they are most often benign, but based on location, symptoms, and size, they do have potential risks: If a lipoma develops along the neck, it could pose a risk to breathing or swallowing. Painful lipomas can affect day-to-day activities, posture, or exercise.

It's unclear what causes lipomas to develop, but genetics is thought to play a significant role. Often, people will note a family history of lipomas, but they can also arise from several diseases and genetic syndromes, including Madelung's disease, Dercum's disease, Gardner's syndrome, and hereditary multiple lipomatosis.

When to See a Doctor

Although very rare, liposarcoma, a malignant lipoma, can occur. If a lipoma increases in size, have it evaluated by your dermatologist to rule out malignancy. Occasionally, patients may perceive a lipoma to be increasing in size when, in fact, the lipoma is stable but an increase in muscle mass behind the lipoma makes it appear more prominent. I routinely ask patients that note a possibly expanding lipoma about new exercise routines to determine the possibility that this may be playing a role in the perceived change in size.

Can These Lumps Be Shrunk or Eliminated Without Surgery?

Lipomas can potentially be minimized or shrunk with steroid injections that cause atrophy of the fatty tissue. Some patients with numerous and/or multiple small lipomas may consider this option for some cosmetic improvement. The challenge with this approach, in my experience, is that it potentially only benefits small lipomas (less than one centimeter in size). This procedure also tends to have a high recurrence rate, simply because it is only shrinking the size but not eliminating the lipoma altogether. Liposuction has also been used to treat lipomas. This would still be considered surgical, but it has a reduced risk of scarring.

If Surgically Removed, What's the Likelihood of Them Recurring?

The likelihood of a lipoma recurrence after surgical excision truly depends on whether the entire lipoma was removed, how the lipoma was removed, whether it was encapsulated or well defined, and whether it had a deeper component that may have involved the fascia or muscle (a deep-seated lipoma). The recurrence rate is around 5 percent after surgery, but this rate may go up based on these factors.

Hidradenitis Suppurativa: A Commonly Misdiagnosed Condition

Patrick Zito, DO, PharmD, a board-certified dermatologist and voluntary assistant professor of dermatology at the University of Miami Miller School of Medicine Dr. Phillip Frost Department of Dermatology & Cutaneous Surgery.

Hidradenitis suppurativa (HS) can be an unpredictable disease. One person may have an occasional small, painful bump in the armpit, while another may have chronic pain, severe scarring, and inflammatory bowel disease. But there is one thing that many people with HS have in common: a long, frustrating road filled with misdiagnoses and failed treatments. On average, it takes seven to 10 years after symptoms appear to get an HS diagnosis, researchers reported in the journal Dermatology. That delay can be devastating: Untreated, this chronic inflammatory condition can worsen, causing severe pain, scarring, odor, and disability.

Understanding HS

HS begins when a hair follicle becomes blocked and forms a small, painful bump. It most often strikes in areas with apocrine sweat glands—such as the armpits and the groin—as well as under and around the

Home Remedies

Many people with HS report success with home remedies that haven't been studied in clinical trials. Here are the most commonly recommended products on the Facebook *Hidradenitis Suppurativa* Support Group...

- **To prevent infection:** Dial antibacterial body soap, apple cider vinegar, honey
- **For pain:** Boil-Ease (over-the-counter), Vicks VapoRub, warm compresses
- **To help a lesion drain:** ichthammol (drawing-out-salve), hydrocolloid bandages, Vicks VapoRub
- **To reduce odor:** white vinegar
- **To reduce inflammation:** turmeric and zinc (both used as topical treatments or taken as supplements), eliminating dairy and yeast from the diet.

breasts. It can progress through three stages (see table below) and can become severe enough to interfere with normal functioning and movement, even causing disability.

People with HS also have a higher risk of a variety of other conditions, including diabetes, squamous cell carcinoma, obesity, metabolic disorders, spondyloarthritis, PAPA syndrome (pyogenic arthritis, pyoderma gangrenosum and acne), polycystic ovarian syndrome, hypertension, dyslipidemia, inflammatory bowel disease, and spondyloarthropathy.

Prevention and Treatment

While there is no cure for HS, early diagnosis and treatment can limit inflammation and skin damage, and lower the risk of systemic conditions. *Management takes a multipronged approach...*

- **Lose weight if necessary.** While HS strikes people of any body weight, it is more prevalent among people with obesity. While the relationship is complicated—obesity may occur with HS but not cause it—researchers

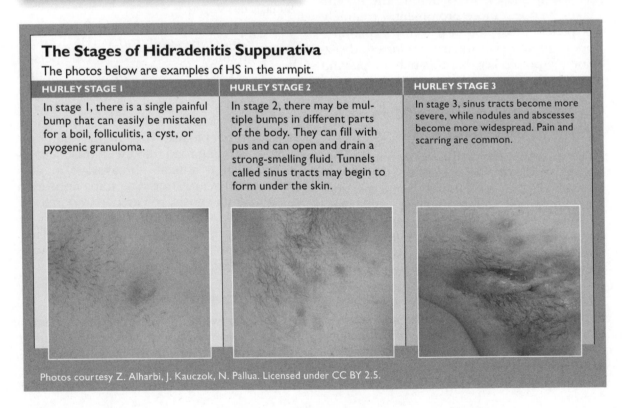

The Stages of Hidradenitis Suppurativa

The photos below are examples of HS in the armpit.

HURLEY STAGE 1	HURLEY STAGE 2	HURLEY STAGE 3
In stage 1, there is a single painful bump that can easily be mistaken for a boil, folliculitis, a cyst, or pyogenic granuloma.	In stage 2, there may be multiple bumps in different parts of the body. They can fill with pus and can open and drain a strong-smelling fluid. Tunnels called sinus tracts may begin to form under the skin.	In stage 3, sinus tracts become more severe, while nodules and abscesses become more widespread. Pain and scarring are common.

Photos courtesy Z. Alharbi, J. Kauczok, N. Pallua. Licensed under CC BY 2.5.

in Denmark found that the number of patients reporting HS symptoms after weight loss from bariatric surgery decreased by 35 percent. They concluded that a weight loss of more than 15 percent was associated with a significant reduction in disease severity.

- **Don't smoke.** Researchers recently discovered that deficiency in a cell-communication system called the Notch pathway likely plays a causal role in HS. Smoking suppresses Notch signaling, which is why smokers with HS have more affected body areas than nonsmokers.

- **Use antibacterial washes.** HS nodules are highly prone to infections. To reduce the risk, use antimicrobial washes such as *chlorhexidine* (Peridex, Hibiclens) or *benzoyl peroxide* (an ingredient in a wide variety of anti-acne products). Some dermatologists recommend bleach baths, where you soak in a 0.005 percent diluted bleach solution for five to 10 minutes twice per week. (Never put full-strength bleach on your skin.)

- **Lifestyle.** Avoid irritating your skin by keeping high-risk areas cool and dry, wearing loose-fitting clothing, and replacing shaving with clippers, waxing, or laser hair removal.

In-Office Procedures

Depending on your specific condition, your dermatologist may suggest an in-office procedure to address the nodules or abscesses…

- **Steroid injections** can reduce inflammation and the size of non-infected nodules.

- **Abscesses** can be drained in the office, but there is a high rate of recurrence.

- **Your dermatologist or a plastic surgeon may "deroof" an abscess** by removing the skin that covers it or may excise the whole lesion and any tunnel.

- **Laser surgery can help treat lesions and scars in some patients** whose disease is otherwise stable and medically managed.

- **Laser hair removal** can prevent outbreaks by destroying the hair follicles in high-risk areas.

While these procedures can address the disease in a particular location, they don't prevent flares from appearing on other parts of the body or address underlying inflammation, so medical management is important even when these are successful.

Medications for HS

A variety of medications show promise in managing HS…

- **Creams.** Topical antibiotics such as *clindamycin* (Cleocin T, Clindagel) and *dapsone* (Aczone) can help treat infection and reduce inflammation. A topical corticosteroid such as *triamcinolone* (Cinolar, Kenalog, Triderm) can reduce local inflammation, but it should be used only for short periods of time (up to two weeks) to avoid damaging the skin. Topical *resorcinol* (Resinol, R A Acne) can open clogged hair follicles and reduce inflammation.

- **Oral antibiotics.** A class of drugs called tetracyclines have both antibacterial and anti-inflammatory properties. A common first choice is *doxycycline* (Vibramycin, Doryx, Oracea, Acticlate, Atridox, Doxy). This medication can cause severe nausea, so let your doctor know if you need to try a different drug.

- **Hormonal medications.** HS strikes follicles with associated apocrine glands. Apocrine glands are inactive until hormonal changes at puberty. Drugs that block the effects of androgens such as *testosterone* help many people with HS.

These include *spironolactone* (Aldactone) and *finasteride* (Proscar, Propecia). Birth control pills can also help women who have menstrual-related flares.

- **Metformin** (*Glucophage*), which is commonly used to treat diabetes, can reduce HS-related inflammation. One small study found that about 70 percent of people who took metformin had improvement in their symptoms and quality of life.

- **Biologics.** For moderate to severe disease, biologic medications are very promising. In fact, the only medication specifically approved to treat HS is *adalimumab* (Humira). Studies show that people who received adalimumab injections have "noticeably fewer abscesses (lumps with pus) and nodules (hard, deep lumps)," the American Academy of Dermatology reports.

Access to Quality Care

Not all dermatologists treat HS, so you may need to shop around. Look for a board-certified dermatologist who is familiar with the latest advances in HS. (Doctors who have more recently completed medical school may be more up-to-date on the latest advances in treating this disease.)

How to Treat the Pesky Bumps of Hives

Anna R. Wolfson, MD, an allergist and clinical researcher at Massachusetts General Hospital and instructor of Medicine at Harvard Medical School. Dr. Wolfson is a physician faculty member at the Massachusetts General Hospital (MGH) Hives (Chronic Urticaria) Program. She is also the director for Quality and Safety of MGH Allergy and Immunology.

Hives, or urticaria, are itchy red bumps that arise when a substance or illness triggers white blood cells in the skin to release histamine. In its attempts to get rid of the offending substance, histamine causes several unpleasant symptoms including swelling, itching, and hives.

While many allergic skin conditions cause itching and redness, hives are uniquely fleeting in nature: A single hive will usually not last longer than 24 hours. New ones may, and often do, appear in the same location or on different parts of the body, but if you were to circle any given hive and check back the next day, it would likely be gone.

You can also tell if you have a hive by pressing on it: It will turn white.

That's different from contact dermatitis, an itchy rash that develops after touching a product to which you're allergic and lasts for several days, or mosquito bites, which resemble hives but last longer.

Know Your Triggers

Several triggers activate the histamine response responsible for acute hives...

• **Drug allergies.** Medication-related hives usually pop up in the first few days of taking a drug. Common culprits include penicillin and other antibiotics (including those containing sulfonamides, also called sulfa drugs), ibuprofen, aspirin and other nonsteroidal anti-inflammatory drugs, anticonvulsants, and chemotherapeutic drugs. New drugs are the most likely culprits. A medication you have been taking for a year or more is an unlikely trigger for a drug allergy.

• **Food allergies.** More than 10 percent of U.S. adults have a food allergy, according to a recent *JAMA Network Open* study. Shellfish ranks number one. Other common triggers are peanuts, tree nuts, fish, wheat, sesame, soy, egg, and dairy. Many adults with food allergies have had them their entire lives, but about half of food-allergic adults developed one or more of these allergies as an adult.

• **Infections.** Viral infections such as the common cold, mononucleosis, or even COVID-19 can trigger hives because the immune system kicks in to fight the virus and, in the process, inadvertently activates the histamine-producing mast cells. They can develop at any point in the course of the infection and sometimes even after it has resolved.

• **Stressors.** Intense stress, exposure to extreme cold or heat, and exercise can also trigger hives, especially in people who are already prone to them. They may cluster in areas where there's physical pressure, like where your pant waistband sits on your hips, under a bra, or where backpack or purse straps hit the shoulder.

Chronic Hives

These triggers above are responsible for acute cases of hives, meaning they last a short time. In about one percent of the global population, though, hives last six weeks or longer. These are called chronic hives, or chronic spontaneous urticaria (CSU). The diagnosis of CSU is made based on the history and often without any confirmatory testing. Patients are often frustrated, not to mention itchy, uncomfortable, and embarrassed that the hives are so persistent.

Holistic Approach

Nonpharmaceutical therapies exist, but their success can be hit or miss, and none have been proven to be consistently effective in studies, so medical management as described below in main article is recommended.

● **Quercetin.** This antioxidant, found in apples, berries, broccoli, capers, cauliflower, grapes, and tea, plus several nuts and seeds, can inhibit histamines. It's available as a supplement. Ask your doctor about dosing.

● **Low-histamine diet.** A small number of people do well by omitting foods that naturally contain histamine, such as fermented dairy products (yogurt, kefir, and aged cheese) and fermented vegetables (sauerkraut), cured meats, alcohol, tomatoes, eggplant, and spinach.

● **Acupuncture** has been used successfully in various skin conditions to decrease the urge to itch, but more research is needed to see if it can improve hives. That said, it can relieve stress, which may help hives patients, especially those who find that stress causes their condition to flare.

—Dr. Anna R. Wolfson

Rarely, chronic hives can signal an autoimmune condition such as lupus, rheumatoid arthritis, diabetes, or a thyroid condition. (Other symptoms, such as weight loss or joint pain, will usually also be present if this is the case.) An allergist can diagnose and manage CSU.

Treating Acute Hives

If hives are accompanied by other allergic reactions, such as throat swelling, difficulty breathing, nausea, vomiting, abdominal pain, or painful, itchy swelling of the eyes, lips, hands, feet, or genitals, you should seek urgent medical attention.

If they aren't accompanied by worrisome symptoms, they can usually be treated at home. Antihistamines are the cornerstone of treatment. While *diphenhydramine* (Benadryl) is most commonly associated with hives

treatment, it's not the best option. It's sedating and lasts for only a few hours. Longer-acting, over-the-counter antihistamines like *fexofenadine* (Allegra) or *cetirizine* (Zyrtec) are more effective. They block the histamine release responsible for the hives for 12 to 18 hours. Skip the decongestant version of these medications, which are marked with a "D," (Zyrtec-D), as they can cause rapid heart rate and high blood pressure, especially in older adults.

If you don't respond to the antihistamine in a day or two, see your primary care doctor, who may prescribe an oral corticosteroid.

Topical steroids aren't usually effective because an individual hive lasts 24 hours or less, so you'd constantly be playing a game of whack-a-mole trying to get each new one.

Treating Chronic Hives

For chronic hives that don't respond to antihistamines and other first-line medications, a monthly injectable medication called *omalizumab* (Xolair) may be prescribed. Omalizumab limits mast cells' ability to release histamine. It is generally well-tolerated, and it works so well that the authors of a recent *Journal of Allergy and Clinical Immunology* study wrote that it has "virtually revolutionized" the treatment of CSU.

Rosacea May Signal a Deeper Problem

Rajani Katta, MD, a board-certified dermatologist and volunteer clinical faculty member at Baylor College of Medicine and University of Texas Houston Health Science Center. Dr. Katta is the author of seven books and more than 80 medical journal articles and book chapters. Her latest book is *Glow: The Dermatologist's Guide to a Whole Foods, Younger Skin Diet.*

To the casual observer, rosacea—a condition marked by facial flushing, pesky bumps, and broken blood vessels centered on the nose and cheeks—might seem to be a skin-deep problem. But many of the estimated 16 million Americans who cope with it are highly aware that what they put in their bellies directly influences the symptoms on their faces.

Rosacea patients routinely experience flare-ups in response to specific foods (see sidebar at right) and eliminating those foods can reduce symptoms. Now researchers are digging deeper and finding that what's happening in the gut itself may play a role in this chronic condition.

Food and the Microbiome

What we eat directly affects the bacteria, fungi, and other organisms that thrive in the gut microbiome. Within 24 hours of eating a high-fat, high-sugar diet, for example, there are markedly fewer good gut microbes and more plentiful bad ones inhabiting what's commonly referred to as your "gut biome." The good microbes play many roles: They act as police officers who battle invading germs, teachers who train the immune system to know the difference between good and bad substances, and factory workers who take what we eat, particularly fiber, and turn it into short-chain fatty acids that strengthen the inner lining of the gut as well as the skin.

Bad gut microbes outnumbering good gut microbes causes an unbalanced gut microbiome (dysbiosis), which has been linked to gastrointestinal conditions such as celiac disease, Crohn's disease, ulcerative colitis, and irritable bowel syndrome—all of which are also more common in people with rosacea. In one study, researchers found that people with rosacea were 13 times more likely to have small intestinal bacterial overgrowth (SIBO), and that treating the SIBO with antibiotics also resolved the rosacea.

Treat the Gut to Treat the Skin

Think of it this way: Your gut is essentially a garden. For more good microbes to thrive, you need to "fertilize" them with the right foods in addition to avoiding your trigger foods. That means eating more probiotics, also known as good gut microbes, and prebiotics, which nourishes them.

Food and Rosacea

Avoid these common triggers…
- **Hot temperature foods or drinks,** like coffee and tea
- **Spicy foods,** such as hot sauce, cayenne, jalapeno, and red peppers
- **Alcoholic beverages of any kind**
- **Cinnamaldehyde foods,** such as citrus, tomatoes, cinnamon, and chocolate

Eat more of these…
- **Prebiotics** from fruits, vegetables, and whole grains
- **Probiotics,** from yogurt, kefir, tempeh, sauerkraut, miso, and kombucha

—Dr. Rajani Katta

Prebiotics comes from the fiber in fruits, vegetables, and whole grains. Stick with real foods, since supplements offer only questionable benefits.

Probiotics come from foods like yogurt, kefir, tempeh, sauerkraut, miso, and kombucha, all of which contain live microbes that have long demonstrated numerous health benefits. While food sources are best, you can also get probiotics in supplement form. While there are many species of probiotics, look for a supplement with at least 1 billion colony-forming units (CFU) of *lactobacillus* or *bifidobacterium*.

Got the Shakes?

Harvard Women's Health Watch. Health.Harvard.edu/newsletters

Your shaky hand might be essential tremor. Unlike Parkinson's disease, characterized by shakiness while at rest, essential tremor happens during activity—such as when you're writing or holding a glass. The trembling can vary in intensity and affect the hands, head, voice, or other parts of the body.

Essential tremor can be inherited and typically starts in middle age. It also can be caused by certain medications, too much caffeine, muscle fatigue, hyperthyroidism, and other conditions.

There is no cure for inherited essential tremor, but medications such as *propranolol* (Inderal) or *primidone* (Mysoline) may help. Also check with your doctor to rule out other causes.

Help! I Sweat So Much That My Palms Drip

Jenny Murase, MD, assistant clinical professor of dermatology, University of California, San Francisco Medical Center.

Sweat is a natural response to prevent the body from overheating during hot weather, vigorous exercise, or in situations that trigger anxiety or anger. But sweat that's excessive could be a sign of a condition called hyperhidrosis.

People with hyperhidrosis sweat excessively for no apparent reason—often from the palms, feet, underarms, or head. It can run in families or result from another medical condition, such as a thyroid problem, diabetes, or even menopause. *Try these tips…*

•**Use powder or a bit of antiperspirant containing aluminum chlorohydrate** (which plugs sweat glands) any place you're experiencing excessive sweating.

•**If your palms still drip with sweat,** consult a dermatologist, who can prescribe a more potent antiperspirant, such as Drysol, or *glycopyrrolate* (Robinul), an oral medication that reduces sweat and other secretions.

•**Botox can be injected to block nerves that stimulate sweating,** but it is very painful when done on the palms.

•**Another option is iontophoresis,** a procedure that uses electricity to shut down sweat glands. The procedure is usually done several times a week until sweating lessens; then treatments are continued on a regular basis (typically once a week) to maintain results. Check with your insurer to see if this is covered.

Severe cases of hyperhidrosis may require surgery to cut nerves in the chest that send signals to sweat glands. The surgery usually has good outcomes, but there are potential risks involved, such as infection and bleeding.

You May Need a Breath Mint!

Study by researchers at Korea Advanced Institute of Science and Technology, Daejeon, Republic of Korea, published in *ACS Nano*.

A prototype sensor has been developed that can detect hydrogen sulfide, the gas responsible for stinky breath, with 86 percent accuracy. Bad breath can signal intestinal or dental problems and other health issues. Researchers hope to put the sensor into small devices for self-diagnosis.

Surprising Benefits of Sex

Studies have found that sex boosts your body's ability to create antibodies, which help fight off viruses and bacteria…lowers heart attack risk…lessens pain…lowers blood pressure…boosts brainpower…and helps you live longer.

MedicineNet.com

Your Personal Scent

Jude Stewart, content strategist, Stewart + Company, a creative company that specializes in marketing, design and copyrighting, and author of *Revelations in Air: A Guidebook to Smell*. JudeStewart.com

Your personal scent comes from three layers—the surface layer, which can be affected by washing and using deodorants… the middle layer, influenced by diet and environment…and a baseline scent that is as unique to you as a fingerprint. This base layer is the result of a cluster of 50 genes associated with the immune system. When we are attracted to someone, we are attracted to scents produced by this gene cluster that are different from and complement our own set of genes.

INDEX